Quality Management of Hospitals

Quality Management of Hospitals

Dr. Farooq A. Jan (M.D)
Prof Hospital Administration

GenNext Publication

ISBN: 978-93-5663-056-7

First Published, 2022

Published by

GenNext Publication
5, Ansari Road
Daryaganj, New Delhi-110002
Phonc: 011-47034999, 9811692060
E-mail: gennextpublication@hotmail.com

Printed at: Gyan Press, Delhi.

Contents

अखिल भारतीय आयुर्विज्ञान संस्थान
अंसारी नगर, नई दिल्ली-110029

ALL INDIA INSTITUTE OF MEDICAL SCIENCES
ANSARI NAGAR, NEW DELHI-110029

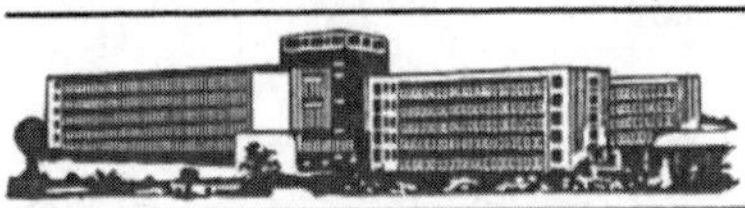

दूरभाष/Tel. No. : 91-11-2658 8389, 2659 4700
फैक्स /Fax No.: 91-11-2658 8641, 2658 8663
ई-मेल/E-mail : ms.aiims@aiims.edu
123dks@gmail.com

डॉ० डी० के० शर्मा/ Dr. D. K. SHARMA
चिकित्सा अधीक्षक/ Medical Superintendent

Foreword

It is indeed a matter of privilege to be sharing my thoughts on the release of an excellent book on 'Quality Hospital Care" authored by Dr. Farooq A. Jan, Professor of Hospital Administration & Medical Superintendent at SKIMS, Srinagar. Quality in hospital care encompasses various dimensions of care, a patient goes through during his journey in a hospital. It is a holistic experience based on the quality of treatment and patient care, and duly includes all those factors which contribute to this care. Quality in clinical treatment is just one facet of it, clean and comfortable environment, good sanitation and hygiene, ease of transport, quality of diet, kind and compassionate communication of staff, quality driven admission and discharge process makes the hospital experience of a patient "the most satisfying one".

I am sure this endeavour of bringing a book on such a vital dimension of hospital care will go a long way in inculcating new arenas of knowledge amongst health care givers and staff and lead to the adoption of best practices by them. I would like to extend my heartiest congratulations and best wishes to the author and contributors who were involved in this great initiative.

20/09/22

(DR. D.K. SHARMA)

Preface

This book has been written for doctors in general and postgraduates of Hospital and Health Administrations, Students of MBA in Hospital Management, Hospital Managers and Medical Administrators in particular. Emphasis has been particularly laid on latest developments and approaches in management of hospitals. Numbers of books on hospital management are available in the market which cover quality in hospitals. In this book not only new topics of current interest have been included but the latest trends in much talked about topics have been discussed.

Dr Farooq Jan
Professor
Hospital Administration &
Medical Supdt
SKIMS

Acknowledgments

I am greatly indebted to my wife Dr Shadab Manzoor who cooperated with me and let me per sue my dreams. I am thankful to my parents and teachers who have given me education. I am thankful to my sons Sarlees and Nibras who were helpful in their peculiar ways. I am also thankful to my friends for encouraging me.

1

History and Evolution of hospitals

The word hospital originates from the Latin word "hospice". In the early Greek and Roman civilizations, the temples of the God were used as hospitals. The Greeks and Romans considered the temples of gods and their priests responsible for providing shelter. Hippocrates universally acknowledged as father of western medicine was born in Greece in 460 B.C. The evolution of hospitals in western world started from charitable guest houses. Origin and development of hospitals in west was closely related with wars and religion. During medieval ages most hospitals were attached to monasteries. After medieval age monastic hospitals suffered a setback and secular hospitals developed. From 16th century hospitals of Europe were gradually spread into North America. Hospitals in early America served quite different purpose from those of today. They were founded to shelter older adults, the dying, orphans and vagrants and to protect the inhabitants of a community from the contagious sick and the dangerously insane. During the eighteenth century medical care in Boston, Philadelphia and New York was provided in the home. It was necessary however in these and other seaport towns to provide refuge for sailors and other shipboard victims of contagious disease who often were unceremoniously left ashore when the ships departed. The towns responded by organizing pest houses, quarantine stations or isolation hospitals to segregate the sick from the town inhabitants and to prevent the spread of disease. Because these facilities were not intended to be used by the local citizenry they were usually located well outside the city limits. The existence of pest houses or isolation hospitals also provided the towns with what seemed an ideal solution for dealing with other individuals whose presence posed a risk to or offended its inhabitants . Over time people with mental illness or those in poor health, the homeless and the petty criminal joined the contagious ill that occupied those facilities. Bellevue Hospital was originally the Poor House of New York city established in 1736 to house the poor, aged, insane and disreputable. In 1789 the Public Hospital Of Baltimore was established for low income populations, people with mental or physical illness and the seafaring of Mary Land. One hundred years later in 1889, it became the now prestigious Johns Hopkins Hospital . Eventually almost every city of any size in early America had a pest house to isolate patients during epidemics. Most cities also had an almshouse for low income populations, sometimes with an added infirmary. Most of the today's county or municipal hospitals were originally combinations of almshouses and infirmaries. The earliest county institution, Eloise Hospital in Wayne County, Michigan was started in 1835 to serve the old, young, deaf, dumb, blind, insane and destitute. It grew to 6000 beds to care for acute and chronic illness and mental diseases and to provide domiciliary services to low income populations. The Kings County Hospital in Brooklyn, Philadelphia General Hospital and Cleveland city Hospital are similar examples. Most hospitals in the United States in the 19th century were disgraceful, dirty, unventilated and contaminated with infections. They were overcrowded and offered little or no medical care. The only nurses available were former inmates or women who could get no other work. As a result they only accelerated the spread of disease . Because visiting was restricted, patients were effectively cut off from outside world. Persons with family or the means to obtain home medical or nursing care shunned hospitals. Certain religious orders however saw the hospitals clients as helpless, so miserable with incurable disease or so maimed by accident that they presented an opportunity for spiritual outlet for those seeking salvation through good works. Religious nursing groups played a major role in the evolution of hospital care. Catholic religious orders were the first groups responsible for kindly and humane nursing performed by fairly well educated, sincere and devoted disciplines. The protestant Nursing movement began in Germany and was brought to Pennsylvania in 1850. It was based on formal training of nurses in religion, nursing and nursing education. The nurse teachers were called deaconesses. By late nineteenth century as society became increasingly industrialized and mobile and as medical practices grew in their sophistication and complexity, the notion that responsible families and caring communities took care of their own became more difficult to apply. The result was a gradual shift toward the professionalization of health care practices that eventually included the development of a full and competitive market for medical services that increasingly took place in hospitals. Nursing played a significant role in the move from home to hospital. Perhaps nursing was the most important single element in reshaping the day to day texture of hospital life.

The University of Pennsylvania school of Medicine was the first and only medical school in America when in 1765 students were enrolled for "anatomical lectures" and a course on "the theory and practice of physik". By organizing a medical faculty separate and distinct from collegiate faculty, Penn's trustees effectively created the first University in North America though the corporate name continued as the college of Philadelphia until 1779. The founder of the School of Medicine was a young Philadelphian physician Joh Morgan. The early faculty including Morgan had earned medical degrees at the University of Edinburgh and supplemented Edinburgh's courses with further study in London. London offered advanced training in Anatomy in private schools owned by men who had become famous in their field with the University of Edinburgh as their model. The University founding faculty introduced two important elements in American Medical Education ie medical lectures supplemented with bedside teaching which for sometime had been provided to apprentice physicians by practitioners at the Pennsylvania Hospital. For more than a century, the pattern of medical education established in 1765 remained relatively unchanged. Not all medical schools, followed Pennsylvania's lead forming academic ties. Bedside teaching was a traditional practice rather than a requirement. But though violated, the standards and procedures introduced by Pennsylvania remained the guiding force in medical education throughout most of the nineteenth century. During this period Pennsylvania enjoyed an uncontrolled preeminence as the leading institution of medical education on the continent.

Florence Nightingale (middle of nineteenth century) was a passionate sanitarian, she puts her emphasis on cleanliness, hygiene, clean air and water. Nightingale training intended to produce young women who would teach sanitary practice and install ideas of higher and good living into patients, hospital workers and doctors. Florence Nightingale by nursing meant little more than the administration of medicine and the application of poultices. It ought to signify the proper use of fresh air, light, warmth, cleanliness, quiet and the proper choosing and giving of diet. In 1859 Florence Nightingale established her famous nursing school hospital in London.

Advances in medical science in the form of anesthesia, sterilization, microscopy gave impetus to further progress in the hospital field. The orgin of the Royal College of Surgeons of England date to the fourteenth century with the foundation of the Guild of surgeons within the city of London. Certain sources date this as occurring in 1368. There was ongoing dispute between surgeons and barber surgeons until an agreement was signed between them in 1493. In 1745 the surgeons broke away from the barbers to form the company of surgeons. In 1800 the company was granted a Royal charter to become the Royal College of Surgeons in London. A further charter in 1843 granted it the present title of the Royal college of surgeons of England. The Royal college of physicians and surgeons of Glasgow is an institute of physicians and surgeons of Glasgow, Scotland. Founded by Peter Lowe after receiving a royal charter by James VI in 1599 as a Glasgow faculty this institution originally existed as a regulatory authority to ensure that physicians, surgeons and dentists were well trained . In the early period it included barbers and apothecaries but they were excluded by 1722. In 1909 it gained the royal moniker and was known as the Royal faculty of physicians and surgeons of Glasgow. By 1962 it was renamed, the Royal College of physicians and Surgeons of Glasgow.

The transformation of hospitals from simple, charitable institutions to complex, technical organizations was accompanied by a parallel growth of private hospital insurance. By 1960's insurance companies such as Blue Cross/BlueShield were flowing money into hospitals. The availability of money through health insurance removed an important constraint from hospital charges. Expanding hospital services and relatively unrestrained reimbursement rates created an inflationary spiral that was to persist for decades. The Hill Burton Act in 1947 provided funds for the construction and expansion of community hospitals. Over 4600 projects to expand existing facilities or construct new ones were initiated within 20 years after its passage. The National Institutes of Health expanded in the 1950s and 1960s stimulating both for profit and not-profit research. Medicare and Medicaid established in 1965 provided money for the care of the aged and the poor respectively. Medicare provided the growing populations of Americans over age 65 years with significant hospital and medical benefits. Thus the group most likely to need hospitalization was assured of hospital care, and the hospitals were assured that they would be reimbursed on the basis of reasonable costs. For all its support however, the cost of hospital care grew even faster. Medicare and to a lesser extend Medicaid had enormous impact on hospitalization rates in the United States. Because the rising Medicare rates became the standards for establishing hospital reimbursement rates in general, Medicare probably did more to fuel the rising costs of hospital care than any other factor. As these programs provided government funding for the hospital care of low income population and older adults, they altered the long standing nature or mission of hospitals by diminishing the traditional charitable or social role of these voluntary institutions. In 1965, the Medicare costs were projected to be $3.1 billion . Five years later however they reached $5.8 billion. Less than 10% could be linked to expanded utilization ; 23% to rapid economic inflation and the remaining two thirds to massive expansions in the hospital pay roll and non pay- roll expenses including profits with a doubling of average patient – care costs between 1966 and 1976.

In 1960's and 1970's rising public expectations for nursing and medical attendance as well as the recognition by nurse and physician reformers that some patient care procedures were unsafe drove recognition of nursing care. In hospitals, Intensive care units grew and machines became ever more prevalent . By 1965 over 90% of large hospitals and 31% of smaller ones had intensive care units staffed by increasingly expert nurses.

Cost containment was the theme of hospitals in 1990's. The burden of power in institutions shifted from care givers to the organized purchases of care, with Medicare and Medicaid becoming a huge governmental influence in all types of hospitals. In private sector, insurance companies began to take a more active role in managing hospital costs. Health maintenance organizations (HMO), which contracted with a network of providers for discounted prices increased in importance. In 1978, the Blue Cross Network purchased the struggling health maintenance organization and became the largest HMO in the state. The focus of care shifted to out patient services, ambulatory care centers for acute care and hospices and nursing homes for chronically ill.

Ernest Codman in 1910 proposed the "end result system of hospital standardization". Under this system a hospital would track every patient if treated long enough to determine whether the treatment was effective. In 1913 Franklin Martin founded the American College of Surgeons (ACS). ACS adopts the "End result system". In 1917 American college of Surgeons developed the "Minimum Standards for Hospitals". In 1951 American college of physicians (ACP), the American Hospital Association (AHA), the American Medical association (AMA), and the Canadian Medical Association (CMA), joined with ACS as corporate members to create the Joint Commission on Accreditation of Hospitals (JCAH) . In 1953 JCAH published "Standards for Hospital Accreditation". The Joint Commission seeks to continuously improve health care for the public by evaluating health care organizations and inspiring them in providing safe and effective care of the highest quality and value.

History of Hospitals in India

In ancient times, it was a tradition to take care of and treat the patients in their homes and for those who had no one to look after them, the state had arranged places where the patients were lodged and treated. The forerunners of the present hospitals can be traced to the times of Buddha followed by Ashoka. The notable of the early hospitals were those built by King Ashoka (273-232 B.C) . Fahien (AD 339-413) who visited India during the times of Chandragupta provides us details about the charitable dispensaries in Pataliputra. Hiven Tsang (AD 629-645) another Chinese traveler provides description of hospitals of that time. According to him in all the highways of the towns and villages throughout India there were hospices, where food, drink and medical treatment was provided to travelers and poor people. These were the Indian counterparts of the western almshouses, monasteries and infirmaries of those times. Mohammedian invasion of India during tenth century brought with it the Greek System of Medicine which came to be known as "Yunani". During 17th century arrival of Christian missionaries brought with it the Modern system of Medicine.

References

1. Gventer B. Risse, Mending bodies, Saving Souls. A history of Hospitals (New York: Oxford University Press, 1999).
2. Paul Starr, The social Transformation of American Medicine (New York: Basic Books, 1982); James H cassedy, Medicine in America: A short History (Baltimore : Johns Hopkins University press, 1991).
3. Starr, The Social Transformation of American Medicine, Charles E. Rosenberg, The care of strangers : The Rise of America's Hospital system (Baltimore: Johns Hopkins University Press, 1987).
4. Daniel Callahan and Angela A. Wasunna, Medicine and the Market: Equity v Choice (Baltimore : Johns Hopkins university Press, 2006).
5. Julie Fairman and Joan Lynaugh, Critical Care Nursing: A history (Philadelphia: University of Pennsylvania Press, 1998).
6. Stevens R. In sickness and in wealth: American Hospitals in the twentieth Century: New York, NY: Basic Books; 1989.
7. Teisberg E O, Vayle E J. The Hospital Sector in 1992. Boston, MA, Harvard Business School; 1991.
8. Louis Kuo Tai Fu (2000). The origins of Surgery.
9. Louis Kuo tai Fu. From Barbers to Surgeons Annals of the College of Surgeons Hong Kong. 4(1), 35-49.
10. Monica. E. Baly. Lorence Nightingale and the development of public health nursing. A Journal of the act and science of Medicine.
11. Nightingale F. Notes on Nursing . London: Duck Worth; 1952 (first Published 1859), p.15.
12. The Joint Commission History. The Joint Commission.

2

Quality in Health Care

Health care services are very complex; on one side new technologies become available very rapidly which make practices obsolete before the process of delivering care can be fully evaluated and variation minimized. On the customer side accessibility, parameters and reimbursement methods are rapidly changing. All these activities demand efficient operations, continuous improvement and update.

Quality management in health sector is important for improving health status of populations, enhancing quality and access, increasing macroeconomic and microeconomic efficiency, strengthening cost and clinical effectiveness and improving quality of care and consumer satisfaction.

Several definitions of quality have been used over the years. Following are some of the predominant ones.

- Freedom from defects.
- Fitness for use.
- The totality of features and characteristics of a product or service that bear on its ability to satisfy given needs.
- The features and characteristics that delight the customer.

Joseph M. Juran has defined Quality management as "meeting or exceeding customer expectations by doing the right things right and doing them the right the first time".

Joint commission on accreditation of Health care organizations, United States, has defined quality of patient care as the "degree to which patient care services increase the probability of desired outcomes and reduce the probability of undesired outcomes, given the current state of Knowledge".

This definition is broad enough to encompass wide variations in individual perceptions of quality and recognizes that outcome of care are not certain.

Avedis Donabedian suggested that assessing quality in health care should include an assessment of structure, process and outcome.

Structure

(a) **Physical facility:-** Scientifically planned and designed for each function of the hospital.
   - (i) General structure i.e. location, architectural pattern, internal and external traffic pattern and facilities.
   - (ii) Location, layout and functional relationships.

(b) **Manpower:**
   - (i) Properly qualified and sufficient manpower for achieving mission of the institution.
   - (ii) Committee composition consistent with institutional mission.
   - (iii) Clearly drawn job descriptions.

(c) **Equipment:**
   - (i) Appropriate technology.
   - (ii) Maintenance
   - (iii) Down time
   - (iv) Utilization

Process

Is the application of knowledge, judgement and skill to improve health status. First standards are established and then degree of adherence to those standards is recorded.

The modern scientific procedures of patient care process in the hospital are:

1. Medical audit
2. Tissue review
3. Mortality meets/death review
4. X-ray review
5. Utilization review
6. Surgical audit
7. Nursing audit etc.

Outcome

Includes:

(1) Clinical outcomes
- Survival
- Recovery

(2) Affiliated outcomes
- Attitude
- Satisfaction
- Disability
- Rehabilitation

It should be clear that structure, process and outcome should not be viewed as strictly causative as they tend to merge in health care i.e. number of intermediate outcomes affect the process itself.

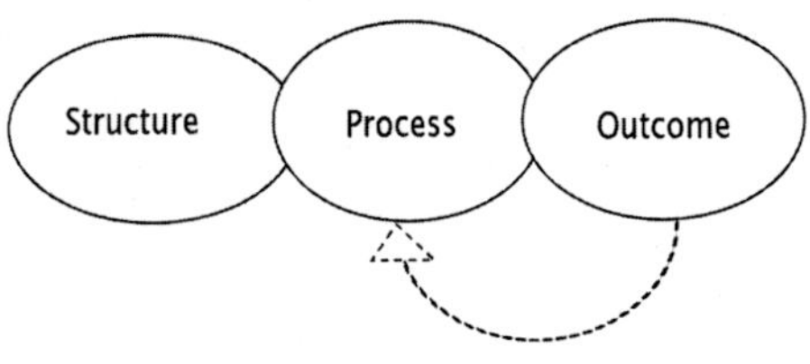

Fig. 2-1: Integrated model of structure, process and outcome.

Quality programs have three main foci: assessing or measuring performance, determining whether performance conforms to standards and improving performance when standards are not met.

Following steps are important for quality improvement:

(i) Leaders must take lead in quality improvement.

(ii) Additional investments in managerial time, capital and technical expertise.

(iii) Health care workers must be assumed to be trying hard, acting in good faith and not willfully failing to do what they know to be correct.

(iv) Communication between customers of health care must be open and carefully maintained.

(v) Modern tools and techniques of quality improvement must be put in use.

Health care organization must organize for quality i.e. quality should get a central place in managerial agenda. Training in quality concepts must be introduced since all staff members must become partners in mission of quality improvement.

Once management is committed to the concept of quality and transformation of culture has begun quality planning follows. Planning emphasizes team formation and building, identification of customer requirement and professional standards, data-based identification of deviation from standards and requirements and identification of opportunities for improvement. After the completion of quality planning organizing quality becomes the second major task for quality management team. During this phase four key elements are emphasized: translating the requirements of customers or professional standards into operational specifications, selecting process performance measures or key indicators, measuring process performance measures or key indicators and planning and implementing the proposed solutions. Structure, process and outcome should be considered important key elements of evaluation. Evaluating quality includes evaluating results of the implemented solutions, holding gains and evaluating team effectiveness.

Challenges to quality improvement:

(i) Lack of political will.

(ii) Lack of awareness and interest among hospital leadership.

(iii) Fear among hospital staff.

(iv) Inadequate trained staff in QM.
(v) Inadequate logistic support.
(vi) Lack of quality management reference material.
(vii) Lack of well organized information system.
(viii) Lack of co-operation from all concerned departments.

References

1. Myer Kutz. Definitions of quality. Total quality management and the Mechanical engineer. Mechanical Engineer Hand book 2nd ed. (72) Jhon Wileyand sons 1998: 2160-2161.
2. Qadiri Ghulam Jeelani. Quality management in Health care. Selected readings in Hospital Administration. 2001; (2): 14-17.
3. "The Role of outcomes in Quality assessment and Assurance," Quality review Bulletin 18(1992) : 356-360
4. Donald. M. Berwick. Sounding board, continuous improvement as an ideal in health care in The Text book of Total Quality in health Care. St. Luece Press Florida. 1997: 31-39.

3

Total Quality Management

Nearly everyone in practice of medicine is highly trained, is usually very well educated and is by far committed to providing high quality of care. Because of all the changes in health care the ways in which quality is perceived, pursued and insured continues to develop. All health care systems are in a state of evolution. Limited resources, changes in insurance coverage, participation, decision making by patient and patient demands and expectations are driving attention to quality today. It remains a challenge to find innovative approaches that improve the quality of health service delivery. Staff needs models of good practice to improve service delivery. Quality is achieved when accessible services are provided in an efficient, cost effective and acceptable manner that can be controlled by the ones providing them.

Evidence of quality problems

Several types of quality problems in health care have been documented through peer reviewed research.

(a) **Variation in Services:-** there continues to be a pattern of wide variation in health care practice including regional variations and small area variation.

(b) **Under use of services:-** Millions of people do not receive necessary care and suffer needless complications that add to costs and reduce productivity.

(c) **Over use of Services:-** Each year a large number of people receive health care services that are unnecessary, increase costs and may even endanger their health. Research has shown that this occurs across all populations. For example a study examining the use of antibiotics for treating ear infections in children on Medicaid found that expensive antibiotics were used far more often than indicated.

(d) **Misuse of Services:-** Too many patients develop complications during the course of their treatment and some die prematurely as a result. For example a study of injuries to patients treated in hospitals in New York State found 3.7% experienced adverse events, 13.6% of these events led to death and 2.6% led to permanent disability. About one-fourth of these adverse events resulted from negligence.

Quality Transformation

Traditional patient care has been a very individual and private affair for clinicians. For them quality means control by others. Clinicians feel powerless in this evolving system and because quality assessment feels invasive and intrusive it can produce resistance. While this seems understandable it is not in health care's best interest to stay stuck in resistance. The changes happening in health care mean that only 15% of health care quality is attributable to performance of individual and 85% is due to performance of systems. A clinician has power in the developing health care system to the extent to which he has knowledge. The knowledge is of his performance and of increases in his performance quality. This power of knowledge allows him within his arena to proactively increase quality of patient care and to share positive outcomes with the influential health care plans.

Management theories and practices to improve quality often have different names and to some extent even different definition but they share same roots. According to current thinking client satisfaction and efficiency happen automatically when organizations focus on improvement in processes and system to improve quality. During this transformation the approaches to quality improvement shift from being reactive to proactive. Rather than only inspecting and controlling, organizations build quality into the design of their services or products and into their work processes and systems. Through strategic quality management there is mobilization of staff at all levels of the organization to be responsible for quality and its implementation instead of reliance on a quality department or programme.

Quality is definitely in the eyes of the beholder. It needs to be considered which dimension of quality or perception of quality the other person may have. Administrator makes an effort to improve the level of performance across an entire organization to achieve higher levels of customer satisfaction (cultural quality). Clinical personnel focus on the delivery of medical care and the consistency of incorporating current professional knowledge (clinical quality). Employees, health care purchasers, patients and families assess the quality of their health care delivery based on personal treatment, access to care and medical outcomes (services quality). The commitment to quality improvement must come from the top of the organization, i.e. the Board of Director, CEO. The chair of the quality Improvement committee is best held by a physician. Without this leadership the program tends not to move forward and lacks commitment of a key group, the physicians. A physician must be the one carrying the message to his peers. The bottom line is that everyone in the organization can participate in improving some aspect of quality from organizational efficiencies in the clinic's operations to service and clinical quality.

Quality improvement teams should initially focus on;

(a) Highly prevalent conditions with significant effects on morbidity and mortality

(b) Conditions in which improving quality of service delivery will be efficacious (spend effort in the wisest manner)

(c) Conditions for which interventions are cost effective (spend money in the wisest manner)

(d) Conditions for which interventions are under control of health plan or provider or for which variation can be controlled i.e. it is easier to control how my team performs a treatment than it is to control patient compliance.

There are different approaches to diagnose quality related problems and to improve quality.

1. Quality Assurance Approach

Quality improvement or quality assurance involves the

development of criteria, standards and tracking methods to ensure that a facility is providing quality services to its customer on an ongoing basis. The process is supposed to detail in what areas a facility can be considered excellent, average or below acceptable standards and practices. Quality improvement programs may be stated clearly, but they cannot be organized and carried out as simply. There are many variables that have a direct impact on how a particular department operates on a daily basis. The status of one's budget, existing staffing levels, condition and age of the facility and its equipment, knowledge level of the staff and the expectations of the senior management staff are significant variables. These variables in turn directly affect how well quality improvement is made and how well existing quality is maintained. Tracking these variables that is comparing current operations against standards based on these variables is a fundamental part of any QA program. If the variables are ignored, a quality improvement program is not going to succeed.

Stages in Implementing a QA programme are:

Stage 1: Situation Analysis.– First step in implementation of QA programme is situational analysis which is done to understand local staff and client perceptions towards quality of health services through a series of focus group discussions and exit interviews.

Stage 2: Developing a quality culture.– Interdisciplinary quality action teams need to be formed which would undergo a programme of intensive orientation and training in QA skills.

Stage 3: Setting quality indicators and standards.– This involves identification of the event to be measured which is called Indicator. Indicator in Quality management is a measureable element in the structure, process or outcome of care whose value suggests one or more dimension of quality of care. Next step is to establish a benchmark which is optimal goal or best practice associated with that event. Once that goal has been determined the event is measured on a routine and periodic basis and the outcome of that measurement is compared to the established goal. Two types of bench marking have been identified. Competitive bench marking is the comparison of an organization to competitors that produce the same product or service. Comparing the performance of one hospitals surgical services to another hospitals surgical services is competitive bench marking. Competitive bench marking does not mean that the objects of comparison are in the same market. By definition one of the hospitals must provide the best surgical services. The best surgical services may not be provided by a local competitor. World-class benchmarking is the comparison of an organization to another organization outside the industry. For example a hospital may compare its billing process to a billing process of a utility company, if the utility's billing process is recognized as the best billing process. Although the clients of the two organizations are very different there still may be procedural lessons to be learned from the utility that are transferable to the hospital. Similarly health care organizations have been much slow to embrace information technology as a path to more efficient delivery of results and data. Bar coding used throughout many industries for materials management is not as prevalent in health care organizations, despite the large number of supplies that move through a hospital or other health care organizations at any given time. In health care, benchmarking typically has been applied to clinical practices rather than to business activities.

Stage 4: Institutionalizing the Quality Assurance system.– QA system has to be formalized by signing service level agreements containing explicit quality specifications. Organizations have to prioritize and classify indicators, prepare data collection instructions, prepare a deviation from standards form and use it to plot progress when a particular benchmark/standard is not met.

Underlying this approach is the " Bad Apples" view: find the bad apple and get rid of it." Such an approach to measuring and insuring quality has, understandably led to much resentment and focuses on meeting minimal standards (then stopping the assessment) rather than on improvement of quality on a continuous basis. A more mature and developed approach than quality assurance alone is "Total Quality Management." It uses QA as its first step and seeks to implement the result of QA into a more comprehensive and continuous effort to improve quality.

2. Total Quality Management

Quality improvement is the effort to improve the level of performance of a key process within an organization. Opportunities to improve care and service are found primarily by examining the systems and processes by which care and services are provided. The goal is to not merely meet standards of care but to exceed them. Performance assessment or measurement (QA) is a necessary step but is not the end-it is the first step in a continuous cycle of improving quality (Continuous Quality Improvement).

CQI is defined as the use of incremental and breakthrough quality management techniques to constantly improve processes, products or services provided to internal and external customers and thus achieve higher levels of customer satisfaction. Total Quality management (TQM) is defined as a structured systematic process for creating organization wide participation in planning and implementing continuous improvement in quality. Total organizational commitment is woven throughout the fabric of the organization, appearing in strategic planning, allocation of resources, role expectations, reward structures, performance evaluations, and the role of the organization in the community. An ongoing comprehensive self assessment system supports and promotes continuous improvement in the quality of patient care. Traditionally quality in health care has been defined by physicians and hospitals in professional and technical terms. However with the reemergence of quality as a major issue in health care, payers and patients are demanding participation in new definitions of quality that will include customer perception and satisfaction with the quality of care received. Definitions and measures contribute in the setting of expectations of the system and provide a method of monitoring the results; however organizations must seek to make quality an integral part of the delivery process. A variety of phrases have been used to define philosophy of total quality management. The principles of the philosophy are described in what are known as Deming's Fourteen points. The burden of effective implementation of TQM falls squarely on top management. Demings fourteen points constitute a road map for management to follow in order to enhance competitive position over the long run. These points have also been called "The Fourteen obligations of top management" and are summarized as follows:

1. **Create constancy of purpose:** Management must believe that the organization will be in business for a long time and therefore develop a strategy that is based on long term thinking. Board plays an important role in creating constancy of purpose by establishing the time frame and criteria by which the chief executive officer will be evaluated. There are additional ways to establish constancy of purpose in an organization (1) innovation, (2) research and education (3) continuous improvement of products and services (4) maintenance of plant and equipment.
2. **Adopt the new philosophy:** Adopting a new philosophy means transformation of management and obtaining appropriate technology.
3. **Cease dependence on mass inspection:** Competitive position can only be enhanced when the root causes of problems are identified and appropriate remedial actions taken upstream in the process. Continuous improvement occurs through the design and redesign of patient care systems and not by blaming individual workers within the health care organization. The problem in many hospitals is that all or most deviations are considered special, which ignores a common observation that 85% or more of variation in systems is from random causes. Employees who are held accountable for common – cause variation can easily become demoralized, angry and disconnected from their work. It is the job of management to redesign the system to reduce variation. One way of accomplishing this is through the development and use of protocols for activities, procedures, intermediate products and patient groups that will allow medical and clinical staff to concentrate on improvement rather than correction.
4. **End the practice of awarding business on price tag alone:** Hospital administrators should consider the implications on quality and productivity before substituting cheaper material and less skilled labour for more costly one on the basis of price tag alone.

5. **Improve constantly and forever the system of service:** Improvement is not a one time effort. Management is obligated to improve continually. Quality as per Deming "must be built in at the design stage" and teamwork is essential to the process. The staff members must as a team always consider what kind of service they can perform for their customers and how they can improve their present service.
6. **Institute training and retraining:** Training and education are essential to continuous improvement and establishing constancy of purpose. Management must encourage and provide for continuing education to assure that employees can perform their jobs correctly and to enhance professional development and employee satisfaction.
7. **Institute leadership:** Leadership is the job of management. It is management's responsibility to discover the barriers that prevent workers from taking pride in what they do and to continually seek ways to provide employees with the tools to do an effective job.
8. **Drive out fear:** Fear of failure, fear of embarrassment and fear of blame or retaliation inhibit to capitalize on opportunity and prevent people from asking questions or suggesting new ideas. This can result in loss of quality. People must feel secure and not be afraid to report problems, to ask for additional instructions or to call attention to conditions that interfere with quality.
9. **Break down barriers between departments:** Continuous improvement on an organization wide basis requires a system that fastens teamwork and a common departmental/ organizational vision. This vision is built on the mission of the organization that has quality as a primary goal. Top management's role in fostering team work means dismantling systems that destroy teamwork.
10. **Eliminate slogans, exhortations and targets for the work force:** Management can generate frustration and resentment in employees by proclaiming slogans like "zero defects" etc. Slogans contain an implicit supposition that employees could if they tried do better. People especially professionals may be offended by this suggestion.

11. **Eliminate numerical quotas:** Work standards such as "measured day work" or rates have been a part of American work ethic for decades. Deming stated that work standards impede quality more than any other single working condition. Work standards place a cap on productivity improvement and are totally contrary to the concept of continuous improvement.
12. **Remove barriers to pride of workmanship:** Top and middle managers must delegate as much authority as possible to their subordinates to foster their autonomy. The systems that evaluate the performance of people on a regular basis must be changed. Health care institutions should make use of "employee involvement programs and quality circles".
13. **Institute a vigorous program of education and retraining:** Closely related to point 6. It essentially means people are assets not commodities.
14. **Take action to accomplish the transformation:** Top management must agree on the direction to take action. They must feel pain and dissatisfaction with past performance. Management at all levels must constantly study the process it controls, ask how it might be improved, organize an appropriate team to address the issues, determine what data are necessary, collect the data, implement change and evaluate what occurred. This is known as the Shewhart cycle or the Deming cycle.

Pyramid of Continuous quality improvement involves cultural, technical, strategic and structural dimensions.

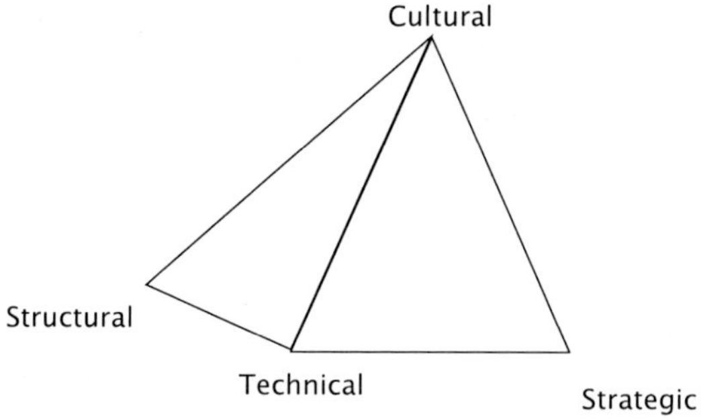

Fig. 3.1: Pyramid of continuous improvement

Cultural dimension refers to the underlying beliefs, values, norms and behaviors of the organization that support or serve as a barrier to organization wide improvement. The technical dimension refers to the extent to which employees have received training in CQI tools and group decision making processes to support quality improvement efforts. The strategic dimension refers to the extent to which the organization's quality improvement efforts are focused on key strategic priorities and on the organization's overall strategic plan. The structural dimension refers to the specific organizational entities such as co-ordinating committees, councils, task force, work groups and reporting/ accountability mechanisms used in the organizational quality improvement efforts.

Integration of QA and TQ

While QA is seen as an activity to fix blame, TQ searches for root causes of the problems in processes within the health care system rather than among the ranks of its employees. QA on one hand does not extend beyond meeting standards thereby making the system static and reactive while on the other hand TQ process continuously seeks opportunities for improvement and is proactive. In QA the coordinator or the department is the main driver while focused and combined efforts of all departments and employees drive TQ. Health care organizations can integrate TQ with QA by using the positive aspects of QA as a foundation for developing a comprehensive systems approach to health care quality issues. Successful implementation of TQ system offers resolution to many current barriers obstructing effective quality management for the health care organization. Quality in health care has multiple dimensions that dictate the need for an integrated quality management systems (IQMS). These dimensions include clinical quality, patient and customer service, appropriateness of care, cost effectiveness and efficiency, reduction of clinical risk and patient and employee safety.

The UK NHS quality proposals require all NHS organizations to develop an integrated approach to quality. In other countries, health care organizations are also working to ensure that the many different quality methods and systems used in health organizations do not duplicate or conflict with each other.

Seven components of integrated quality development approach which characterizes the hospitals programme and which can guide other in their quality journey are:

1. Four coordinated organization wide programmes to develop professional competencies, organization and processes, and a new role for patients.
2. Three dimensional definition of quality (patient, professional and management quality)
3. Patient pathway and process development
4. Quality data gathering
5. Team quality projects.
6. Patient focused system development and
7. Creating soulful spirals.

The aim of "Integrated quality development (IQD) is to develop the capability of a service better to meet the wants and needs of patients and to use fewer resources in doing so. It is an approach which provides a common language, simple methods and frame work for professionals and managers to work together to improve their services. It integrates the professional, management and patient quality perspectives and views the organization of services to a patient as a system made up of processes. The IQD approach recognizes that people have a right and a wish to grow as people from giving service to develop their technical and their human potential. The programme requires to recognize that the individual professionals competence is no longer the only source of quality. In modern health care, quality also depends on the contributions of other employees and on how these contributions are coordinated. Another challenge that the programme brought was to understand and bring about a change in role for managers from one of controlling to one of empowering. The managers role becomes one of motivating professionals to improve quality and ensuring that they know how to use organizational quality methods to understand and gain control over systems of care which they work in and contribute to.

Component 1-Four coordinated sub-programmes

The integrated quality development approach is to establish four sub-programmes and to coordinate these. These sub programmes are to develop professionals, managers, and the organizations but also to develop the patient's role.

Separate but coordinated programmes for each are:

Professional development:

- Education and practice development
- Updating
- Peer review
- Evidence based guidelines
- IT supported practice
- Inter professional working skills & culture

Management development:-

- Managing change to professional practice
- Education in quality management
- Quality measurement
- Managing empowerment
- Matrix management of projects
- Systems thinking and acting

Organization development:

- Responsibility and recognition of structure
- Matrix structure for process and professions
- Application of improvement science process/systems
- Variation
- People and teams.

Patient development:-

- Information about condition and options.
- Expectations
- Develop interdependence and self care as appropriate
- Ability to help improve service.

Component 2- Integrated quality definition

The integrated definition combines three elements:

- Patient quality i.e. what patients want.
- Professional quality i.e. what professionals want.

- Management quality using fewest resources without waste, errors or delay within policy and legal regulations.

Component 3- patient pathway and process development

Research has found that one of the most effective methods to improve quality is to form teams to describe and improve processes. In professional services there are many processes, but the most important are different patient pathways-all processes should contribute to these primary processes in some way. The idea is to describe patient's journey through out the service system i.e entry, first contact, assessment, intervention, follow-up etc. This is the easiest way to reveal the service system acting on the patient, to see where things go wrong and to decide where to concentrate improvement efforts. A true map of the pathway flow process is the basis for changing the process.

Component 4- quality data gathering

Gathering and using data are essential for monitoring and improving quality in modern professional services. It has been seen that hospital personnel usually do not have the skills to gather and use quality data or do not see the need to do so. Information management systems for automatic data capture and analysis usually are not available. Quality data is essential to quantify problems, gather data to be more certain about possible causes of complex problems and to evaluate quality interventions.

Component 5 – team quality projects

Multidisciplinary quality project teams are one of the most effective ways to improve quality in health services as long as they are well managed and well led. The nine phase team quality improvement sequence (TQIS) is

1. Choosing the problem.
2. Formulating the problem.
3. Guessing the cause of the problem.
4. Gathering data.
5. Analysis of data.
6. Planning the solution.

7. Implementing change.
8. Evaluating results.
9. Closing or continuing.

Component 6- patient focused service systems

In addition to concentrating on improving professional competence a service system approach recognizes that the patients experience is the result of many direct and indirect influences.

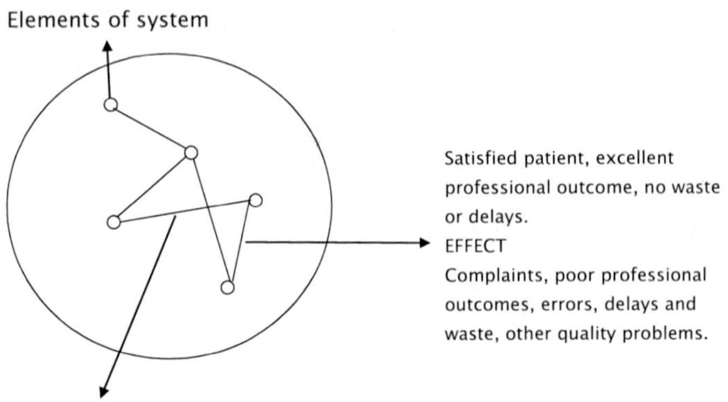

Fig. 3.2: Interaction between elements of system

Component 7- developing the soul and spirit of quality

This approach recognizes the importance of motivation, values and morale to professional service quality. There was a need to develop technical excellence but also to develop the humanity of service and the spirit of quality. Professionals expect fulfillment from their work and opportunities to grow.

The soulless spiral results in complaints leading to personnel withdrawing from and losing satisfaction from their work. People leave and put more stress on those remaining, leading to drop in quality sending the spiral of morale down wards. The upward spiral is where personnel grow through achieving recognized improvements.

References

1. Katherine Crasson. Improving Health care Quality AHRQ Publication No. 02-P032 September 2002, http://www.ahrq.gov/news/qualfact.htm.
2. Robert Cole. Quality Assurance in health care. Policy briefings for health sector Reform. Liverpool School of Tropical Medicine No 1 March 2000.
3. Jennifer Kenricks. Department of Family Medicine Quality Assurance. Research and faculty development. Department of Family Medicine Medical college of Georgia, 2005
4. Robert R. Casolou. Total Quality management in health care. Journal of Hospital and health care Administration 1991; 36(1) : 134-146.
5. Norman Velter. Effects of changes: Quality assurance in the Hospital, from centre of excellence to community support, 1st Edition chapman and Hall: 1995; 10: 183-202.
6. Stephen M. Shortell. Assessing the evidence on CQI: Is the glass half empty or half full. Journal of hospital and health services Admn. Special issue 1995; 40(1) : 4-24
7. Bryan S. Tindill, Douglas W. Stewart: Integration of Total quality and Quality assurance in the Text book of Total Quality in healthcare by A.F. Al Assaf, June A Schmele; St Lucie Press: 2000; 9:209-220
8. Robert C. Camp. Benchmarking (Milwavkee, WI: ASQC Quality press, 1989)
9. Craig Anderson, Peggy A Rivenburgh, " Bench marking," in Mara M. Melum and Marie K. Sinaris, Total Quality Management: The Health care Pioneers (American Hospital publishing; 1992)
10. David Casarett, Jason H.T Karlawish, Jeremy Sugarman. Determining when quality improvement Initiatives should be considered Research. JAMA : 2000; 283(17): 2275-2280.
11. Humberto de Moraes Novaes. Quality in hospital care. World Health forum; Volume 14: 1993
12. Robert D. Harris. Returning to the Basics: The bottom line to Quality improvement. Hospital topics; 1989; 19-23
13. John Ovretveit: The Norwegian approach to integrated quality development. Journal of Management in Medicine Vol. 15 No.2 2001. 125-141.

4

Tools of Quality Management

A Particular method being used by quality specialists for a particular purpose is referred to as a quality tool. A quality strategy differs from a quality tool in being an overall approach an organization takes over a period of time. Thus a programme for inspection of hospitals is a strategy and a particular method for carrying out inspection is referred to as a tool.

(A) Technical tools

(a) Quality function deployment (QFD): If quality is defined by the customer, QFD is the tool to assure that the customer's vision of quality is captured, defined, deployed through the enterprise and linked to the activities of the enterprise. QFD possesses a fairly extensive research and literature base. A few of the benefits stemming from the use of QFD are:

- More satisfied customers.
- More efficient use of resources since the team works on important things first.
- The ability to present and evaluate data on requirements, alternatives, competitive position, targets, possible sources of interrelations and priorities.

A comprehensive QFD analysis ensures that we have addressed all customer needs, that every one who works in the process understands what is important to the customer, and that every one understands why each performance measure is tracked.

(b) Seven Management and Planning (7MP) tools

The 7 MP tools are:

1. Affinity diagram.
2. Tree diagram.
3. Prioritization matrix.
4. Interrelation ship digraph.
5. Matrix diagram.
6. Activity network diagram.
7. Process decision program chart.

Affinity diagram (affinity chart) also known as the K-J Method in honour of its developer Kawakito Jivo is useful for generating and grouping ideas and concepts. This tool uses Paper or cards to generate and collect team ideas. These are then arranged into groupings and assigned a descriptive header. The number of cards under each header indicates the breadth of team consensus on the issue.

Tree diagram (also known as the schematic diagram) By tree diagram a complex project is broken into manageable tasks. Each element is divided into a list of self contained tasks that may be assigned to one or more sub teams or individuals. The tree diagram is used to identify the best solution. After the team has identified the best solution for addressing the problem statement, a recommendation is made to the quality council. The purpose of communication is to gain the sanction of executive level management so that they may demonstrate their commitment to the overall TQ process. The dissecting process continues until the team reaches the point where tasks are defined well enough that they can be assigned to some one.

Prioritization matrix This tool makes it easy for the team to focus on important items. Pair wise comparisons are made to determine the over all relationship of a large number of elements.

Interrelationship digraph. (1D) or relations diagram. It helps to discover relationships and dependencies between different activities. Using graphical techniques relationships are identified one by one and driver tasks as well as out come tasks are identified.

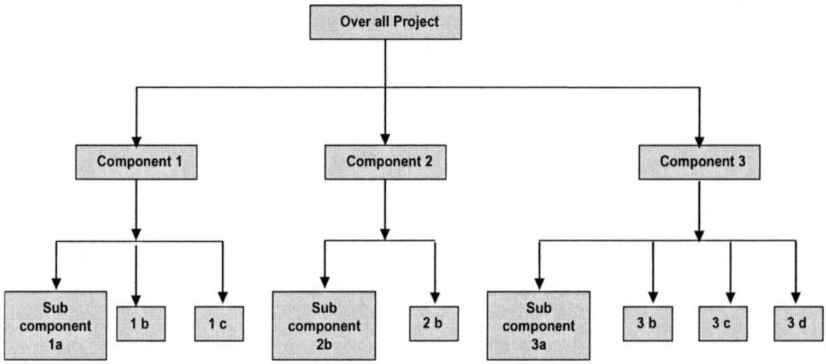

Fig. 4.1: Tree Diagram

Matrix diagrams. Matrix diagrams allow to display relationship and responsibilities in concise and efficient manner. They may appear similar to interrelationship digraph but are used for assignments not assessments.

Activity network diagrams. Is a way to schedule project tasks. The tasks are arranged in anticipated flow order (sequential, parallel or a combination). Times are assigned to each task and the result is an ordered diagram that shows predecessor/ successor relationships, total task times and the critical path.

Process decision program chart (PDPC) In PDPC after exploring likely problems for each step, contingency countermeasures are planned for each potential problem and the best choice from the options is selected. The team begins as with tree diagram but instead of breaking each of the second level items down into more tasks the team leader takes each second level item and asks, what could go wrong with this ? The various failure scenarios based on data, past experience are written on individual cards to form the third level of tree. Next the fourth level of diagram is used to describe various contingencies that the team could utilize to minimize the impact of each failure scenario. The symbol X is typically used to mark those that are impractical, while the symbol O is used to mark those that should be implemented.

Failure mode & effects analysis: (FMEA) is a slightly more sophisticated version of contingency planning. In FMEA steps, failure scenarios and contingency plans are typically described in more detail and the resulting information is displayed in tabular form. The key refinement is that each failure mode is then rated based on likelihood of occurrence and severity. These rating scores follow a pareto distribution and direct the planning groups attention toward the most likely and most severe potential failures.

(C) SPC, SQC, and 7QC Statistical process control (SPC) is the application of statistical methods to identify when a process may have been influenced by a special cause of variation. While SPC deals with in process measures often our only significant way to measure the process result is by measuring the performance of the finished product. As with in process measures final performance variation is a function of the variation resulting from normal and special causes. Often this approach is called statistical quality control (SQC). The same charts and approaches are often used. SQC should not be used as a substitute for SPC. Since SPC is directed at process, it offers faster detection and correction of Problems. Many of the tools for this job are grouped with SPC/SQC in what are called the seven quality control tools (7QC).

(1) SPC/SQC
(2) Histograms.
(3) Scatter diagram.
(4) Pareto charts
(5) Fish bone diagram.
(6) Check sheets.
(7) Defect Maps.

Histogram

Histogram is a modified bar graph where the data on the X-axis are continuous and thus the bars are adjacent to one another. It is a graphic summary of variation in a set of data. It enables us to see patterns that are difficult to see in a simple table of numbers.

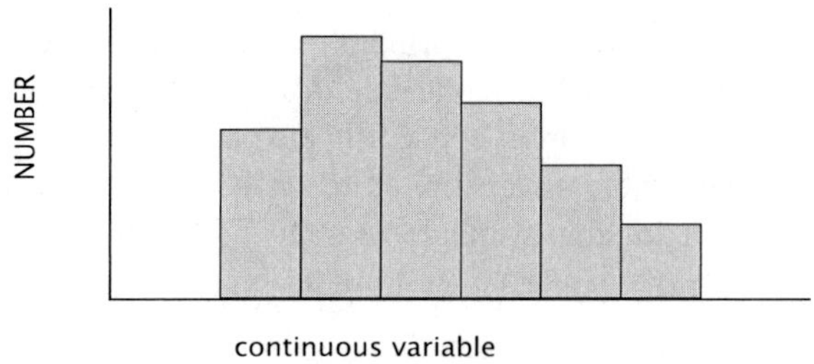

Fig. 4.2: Histogram

Scatter diagram

The technique is useful in displaying data from two variables that may relate to each other. The data collected is plotted on a graph with one variable on X-axis and the other on Y-axis.

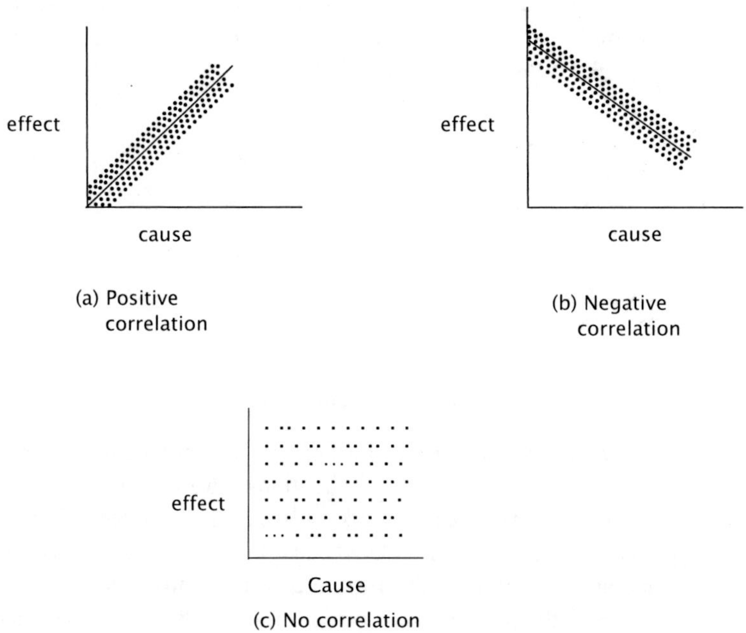

Fig. 4.3: Scatter Diagram

Pareto chart: The Pareto principle is defined as the separation of the vital few issues that contributed to a problem from the less important issues. The Pareto concept is also known as the 80-20 rule i.e. most of the problems are linked to only a few causes. One can analyze data utilizing this principle with the aid of bar and line graphs.

- Identify the quality problem to be studied.
- Select data collection method.
- Categorize your data according to the type.
- Plot the frequency of each category of problem on a bar graph and arrange the categories in order of descending frequency from left to right on horizontal axis. Two vertical axis are designated. The left axis is divided into equal intervals based on the highest frequency while the right vertical axis is divided into percentages from 0-100%.
- Add the percentage values of the bars and calculate the cumulative total for each bar. Plot these totals on the same graph but as a line graph.

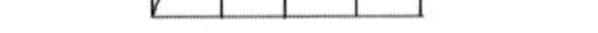

Fig. 4.4: Pareto Chart

Fish bone diagram or cause and effect diagram are tools to help organizations analyze problematic situations. Problematic situations are set equal to effects. Then by working backward from the effect and asking why? a diagram of interrelated causes is constructed. Cause and effect diagrams are constructed by the quality improvement team in few steps. Once the problem is selected for study its causes are listed. The list of the causes is then classified into categories and subcategories which are displayed on a diagram with arrows directed towards the main problem. The final diagram represents a fish skeleton and is therefore referred as fish bone diagram. It is also called Ishikawa diagram.

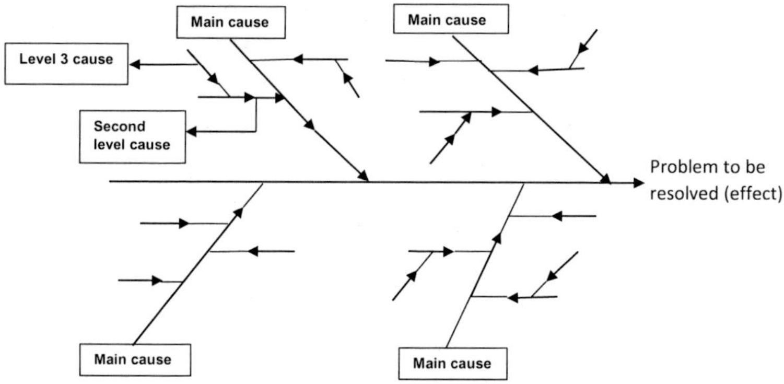

Fig. 4.5: FISH Bone Diagram

Check sheets

Check sheet is a data recording form that has been designed to readily interpret results from the form itself. It needs to be designed for the specific data it is to gather. It is used for the collection of quantitative or qualitative data and is adaptable to different data gathering situations.

Defect Maps

In defect maps locations of the defective devices are stored. Defect maps are fundamental for defect tolerant computing and are fundamental to bridge the manufacturing and system design stages.

Other TQM technical tools.

Brain storming: In this technique a group of individuals meet to generate a list of ideas regarding a topic. Discussion is then encouraged to clarify each idea and its objective. Duplication is eliminated and ideas are sorted into related subtopics. The final list is then used for the purpose intended.

Brain writing: Brain writing differs from brain storming in that after writing the ideas on a piece of paper each member modifies his own list after reading the ideas of other members. It provides all members an equal opportunity to participate and eliminate ideas that are not well thought out.

Event log: logs are used to keep track of a sequence of events and/ or periods of time during which such events occur in order to chart trends. Logs are drawn as tables with columns and rows.

Pie- chart: Is a graphic representation of data elements that are part of a whole. The segments of the pie chart must add up to 100% of whole and should not exceed six so as to avoid a cluttered appearance. If one or more categories have a value of zero then pie charts should not be used.

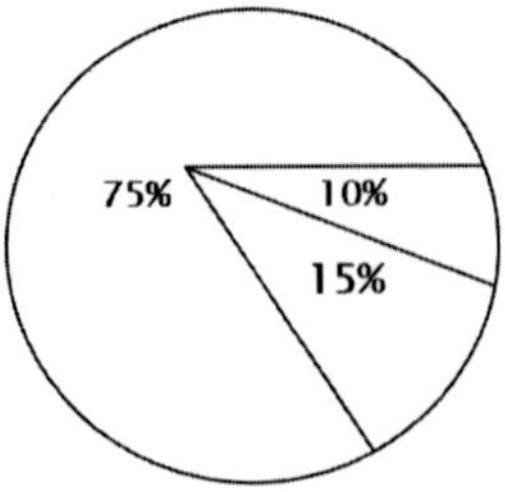

Fig 4.6: Pie-chart

Check lists: A check list contains items that are important or relevant to a specific issue or situation. Check lists are used under operational conditions to ensure that all important steps or actions have been taken. Their primary purpose is for guiding operations, not for collecting data. Generally used to check that all aspects of a situation have been taken into account before action or decision making.

Control chart: Control charts are a method of statistical process control. They enable the control of distribution of variation rather than attempting to control each individual variation. Upper and lower control and tolerance limits are calculated for a process and sampled measures regularly plotted about a control line between the two sets of limits. The plotted line corresponds to the stability/trend of the process. Action can be taken based on trend rather than on individual variation. A process is said to be in control if trend falls within the upper and lower control limit. The process is out of control if trend falls outside UCL or LCL or if at least three consecutive points on the process trend line fall below or at least three consecutive points falls above the average even though the process trend line is between the UCL and LCL.

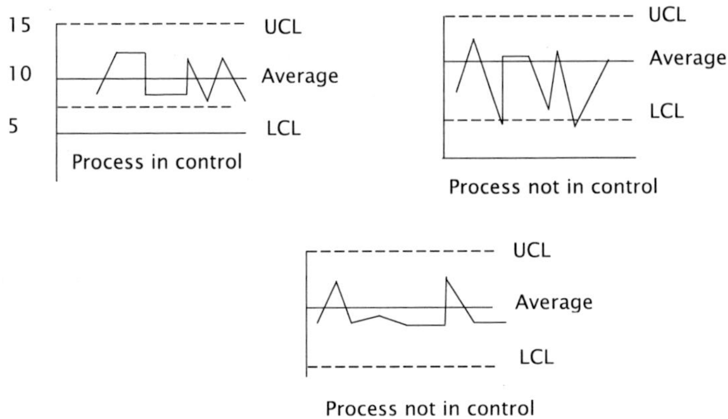

Fig 4.7: Control Chart

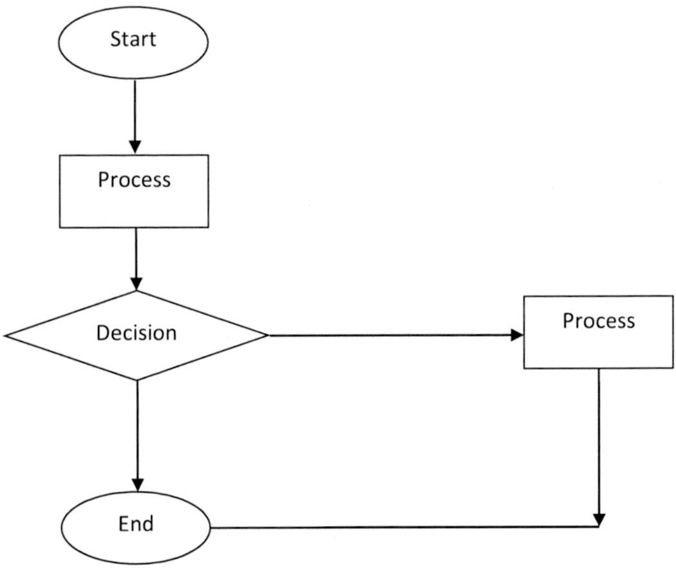

Fig 4.8: Flow Chart

Flow chart

Pictures, symbols or text coupled with lines, arrows on lines show direction of flow. It enables modeling of processes; problems/ opportunities and decision points etc. Develops a common understanding of a process by those involved. No particular standardization of symbology is required as communication to a different audience may require considerable time and explanation. Oval represent beginnings, diamonds represent decision points circle connector, rectangle process etc.

Quality Circles

Quality Circles are group of employees who meet voluntarily to solve their own work related problems in an organized way. Successful utilization of quality circles requires a long term commitment. Members of quality circles need to have adequate knowledge of the subject and need to know how to evaluate and improve process and product quality.

Bar chart: Which are found in pareto charts and histograms help give a visual sense of weight to the problem at hand. It differs from histogram in that bars are not adjacent to each other i.e. data on X- axis is not continuous.

Line graph: shows how a process performs over time. Add a arrow pointing up or down to orient people's attention and you have got an immediate grasp of any process issue.

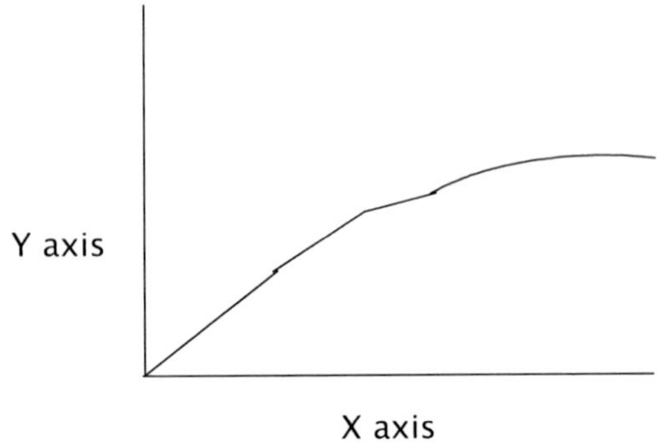

Fig 4.9: Line Graph

Nominal group Technique

Once the list of ideas is generated then prioritizing or ranking is done by nominal group technique. The ideas are then used to improve the process. The ranking can be done by multiple voting, weighted voting or rank ordering. In multiple voting, group arbitrarily chooses the number of votes each member may have while in weighted voting technique each group member is allowed a set number of votes which is usually 1.5 times the number of ideas to be voted on.

Decision matrices are helpful where the criteria are multi-dimensional. In a two dimensional matrix, options are listed as rows while as specific criteria are listed as columns. The intersection of rows and columns are used to capture the group's opinion about how each option rates on the specific criteria.

Six sigma

Sigma is a measure of statistical variation. Six sigma indicates near perfection and is a rigorous operating methodology aimed to ensure complete customer satisfaction by ingraining a culture of excellence, responsiveness and accountability within an organization. Such programs also incorporate a strong system for gathering customer feed back. Six sigma entails five key steps.

- Identify the customer requirements, clarify the problem and set goals.
- Select what needs to be measured, identify information source and gather data.
- Develop hypotheses, identify the variables and causes.
- Generate solutions and put them into action, either modifying existing processes or developing new ones.
- Develop monitoring processes for continued high quality performance.

Six sigma can

- Make processes more rigorous by using hard, timely data, not opinions or gut feel to make operating decisions.
- Cultivate customer loyalty by delivering superior value.
- Achieve quantum leaps in product performance.
- Reduce variation in service processes such as offering a consistent high quality service experience.

- Improve financial performance, through cost savings from projects, increased revenue from improved products and expanded operating margins.

The five objectives of six sigma are:

1. To satisfy the customer
2. To lift internal performance.
3. To enable better performance by better design.
4. To improve the quality of purchased supplies.
5. To reduce costs.

Six main benefits of the sigma break through strategy are remarkable improvements in.

1. Processes.
2. Products & services.
3. Investor relations.
4. Design methodology.
5. Supplier relationships.
6. Training and recruitment.

While TQM focuses on improvement in individual operations with unrelated processes six sigma focuses on making improvement in all operations within a process producing results more rapidly and effectively.

The main objective of six sigma methodology is the implementation of measurement band strategy that focuses on process improvement and variation reduction through the application of six sigma improvement projects. This is accomplished through the use of two six sigma sub methodology: DMAIC and DMADV. The six sigma DMAIC process (define, measure, analyze, improve, control) is an improvement system for existing processes falling below specification and looking for incremental improvement. The six sigma DMADV process (define, measure, analyze, design, verify) is an improvement system used to develop new processes or products at six sigma quality levels.

Specific process planning Methods in health care. The importance of quality in health care led to the development of specific adoptions for health care.

Critical paths: or care paths are multidisciplinary high level process design efforts that specify key milestones in the care process for patients in given diagnostic category. It not only reduces average length of stay but improves quality of care, patient and attendant satisfaction and coordination between team members.

Clinical guides lines: clinical guide lines outline the process of clinical decision making and thereby focus discussion on potentially unnecessary variation in clinical practice.

In order to make quality in health care a success each health care organization should have a annual quality plan same as they have annual budget. A health care organization might ask each department or service to set specific improvement goals which would then be categorized and summarized to form organization wide goals. Japanese developed Hoshin planning which places quality firmly at the centre of all organizations plans. Hoshin planning rests on two critical assertions: one that central goal of any organization must be to meet the needs of its customers, and second that to be successful the organization must achieve alignment between organizational and personal goals. Implementation of hoshin planning in health care is hindered by confusion over multiple customers, lack of information about the true needs and expectation of these customers, and the tradition of not involving staff in strategic planning.

A review of the clinical application of CQI in United States found 41single and 13 multi-site studies mostly using practitioner before and after measures. Accepting the scientific weaknesses of the studies the review concluded that there was some evidence that improved quality and economic efficiencies were achieved. One policy evaluation of a 24-pilot United Kingdom National CQI based improvement programme explained the wide range of short term and long-term results as due to "the power of physicians, the inertia built into established ways of working and the effort needed to implement new work processes." Recommendations included stimulating change at individual, team, organization and systems levels simultaneously and need for personnel to feel that they too as well as patients benefit from improvement. Some studies have shown application of TQM difficult in health sector because of three different management hierarchies as opposed to one in industries. Professionals show resistance to management because it narrows their autonomy.

Approaches to improve quality in hospitals

The various quality strategies are increasing resources, large scale reorganization, strengthening management, formulating standards, patient empowerment, quality management system, accreditation etc. There is no scientific evidence that one type of strategy is better than another. There is little research assessing the effectiveness of one or more hospital or national quality strategies. The lack of evidence is largely a result of the difficulties of evaluating this type of intervention and of proving that the results are due to the strategy and not to other changes. In sum no one quality strategy can be recommended over another.

The main recommendations by WHO Regional office for Europe's Health Evidence network (HEN) are:

1. Hospitals should decide which approach to adopt after making an assessment of their quality and safety status and listing the different strategies which might be appropriate to their situation.
2. When reviewing types of strategies, hospitals and governments should question the claims of proponents of any one approach because there is no strong evidence of effectiveness of any strategy. They should recognize the value of extensive experience as a form of evidence but also the commercial nature of the growing quality industry in health care.
3. Decision makers should be aware that the same strategy applied in a different place may well yield different results, even if fully implemented. Attention needs to be paid to financial, cultural and other conditions surrounding implementation.
4. Having chosen one type of quality strategy one should review it regularly and adapt it to changing situations and the responses of the interested personnel. Efforts should be made to assess whether any lack of results is due to the wrong strategy, poor implementation or the time required for results to become measurable. Close monitoring using a range of types of information can assist this assessment.

5. It is possible that applying a consistent quality strategy over time is more likely to be effective than changing to another approach. Flexibility without sudden radical change appears to be important.
6. Quality experts with wide experiences can be useful, but need to be chosen with care. One or more independent experts should be used to give independent feed back for regular reviews of a strategy.
7. Researchers need to pay more attention to describing the strategy actually carried out, assessing the depth of implementation and considering alternative explanations for the apparent results of a strategy.

References

1. Myer Kutz. Total quality management and the mechanical engineer in Mechanical engineers Hand book .72; 2159-2176. 1998 John Wiley and sons, inc.
2. Paul E. Plsek. Techniques for managing quality. Journal Hospital and Health services Admn. Special CQI issue 40:1 spring 1995.
3. J T Burr. The tools of quality; quality progress Nov. 1990.
4. Bioblos Jim. " Six sigma Meets the service Economy." Harvard Management update 2002, PP 1-4.
5. Brey fogle, Forrest; III. Implementing six sigma; Smarter solutions using statistics 2nd e d / John Wiley and sons, 2003.
6. Short tell SM, Bennett Cl, Byck GR. Accessing the impact of continuous quality improvement on clinical practice: what will it take to accelerate progress? Milbank quarterly, 1998, 76: 593-624.
7. Ham C, Kipping R, Mcleod H. Redesigning work processes in health care: lessons from the NHS. Milbank quarterly 2003, 81, 3: 415-428.
8. What are the best strategies for ensuring quality in hospitals? World Health Organization 2003.

5

Indicator in Quality Improvement

Indicators are defined as specific criteria used to measure the quality of care. Indicator is a measurable element in the structure, process or outcome of care whose value suggests one or more dimensions of quality of care. Indicators of care can be divided into three categories: structure, process and outcome. Structure indicators are those that focus on the physical facilities and resources of an institution. Process indicators look at departmental functions that in themselves do not ensure a good outcome but that, when done well increase the likelihood of a positive outcome. Outcome indicators include patient complaints, deaths, discharges etc.

The quality of health care is on the agenda in most countries, however there is no mandatory national system to track the quality of care delivered to the citizens. Health care in the aggregate is the largest enterprise in the United States, employing more people than any other industry, consuming nearly 15% of the gross domestic product and having expenditures of more than $1.2 trillion a year. Given this, it is remarkable how little is known about the quality of US health care. Whatever little is known it shows serious lapses and systematic quality problems. Hospitals need to have quality improvement as their primary business strategy. Providers increasingly wish to know how well they are performing and to have effective means of assessing and improving the quality of care they provide. For this they require measures that are meaningful, interpretable and of demonstrable value in helping to improve quality. Indicators for performance and outcome measurement allow the quality of care and services to be measured.

In 1984 leaders of seven Maryland Hospital Association met and agreed to share data. Using grant from the Robert Wood Johnson Foundation, Maryland Hospital Association (MHA) began in 1987 to test its model of indicators and assessment tools for use of hospitals outside the state. Today Maryland Quality Indicator Project is a registered trademark with more than 225 hospitals in States and more than 1000 US health Care organizations using its data mining services. In addition more than 300 health care institutions in nine countries abroad are associated with it. The International Quality Indicator Project (IQIP) comprises sets of performance indicators for four different pattern care settings-acute care, psychiatric care, long term care and home care. Each indicator set has numerous measures for which a facility can submit data and receive comparative feed back. It is common for new participants to select a handful of measures for the first few reporting periods, then add more measures as the facility gains experience in the IQIP and the data collection process.

The Agency for Health care Research and Quality (AHRQ) makes use of administrative patient data and has four models measuring various aspects of quality. Preventive quality indicators identify e.g. hospital admissions that evidence suggests could have been avoided at least in part through high quality out-patient. In-patient quality indicators reflect quality of care inside hospitals including inpatient mortality for medical conditions and surgical procedures, patient safety indicators reflect quality of care inside hospitals but focus on potentially avoidable complications and iatrogenic effects and pediatric quality indicators reflect quality of care inside hospitals and identify potentially avoidable hospitalizations among children. In 2000, the National Indicator Project was established in the Danish health care system. From 2000 to 2002 disease specific quality standards, indicators and prognostic factors have been developed for six diseases: stroke, hip fracture, schizophrenia, acute gastrointestinal surgery, heart failure and lung cancer. Indicators and standards have been based on scientific literature to assure the highest strength of evidence. If there is no scientific evidence available and the clinical problem in relation to disease is very important indicators and standards are determined by consensus among experienced and competent clinical experts. For each disease six to ten indicators were determined relating to structure, process and outcome of care. To secure the comparability of the collected data at the hospital and national levels, prognostic factors were identified in relation to the defined indicators and standards. These prognostic factors are used as explanation variables and to adjust for case mix. This is important as it then becomes possible to evaluate whether a favorable or unfavorable outcome is due to the health care system or due to conditions over which the health care system has no influence e.g. conditions related to the patient or the disease. Indicators, Standards and prognostic factors are implemented in all hospital units in Denmark. There is mandatory participation for all hospitals and relevant clinical departments and units treating patients with the six diseases. This requires development of an organization at the clinical units; hospital and country levels to ensure that the data collected are reproducible and correspond with the definitions determined by the indicator groups. Care is taken to ensure that the implementation of the project is incorporated into the daily work of the units and that structure of the project follows the daily structure in management and consultancy. Clinical indicators for stroke are illustrated in table 5-1.

Table 5.1: Clinical indicators for stroke

Indicator Concept	Indicator
Organization of treatment	Proportion of patents treated/rehabilitated in stroke units
Secondary prophylactic treatment	Proportion of patients treated with platelet inhibitors
	Proportion of patient treated with anticoagulants
Diagnostics	Proportion of patients who undergo a CT/ MRI scan
Assessment by a physiotherapist	Proportion of patients assessed by a physiotherapist
Assessment by an occupational therapist	Proportion of patient assessed by an occupational therapist
Assessment of nutritional status	Proportion of patients who have their nutritional status evaluated
Mortality	30 days and 3,6 and 12 months mortality

Adopted from International Journal for Quality in health care 2004. Vol. 16, supp 1.

The project aims to document and develop the quality of health care. It aims to assess the health care system as an organization and does not focus on individuals. It is not the aim of the project to find scapegoats but to bring forth the best possible basis for improvement of quality and development of quality in the health care system. At the same time a qualified basis has been created for a dialogue between the health care providers, managers, the political system and patients founded on evidence based documentation.

Patient satisfaction has also been used as an indicator of quality care in independent health facilities. Although patient ratings cannot substitute for expert on spot assessments, they are important part of a quality management program and provide additional complementary information about components of quality care. In US National Quality Forum (NQF) has been established as a private, not–for-profit, open membership, public benefit cooperation for the purposes of developing consensus about standardized health care performance measures, reporting mechanisms and a national strategy for heath care quality improvement. The new assertiveness of consumers as well as that of providers has challenged the traditional roles of physicians and health care provider organizations in establishing quality improvement and in determining quality improvement priorities. At this time the myraid health care stake holders have divergent views about who should determine quality standards, how performance measures or standards should be set, and who should be allowed access to data about compliance with standards. Standards are more likely to be accepted and implemented if representatives of those who will have to implement and use the standards are involved throughout their development. The idea of establishing a unique public private organization to promote a national agenda for health care quality improvement was advanced by the President's Advisory Commission on Consumer Protection and Quality in the health care Industry in U.S. In pursuing this strategy, the NQF does not anticipate that it will develop new quality performance measures. Many research, accreditation and over-sight organizations as well as commercial interests have developed measures or are developing new performance indicators. The NQF sees a greater need at this time for weighing the evidence behind existing measures and endorsing those that are both evidence based and linked to national priorities for health care quality. NQF is unique in blending consumer, purchaser and provider perspectives on an equitable basis and then using the combined market power of both the public and private sectors to leverage quality improvement. Care is taken that standards have five attributes i.e. openness, balance of interest, due process, an appeals process and consensus. Priorities of health care consumers are better addressed. It includes those parts of health care system that consumer directly interface with i.e. hospitals, out patient clinics and individual care givers.

Bench marking is not solely a measurement technique but goes deeper to understand why there are performance differences between seemingly similar processes. Knowing why something is better is the key to improving processes. Internal benchmarking compares similar processes and services within the organization. While this is a good way to reduce unnecessary variation we may not uncover substantially better practices simply by looking within our own organization. Competitive benchmarking is the comparison of an organization to competitors that produce the same product or service. For example, comparing the performance of one hospital surgical services to another hospital's surgical services is competitive benchmarking. It does not mean that the objects of comparison are in the same market. But that one of the hospitals must provide the best surgical services. World class benchmarking (generic benchmarking) is the comparison of an organization to another organization outside the industry. Functional benchmarking compares performance against those who are the best in the industry, but not direct competitors. It is also called group benchmarking. The absence of direct competition opens up a better channel for detailed sharing across organization.

References

1. C.David Burkland. Quality Assurance and Continuous Process Improvement in Emergency Medicine Vol. II 176; 1697-1701. 1998 W.B Saunders Company.
2. Kenneth W. Kizer. Establishing Health Care performance standards in an Era of consumerism. JAMA, Sept 12:286 (10); 1213-1217. 2001.
3. Jan Mainz, Birgilte Randrup Krog, Bodil Bjornshave and Paul Bartels. Nation wide continous quality improvement using clinical indicators: the Danish National Indicator Project. International Journal for quality in Health Care. 2004 volume 16, supplement 1: 145-150.

4. Thomson RG, MC Elroy H, Kazand Jlan VA. Maryland Hospital quality Indicator project in the United Kingdom: an approach for promoting continuous quality improvement. Quality Health care 1997; 6: 49-55
5. Mainz J. Defining and classifying clinical indicators for quality improvement International Journal Quality Health Care 2003; 15: 523-530.
6. Palmer RH, Reilly MC. Individual and institutional variables which may serve as indicators of quality of Medical care 1979; 17: 693-717
7. Jerod Loeh. Leading indicator. Modern Health care August 15, 2005.
8. Christel A, Wood Ward. Patient satisfaction as an indicator of quality care in independent health facilities: Developing and assessing a tool to enhance public accountability. American journal of Medical Quality, Vol. 15, No.3, 94-105(2000).
9. Cleary PD, Edgman- Levitan S. Health care quality: incorporating consumer perspectives. JAMA. 1997. 278:1608-1612.
10. Schuster MA, Mc Glynn EA, Brook BH. How good is the quality of health care in the United States? Milbank Q 1998; 76: 517-563.
11. The President's Advisory Commission on consumer protection and quality first: Better health care for all Americans. Washington DC. US Dept. of Health and Human Services 1998.
12. Paul. E.P. Techniques in Managing Quality. J. Hospital and Health Services Admn. 40(1) 1995: 50-79.

6

Hospital Accreditation

Quality issues began to be addressed in hospitals during early 1900s. In 1913 American college of surgeons (ACS) was founded and in 1918 Hospital standardization program was established by ACS for hospital where surgery was performed. Eventually it evolved into Joint Commission on Accreditation of Health care Organizations (JCAHO) which is still key accrediting agency for hospitals.

Accreditation is defined as the process by which an agency or organization evaluates the degree to which an institution meets certain predetermined standards.

C.E Lewis defines accreditation as a professional recognition of facilities that provide high quality care.

Accreditation is a voluntary process for introduction of formal quality assurance system into hospital programme in which hospitals invite survey by the commission.

Four basic elements of accreditation are:

I. It is voluntary.

II. Standards are laid.

III. Compliance is measured by external review.

IV. Rating.

Models of Accreditation

There are three models of accreditation

I. Standard based:- This model emphasizes on the availability of basic health facilities i.e., space and equipment requirements and human resources.
II. Quality assurance based:- Ranking is based on satisfying some basic indicators of quality in those institution that are striving to improve quality.
III. Citizens charter based:- In this model criteria of assessment is geared towards people-centric indicators. It emphasizes on evaluating health systems from indicators such as user friendliness, providing information to users about services available, setting up procedures for redressal of grievances.

Standards

Standards represent a degree of excellence, serve as a basis for comparison and are a minimum with which a community may be content. 50% of the standards are designated as core standards or minimum standards and are necessarily to be met for an organization to be accredited. Criteria for identification of care standard include; the standard reduces the risk that the rights of the patient will not be respected, standard reduces risk point in the clinical care process or the standard reduces risk in the patient care environment. Beyond the minimum there are desirable or optimum or reach standards. A hospital while meeting a minimum standard should seek to achieve a desirable or optimum standard. Standards can be explicit or implicit. Explicit criteria are written down and the work under study is checked against them. Implicit criteria on the other hand exist only in the mind of the evaluator and nothing is written down. Assumption is made that evaluators can distinguish between good and bad based on their experience and knowledge. Ideally standards should be explicit as these allow assessment of care to be based on clearly delineated agreed upon benchmarks.

Accreditation body

For proper development and implementation of quality, authority and responsibility should be vested in an autonomous body or commission which should be nonpolitical.

The composition of this body should be

I. Representation of public sector especially the ministries of health and social security and the private sector.

II. Experts from the field of hospital administration, finance, law, hospital engineering and medicine.

III. Representation of the most distinguished medical councils and academies.

IV. Representation from the voluntary organizations.

Accreditation body should be supported by a proper secretariat and as an alternative to use of subjective criteria by physicians in assessing the quality of medical care, accreditation body relies on precise criteria that makes assessment easier and simple.

Functions of the accreditation body include

1. Granting accreditation to the hospitals meeting specified requirements.
2. Periodic inspection for evaluating hospital performance.
3. Inspection of hospitals from time of construction to the time of commissioning as per approved plan.
4. Temporary/permanent cancellation of accreditation if the hospital fails to meet the prescribed standards.

The various standards laid down by Joint Commission for international accreditation are based on following:

PATIENT-CENTERED STANDARDS

(1) Access

- Patients have access to the health care organization's services based on their identified health care needs and the organization's mission and resources.
- The organization has a process for admitting patients to the organization.
- Patients with emergency or immediate needs are given priority for assessment and treatment.

(2) Continuity

- The organization designs and carries out processes to provide continuity of patient care services within the organization and coordination among health professionals.
- During all phases of care there is a qualified individual identified as responsible for the patients care.
- Information about the patient's care and response to care is shared among medical, nursing and other care providers during each staffing shift, between shifts and during transfers between units.
- Patient record is available to the care providers to facilitate the exchange of information.

(3) Discharge, Referral & follow up

- A process is in place to appropriately refer or discharge patients.
- The organization co-operates with health care practitioners and outside agencies to ensure timely and appropriate referrals.
- Patients and their attendants are given understandable follow-up instructions at referral or discharge.

(4) Transfer of patients

- There is a process to appropriately transfer patients to another organization to meet their continuing care needs.
- The receiving organization is given a written summary of the patient's clinical condition and the interventions provided by the referring organization.
- The transfer process is documented in the patient record.

(5) Patient and Family rights

- The organization is responsible for providing processes that support patient's and his attendant's rights during care.
- The organization informs patients and families about its care and services and how to access those services.
- Care is considerate and respectful of the patient's personal values and beliefs.
- Care is respectful of the patient's need for privacy.

- The organization takes measures to protect patient's possessions from theft or loss.
- Patients are protected from physical assault.
- Venerable children, disabled individuals and the elderly receive appropriate protection.
- Patient's information is confidential and protected from loss or misuse.
- The organization supports patients and families rights to participate in the care process.
- The organization informs patients and families about how they will be told of medical conditions and treatments and how they can participate in care decision to the extent they wish to participate.
- The organization informs patients and families about their rights and responsibilities relating to referring or discontinuing treatment.
- Staff are educated about their role in identifying patient's values and beliefs and protecting patient's rights.
- All patients are given information about their rights in a manner they can understand.
- Patient informed consent is obtained through a process defined by the organization and carried out by trained staff.
- Patients and families receive adequate information about the illness, proposed treatment and care providers so that they can make care decisions.
- When someone other than the patient gives the informed consent, that individual is noted in the patient's record.
- The organization has a committee to oversee all research in the organization involving human subjects.
- The organization provides patient care within business, financial, ethical and legal norms that protect patients and their rights.

(6) Assessment of patient

- All patients cared for by the organization have their health care needs identified through an established assessment process.

- Assessments are completed in the time frame prescribed by the organization.
- The initial medical assessment is documented in the patient's record within the first 24 hours after the patient's entry.
- The initial medical assessment is documented before anesthesia or surgical treatment.
- All patients are reassessed at appropriate intervals.
- Qualified individuals conduct the assessment and reassessments.

(7) Laboratory services

- Laboratory services are available to meet patient needs, and all such services meet applicable local and national standards, laws and regulations.

(8) Radiology services

- Radiology services are available to meet patient needs and all such services meet applicable local and national standards, laws and regulations.
- Medical, nursing and other individuals and services responsible for patient care collaborate to analyze and integrate patient assessments.

(9) Care of patients

- Policies and procedures, and applicable laws and regulations guide the uniform care of all patient's.
- The care provided to each patient is planned and written in the patient's records.
- Polices and procedures guide the care of high risk patients and the provision of high risk services.
- Policies and procedures guide the care of emergency patients.
- Policies and procedures guide the use of resuscitation services throughout the organization.
- Policies and procedures guide the handling, use and administration of blood and blood products.
- Policies and procedures guide the care of patients on life support who are comatosed, who are on dialysis, vulnerable

elderly patients and children, patients with a communicable disease and immuno- suppressed patients.

(10) Anesthesia care

- A qualified individual conducts a pre-anesthesia assessment.
- Each patient's anesthesia care is planned and documented.
- The risks, potential complications and options are discussed with the patient, his or her attendants.
- The anesthesia used and patient's physiological status during anesthesia administration is documented in the patient's record.
- Each patient's post anesthesia status is monitored and documented.

(11) Surgical care

- Each patient's surgical care is planned and documented based on the results of the assessment.
- The risks, benefits, potential complications and options are discussed with the patient and family.
- Each patient's physiological status is continuously monitored during and immediately after surgery and written in the patient's record.

(12) Medication use

- The pharmacy service and medication use in the organization comply with applicable laws and regulations.
- An appropriate selection of medications for prescribing or ordering is stocked or readily available.
- Medications are stored properly.
- Prescribing, ordering and administration of medications are guided by policies and procedures.
- The organization identifies those qualified individuals permitted to prescribe or order medications and those permitted to administer medications.
- An appropriately licensed pharmacist, supervises the storage, preparation and dispensing of medications.

- Medication prescription or order are verified.
- System is used to dispense medication in the right dose to the right patient at the right time.
- Patients are identified before medications are administered.
- Medication effects on patients are monitored
- Medication prescribed, administered and its adverse effects are recorded.
- Medication errors are reported through a process and within time frame defined by the organization.

(13) Food and nutrition Therapy

- All patients receive an order for food or other nutrients based on their nutritional status.
- Food preparation, handling, storage and distribution are safe and comply with laws, regulations and current acceptable practices.

(14) Patients and Family Education

- Each patient and his family must receive education to help them give informed consent, participate in care processes and understand any financial implication of care choices.

Health care organization management standards

1. Quality Leadership

- Those responsible for governing and leading the organization participate in planning and monitoring a quality management and improvement program.

2. Quality Design

- The organization designs new and modified systems and processes according to quality improvement principles.

3. Data collection for Quality Monitoring

- The organization's leaders identify key measures to monitor the organization's clinical and managerial structures, processes and outcomes.

4. Analysis of Data

- Individuals with appropriate experience, knowledge and skills systematically aggregate and analyze data in the organization.

5. Quality improvement

- Improvement activities are undertaken for the priority areas identified by the organization's leaders.
- Assignments are made and support provided.
- Staff are trained, appropriate policy changes made and necessary resources allocated.

6. Prevention and control of infections

- The organization establishes the focus of the nosocomial infection prevention and reduction program.
- The organization identifies the procedures and processes associated with the risk of infection and implements strategies to reduce infection risk.
- Gloves, masks, soap and disinfectants are available and used correctly when required.
- The infection control process is integrated with the organization's over all program for quality management and improvement.

7. Governance of the organization

- Governance responsibilities and accountabilities are described in by laws, policies and procedures, or similar documents that guide how they are to be carried out.

8. Leadership of the organization

- A senior manager or director is responsible for operating the organization and for complying with applicable laws and regulations.
- The organization's clinical and managerial leaders are identified and are collectively responsible for defining the organization's mission and creating the plans and policies needed to fulfill the mission.

9. Direction of Departments and Services

- One or more qualified individuals provide direction for each department or service in the organization.
- Directors identify in writing the services to be provided by the department.
- Directors provide orientation and training for all staff of the department or service appropriate to their responsibilities.

10. Facility Management and Safety

- The organization complies with relevant laws, regulations and facility inspection requirements.
- The organization inspects patient care buildings for fire safety and has a plan to reduce evident risks and provide a safe physical facility for patients, families, staff and visitors.
- The plan includes prevention, early detection, suppression, abatement and safe exit from the facility in response to fire and non-fire emergencies.
- The organization develops a plan to respond to likely community emergencies, epidemics, and natural or other disasters.
- The organization has plan for the inventory handling, storage and use of hazardous materials and the control and disposal of hazardous materials and waste.

11. Medical equipment and utility System

- The organization plans and implements a program for inspecting, testing and maintaining medical equipment and documenting the results.
- Portable water and electrical power are available 24 hours a day, seven days a week, through regular or alternate sources to meet essential care needs.
- Designated individuals or authorities monitor water quality regularly.

12. Staff Education

- The organization educates and trains all staff members about their roles in providing a safe and effective patient care facility.

13. Staff Qualifications and education.

- Each organization defines the desired education, skills, knowledge and other requirements of all staff members.
- Each staff member's responsibilities are defined in a current job description.
- The organization maintains a record of the current professional license, certificate or registration when required by law, regulation or by the organization of every medical staff member.

14. Patient clinical record

- The organization initiates and maintains a clinical record for every patient assessed or treated.
- Aggregate data and information support patient care, organization management and the quality management program.

Accreditation of Health Services in India

Accreditation of health services has never been taken seriously in India though some efforts were made in late eighties and early nineties. The Bureau of India Standards (BIS) and National Institute of Health and Family Welfare had laid down standards for hospitals of different bed strengths but these standards were urban oriented. Different states have tried to lay down standards but there is no uniformity. Any effort toward accreditation in India should consider uniformity of standards.

The relationship of accreditation bodies with the to-be-accredited institutions should be evaluative, educational, consultative, inspectorial and judgmental with punitive powers. Medical tourism in India is at present worth $333 million and is expected to grow to $2.2 billion by 2010. Considering this and the increased pressure from insurance sector seeking grading of hospitals, there would be an exceeding emphasis on quality of hospitals making role of accreditation bodies more stringent. Through these standards on price, service and quality India can be promoted as a health value destination. More important than ranking of hospitals would be survey of facilities i.e. facility-survey model which would be pertinent in putting in place the basic facilities required for providing care. The most relevant model for

Indian health system would be people-centric model, which would ensure acceptability, accessibility, accountability and allocative efficiency. This would monitor utility of the health available services and orient the health system towards performance management.

The accreditation process should begin with minimum or moderate level standards and over a period of time expand to higher ideal level standards addressing all the dimensions of health care.

There has been mushrooming of private hospitals and nursing homes in India but they do not maintain any standards of services and charge exorbitant fee. There is a need to regulate the growing number of private hospitals and to keep a track of their operations. A central body under the ministry of science and technology namely National Accreditation Board for Testing and Calibration of Laboratories (NABTCL) laid down norms for pathological laboratories. Many laboratories have applied for accreditation in India.

National Accreditation Board for Hospitals and Health Care Providers

National Accreditation Board for Hospitals and health care providers (NABH) is a constituent board of Quality Council of India set up to establish and operate accreditation programme for health care organizations. The board is structured to cater to much desired needs of the consumers and to set benchmarks for progress of health industry.

Accreditation is a public recognition of the achievement of accreditation standards by a health care organization, demonstrated through an independent external peer assessment of that organizations, level of performance in relation to the standards. Accreditation benefits all stake holders. Patients are the biggest beneficiaries. Accreditation results in high quality of care and patient safety. The patients get services by credential medical staff. Rights of patients are respected and protected. Patient satisfaction is regularly evaluated. The staff in an accredited hospital is satisfied lot as it provides for continuous learning, good working environment, leadership and above all ownership of clinical process. Accreditation to a hospital stimulates continuous Improvement. It also provides opportunity to health care unit to benchmark with the best.

National Accreditation Board for Hospitals (NABH) is a constituent board of Quality Council of India (QCI). NABH has been set up with the co-operation of Ministry of Health and Family Welfare (Government of India) and Indian Health Industry to establish and operate accreditation for hospitals and health care providers. The NABH standards for hospitals were released in December 2005.

Accreditation is an external review of quality with four principal components.

1. It is based on written and published standards.
2. Reviews are carried by professional peers.
3. The accreditation process is administered by independent body.
4. The aim of accreditation is to encourage organizational development.

The Standards focus on:

- Patient safety
- Staff and employee safety.
- Environment and community safety.
- Information, education and communication.

STANDARDS

Chapter 1; access, assessment and continuity of care (AAC)

AAC 1 : The organisation defines and displays the healthcare services that it provides.

Objective Elements

(a) The healthcare services being provided are defined and are in consonance with the needs of the community. C
(b) Each defined healthcare service should have diagnostic and treatment services with suitably qualified personnel who provide out-patient, in-patient and emergency cover. C
(c) Scope of the healthcare services of each department is defined. C
(d) The organisation's defined healthcare services are prominently displayed. C

Against each element is shown an alphabet where C stands for commitment, Core for core element, A for achievement and E for excellence.

AAC 2: The organisation has a well-defined registration and admission process.

Objective Elements

(a) The organisation uses written guidance for registering and admitting patients. C

(b) **A unique identification number is generated at the end of the registration.** Core

(c) Patients are accepted only if the organisation can provide the required service. C

(d) The written guidance also addresses managing patients during non-availability of beds. C

(e) Access to the healthcare services in the organisation is prioritised according to the clinical needs of the patient. A

AAC 3: There is an appropriate mechanism for transfer (in and out) or referral of patients.

Objective Elements

(a) Transfer-in of patients to the organisation is done appropriately. C

(b) Transfer- out/referral of patients to another facility is done appropriately. C

(c) During transfer or referral, accompanying staff are appropriate to the clinical condition of the patient. C

(d) The organisation gives a summary of the patient's condition and the treatment given. C

AAC 4: Patients cared for by the organisation undergo an established initial assessment.

Objective Elements

(a) **The initial assessment of the outpatients, day-care, in-patients and emergency patients is done.** Core

(b) The initial assessment is performed by qualified personnel. C

(c) The initial assessment is performed within a time frame based on the needs of the patient. C

(d) Initial assessment of day-care and in-patients includes nursing assessment, which is done at the time of admission and documented. C

(e) The initial assessment for in-patients results in a documented care plan. A

(f) The care plan is counter signed by the clinician incharge of the patient within 24 hrs. A

(g) The care plan includes the identification of special needs regarding care following discharge. E

AAC 5: Patients cared for by the organisation undergo a regular reassessment.

Objective Elements

(a) **Patients are reassessed at appropriate intervals to determine their response to treatment and to plan further treatment or discharge.** Core

(b) Out-patients are informed of their next follow-up, where appropriate. C

(c) For in-patients during reassessment, the care plan is monitored and modified, where found necessary. A

(d) Staff involved in direct clinical care document reassessments. C

(e) The organisation lays down guidelines and implements processes to identify early warning signs of change or deterioration in clinical conditions for initiating prompt intervention. C

AAC 6: Laboratory services are provided as per the scope of services of the organisation.

Objective Elements

(a) Scope of the laboratory services is commensurate to the services provided by the organisation. C

(b) The infrastructure (physical and equipment) is adequate to provide the defined scope of services. C

(c) Human resource is adequate to provide the defined scope of services. C

(d) Qualified and trained personnel perform and supervise the investigations and report the results. C

(e) Requisition for tests, collection, identification, handling, safe transportation, processing and disposal of a specimen is performed according to written guidance. C

(f) Laboratory results are available within a defined time frame. C

(g) Critical results are intimated to the person concerned at the earliest. C

(h) Results are reported in a standardised manner. C

(i) There is a mechanism to address the recall / amendment of reports whenever applicable. A

(j) Laboratory tests not available in the organisation are outsourced to the organisation(s) based on their quality assurance system. C

AAC 7: There is an established laboratory quality assurance programme.

Objective Elements

(a) The laboratory quality assurance programme is implemented. C

(b) The programme addresses verification and/or validation of test methods. C

(c) The programme ensures the quality of test results. C

(d) The programme includes periodic calibration and maintenance of all equipment. C

(e) The programme includes the documentation of corrective and preventive actions. C

(f) The programme addresses clinicopathological meeting(s). E

AAC 8: There is an established laboratory safety programme.

Objective Elements

(a) The laboratory safety programme is implemented. C

(b) This programme is aligned with the organisation's safety programme. C

(c) Laboratory personnel are appropriately trained in safe practices. C

(d) Laboratory personnel are provided with appropriate safety measures. C

AAC 9: Imaging services are provided as per the scope of services of the organisation.

Objective Elements

(a) **Imaging services comply with legal and other requirements.** Core

(b) Scope of the imaging services is commensurate to the services provided by the organization.C

(c) The infrastructure (physical and equipment) and human resources are adequate to provide for its defined scope of services. C

(d) Qualified and trained personnel perform, supervise and interpret the investigations. C

(e) Patients are transported in a safe and timely manner to and from the imaging services. C

(f) Imaging results are available within a defined time frame. C

(g) Critical results are intimated immediately to the personnel concerned. C

(h) Results are reported in a standardised manner. C

(i) There is a mechanism to address the recall / amendment of reports whenever applicable. A

(j) Imaging tests not available in the organisation are outsourced to the organisation(s) based on their quality assurance system. C

AAC 10: There is an established quality assurance programme for imaging services.

Objective Elements

(a) The quality assurance programme for imaging services is implemented. C

(b) Quality assurance programme includes tests for imaging equipment. C

(c) Quality assurance programme includes the review of imaging protocols. C

(d) A system is in place to ensure the appropriateness of the investigations and procedures for the clinical indication. A

(e) The programme addresses periodic internal/external peer review of imaging results using appropriate sampling. A

(f) The programme addresses the clinico-radiological meeting(s). E

(g) The programme includes periodic calibration and maintenance of all equipment. C

(h) The programme includes the documentation of corrective and preventive actions. C

AAC 11: There is an established safety programme in imaging services.

Objective Elements

(a) The radiation-safety programme is implemented. C

(b) This programme is aligned with the organisation's safety programme. C

(c) Patients are appropriately screened for safety/risk before imaging. C

(d) Imaging personnel and patients use appropriate radiation safety and monitoring devices where applicable. C

(e) Radiation-safety and monitoring devices are periodically tested, and results are documented. C

(f) Imaging and ancillary personnel are trained in imaging safety practices and radiation-safety measures. C

(g) Imaging signage is prominently displayed in all appropriate locations. C

AAC 12: Patient care is continuous and multidisciplinary.

Objective Elements

(a) During all phases of care, there is a qualified individual identified as responsible for the patient's care. C

(b) Patient care is co-ordinated in all care settings within the organisation. C

(c) Information about the patient's care and response to treatment is shared among medical, nursing and other care -providers. C

(d) **The Organisation implements standardized hand-over communication during each staffing shift, between shifts and during transfers between units/ departments.** Core

(e) Patient transfer within the organisation is done safely in a safe manner. C

(f) Referral of patients to other departments/ specialities follow written guidance. C

(g) The organisation ensures predictable service delivery by adhering to defined timelines and informs the patient/ family and/ or caregiver whenever there is a change in schedule. A

(h) The organisation has a mechanism in place to monitor whether adequate clinical intervention has taken place in response to a critical value alert. E

AAC 13: The organisation has an established discharge process.

Objective Elements

(a) The patient's discharge process is planned in consultation with the patient and/or family. C

(b) The discharge process is coordinated among various departments and agencies involved (including medico-legal and absconded cases). C

(c) Written guidance governs the discharge of patients leaving against medical advice. C

(d) A discharge summary is given to all the patients leaving the organisation (including patients leaving against medical advice). C

(e) The organisation adheres to planned discharge. A

(f) The organisation conforms to the defined timeframe for discharge and makes continual improvement. E

AAC 14: The organisation defines the content of the discharge summary.

Objective elements

(a) Discharge summary is provided to the patients at the time of discharge. C

(b) Discharge summary contains the patient's name, unique identification number, name of the treating doctor, date of admission and date of discharge. C

(c) Discharge summary contains the reasons for admission, significant findings and diagnosis and the patient's condition at the time of discharge. C

(d) Discharge summary contains information regarding investigation results, any procedure performed, medication administered, and other treatment given. C

(e) Discharge summary contains follow-up advice, medication and other instructions in an understandable manner. C

(f) Discharge summary incorporates instructions about when and how to obtain urgent care. A

(g) In case of death, the summary of the case also includes the cause of death. C

Chapter 2: Care of Patients

COP.1: Uniform care to patients is provided in all settings of the organisation and is guided by written guidance, and the applicable laws and regulations.

Elements

(a) Uniform care is provided following written guidance. C

(b) **The organisation has a uniform process for identification of patients and at a minimum, uses two identifiers.** Core

(c) Care shall be provided in consonance with applicable laws and regulations. C

(d) The organisation adapts evidence-based clinical practice guidelines and/or clinical protocols to guide uniform patient care. A

(e) Clinical care pathways are developed, consistently followed across all settings of care, and reviewed periodically. E

(f) Care delivery is uniform for a given clinical condition when similar care is provided in more than one setting. C

(g) Multi-disciplinary and multi-speciality care, where appropriate, is planned based on best clinical practices/ clinical practice guidelines and delivered in a uniform manner across the organisation. E

(h) Telemedicine facility is provided safely and securely based on written guidance. C

COP.2 : Emergency services are provided in accordance with written guidance, applicable laws and regulations.

Elements

(a) There shall be an identified area in the organisation which is easily accessible to receive and manage emergency patients, with adequate and appropriate resources. C

(b) Prevention of patient over-crowding is planned, and crowd management measures are implemented. A

(c) **Emergency care is provided in consonance with statutory requirements and in accordance with the written guidance.** Core

(d) The organisation manages medico-legal cases in accordance with statutory requirements. C

(e) Initiation of appropriate care is guided by a system of triage. C

(f) Patients waiting in the emergency are reassessed as appropriate for change in status. C

(g) Admission, discharge to home, or transfer to another organisation is documented. C

(h) In case of discharge to home or transfer to another organisation, a discharge/ transfer note shall be given to the patient. C

(i) The organisation shall implement a quality assurance programme. A

(j) The organisation has systems in place for the management of patients found dead on arrival and patients who die within a few minutes of arrival. C

COP.3 : Ambulance services ensure safe patient transportation with appropriate care

Elements

(a) The organisation has access to ambulance services commensurate with the scope of the services provided by it. C

(b) There is adequate access and space for the ambulance(s). C

(c) The ambulance(s) is fit for purpose and is appropriately equipped. C

(d) The ambulance(s) is operated by trained personnel. C

(e) The ambulance(s) is checked daily. C

(f) Equipment is checked daily using a checklist. C

(g) A mechanism is in place to ensure that emergency medications are available in the ambulance. C

(h) The ambulance(s) has a proper communication system . C

(i) The emergency department identifies opportunities to initiate treatment at the earliest when the patient is in transit to the organisation. A

COP.4 : The organisation plans and implements mechanisms for the care of patients during community emergencies, epidemics and other disasters.

Elements

(a) The organisation identifies potential community emergencies, epidemics and other disasters. C

(b) The organisation manages community emergencies, epidemics and other disasters as per a documented plan. C

(c) Provision is made for availability of medical supplies, equipment and materials during such emergencies. C

(d) The plan is tested at least twice a year. C

COP.5 : Cardio-pulmonary resuscitation services are provided uniformly across the organisation.

Elements

(a) Resuscitation services are available to patients at all times. C

(b) During cardio-pulmonary resuscitation, assigned roles and responsibilities are complied with. C

(c) Equipment and medications for use during cardio-pulmonary resuscitation are available in various areas of the organisation. C

(d) The events during cardio-pulmonary resuscitation are recorded. C

(e) A multidisciplinary committee does a post-event analysis of cardiopulmonary resusitations. C

(f) Corrective and preventive measures are taken based on the post-event analysis. C

COP. 6 : Nursing care is provided to patients in the organisation in consonance with clinical protocols.

Elements

(a) Nursing care is provided to patients in accordance with written guidance. C

(b) The organisation develops and implements nursing clinical practice guidelines reflecting current standards of practice. A

(c) Assignment of patient care is done as per current good clinical/ nursing practice guidelines. C

(d) The organisation implements acuity-based staffing to improve patient outcomes. E

(e) **Nursing care is aligned and integrated with overall patient care**. Core

(f) Care provided by nurses is documented in the patient record. C

(g) Nurses are provided with appropriate and adequate equipment for providing safe and efficient nursing care. C

(h) Nurses are empowered to make patient care decisions within their scope of practice. C

COP. 7 : Clinical procedures are performed in a safe manner.

Elements

(a) Procedures are performed based on the clinical needs of the patient. C

(b) Performance of various clinical procedures is based on written guidance. C

(c) Qualified personnel order, plan, perform and assist in performing procedures. C

(d) **Care is taken to prevent adverse events like a wrong patient, wrong procedure and wrong site.** Core

(e) Informed consent is taken by the personnel performing the procedure, where applicable. C

(f) The procedure is done adhering to standard precautions. C

(g) Patients are appropriately monitored during and after the procedure. C

(h) Procedures are documented accurately in the patient record. C

COP.8 : Transfusion services are provided as per the scope of services of the organisation, safely.

Elements

(a) Scope of transfusion services is commensurate with the services provided by the organisation. C

(b) **Transfusion of blood and blood components is done safely.** Core

(c) Blood and blood components are used rationally. C

(d) Informed consent is obtained for transfusion of blood and blood components. C

(e) Informed consent also includes patient and family education about the donation. C

(f) Blood/blood components are available for use in emergency situations within a defined time-frame. C

(g) Post-transfusion form is collected, reactions if any identified and are analysed for preventive and corrective actions. A

(h) The organisation shall implement a quality assurance programme. A

COP.9 : The organisation provides care in intensive care and high dependency units in a systematic manner.

Elements

(a) Care of patients in intensive care and high dependency units is provided based on written guidance. C

(b) The defined admission and discharge criteria for intensive care and high dependency units are implemented. C

(c) Adequate staff and equipment are available. C

(d) The organisation endeavours to upgrade its physical infrastructure to meet national and international guidelines. E

(e) Defined procedures for the situation of bed shortages are followed.

(f) Infection control practices are followed. C

(g) The organisation shall implement a quality assurance programme. A

(h) The organisation has a mechanism to counsel the patient and/ or family periodically. C

COP.10 : Organisation provides safe obstetric care.

Elements

(a) Obstetric services are organised and provided safely. C

(b) The organisation identifies and, provides care to high-risk obstetric cases, and where needed, refers them to another appropriate centre. C

(c) Persons caring for high-risk obstetric cases are competent. C

(d) Ante-natal services are provided. C

(e) Obstetric patient's assessment also includes maternal nutrition. C

(f) Appropriate peri-natal and post-natal monitoring is performed. C

(g) The organisation caring for high-risk obstetric cases has the facilities to take care of neonates of such cases. C

COP. 11 : Organisation provides safe paediatric services.

Elements

(a) Paediatric services are organised and provided safely.

(b) Neonatal care is in consonance with the national/ international guidelines.

(c) Those who care for children have age-specific competency.

(d) Provisions are made for special care of children.

(e) Paediatric assessment includes growth, developmental and immunisation assessment.

(f) The organisation has measures in place to prevent child/ neonate abduction and abuse.

(g) The child's family members are educated about nutrition, immunisation and safe parenting.

COP. 12 : Procedural sedation is provided in a consistent and safe manner.

Elements

(a) Procedural sedation is administered in a consistent manner . C

(b) Informed consent for administration of procedural sedation is obtained. C

(c) Competent and trained persons administer sedation. C

(d) The person monitoring sedation is different from the person performing the procedure. C

(e) Intra-procedure monitoring includes at a minimum the heart rate, cardiac rhythm, respiratory rate, blood pressure, oxygen saturation, and level of sedation. C

(f) Patients are monitored after sedation, and the same is documented. C

(g) Criteria are used to determine the appropriateness of discharge from the observation/recovery area. C

(h) Equipment and workforce are available to manage patients who have gone into a deeper level of sedation than initially intended. C

COP. 13 : Anaesthesia services are provided in a consistent and safe manner.

Elements

(a) Anaesthesia services are provided in a consistent manner.

(b) **The pre-anaesthesia assessment results in the formulation of an anaesthesia plan which is documented.** Core

(c) A pre-induction assessment is performed and documented.

(d) The anaesthesiologist obtains informed consent for administration of anaesthesia.

(e) **During anaesthesia, monitoring includes regular recording of temperature, heart rate, cardiac rhythm, respiratory rate, blood pressure, oxygen saturation and end tidal carbon dioxide.** Core

(f) Patient's post-anaesthesia status is monitored and documented.

(g) The anaesthesiologist applies defined criteria to transfer the patient from the recovery area

(h) The type of anaesthesia and anaesthetic medications used are documented in the patient record.

(i) Procedures shall comply with infection control guidelines to prevent cross infection between patients.

(j) Intraoperative adverse anaesthesia events are recorded and monitored. A

COP.14 : Surgical services are provided in a consistent and safe manner.

Elements

(a) Surgical services are provided in a consistent and safe manner. C

(b) Surgical patients have a preoperative assessment, a documented pre-operative diagnosis, and pre-operative instructions are provided before surgery. C

(c) Informed consent is obtained by a surgeon before the procedure

(d) **Care is taken to prevent adverse events like the wrong site, wrong patient and wrong surgery.** Core

(e) An operative note is documented before transfer out of patient from recovery . C

(f) Postoperative care is guided by a documented plan. C

(g) Patient, personnel and material flow conform to infection control practices. C

(h) Appropriate facilities, equipment, instruments and supplies are available in the operating theatre. C

(i) The organisation shall implement a quality assurance programme. A

(j) The quality assurance programme includes surveillance of the operation theatre environment. A

COP.15 : The organ transplant programme is carried out safely.

Elements

(a) **The organ transplant program shall be in consonance with the legal requirements and shall be conducted ethically**. Core

(b) Care of transplant patients is guided by clinical practice guidelines. C

(c) The organisation ensures education and counselling of recipient and donor through trained/qualified counsellors before organ transplantation. C

(d) **The organisation shall take measures to create awareness regarding organ donation**. Core

COP.16 : The organisation identifies and manages patients who are at higher risk of morbidity/ mortality.

Elements

(a) The organisation identifies and manages vulnerable patients. C

(b) The organisation provides for a safe and secure environment for the vulnerable patient. C

(c) **The organisation identifies and manages patients who are at a risk of fall**. Core

(d) **The organisation identifies and manages patients who are at risk of developing/worsening of pressure ulcers**. Core

(e) **The organisation identifies and manages patients who are at risk of developing deep vein thrombosis**. Core

(f) The organisation identifies and manages patients who need restraints. C

COP.17 : Pain management for patients is done in a consistent manner.

Elements

(a) Patients in pain are effectively managed. C

(b) Patients are screened for pain. C

(c) Patients with pain undergo detailed assessment and periodic reassessment. C

(d) Pain alleviation measures or medications are initiated and titrated according to the patient's need and response. C

COP.18 : Rehabilitation services are provided to the patients in a safe, collaborative and consistent manner.

Elements

(a) Scope of the rehabilitation services at a minimum is commensurate to the services provided by the organisation. C

(b) Rehabilitation services are provided in a consistent manner. C

(c) Care providers collaboratively plan rehabilitation services. C

(d) There are adequate space and equipment to provide rehabilitation. C

(e) Care is guided by functional assessment and periodic re-assessments which are done and documented. C

(f) Care is provided adhering to infection control and safety practices. C

(g) Care pathways are developed, implemented, and reviewed periodically. E

COP.19 : Nutritional therapy is provided to patients consistently and collaboratively

Elements

(a) Patients admitted to the organisation are screened for nutritional risk. C

(b) Nutritional assessment is done for patients found at risk during nutritional screening. C

(c) The therapeutic diet is planned and provided collaboratively. C

(d) Patients receive food according to the written order for the diet. C

(e) When family provides food, they are educated about the patient's diet limitations. C

COP.20 : End-of-life-care is provided in a compassionate and considerate manner.

Elements

(a) End-of-life care is provided in a consistent manner in the organisation. C

(b) A multi-professional approach is used to provide end-of-life care. A

(c) End-of-life care is in consonance with the legal requirements. C

(d) End of life care also addresses the identification of the unique needs of such patient and family. C

(e) Symptomatic treatment is provided and where appropriate measures are taken for the alleviation of pain. C

Chapter 3 : Management of medication (MOM)

MOM.1 : Pharmacy services and usage of medication is done safely.

Elements

(a) Pharmacy services and medication usage are implemented following written guidance. C

(b) A multidisciplinary committee guides the formulation and implementation of pharmacy services and medication usage. C

(c) There is a mechanism in place to facilitate the multidisciplinary committee to monitor literature reviews and best practice information on medication management and use the information to update medication management processes. E

(d) There is a procedure to obtain medication when the pharmacy is closed. C

(e) The organisation has a mechanism to inform relevant staff of key changes in pharmacy services and medication usage to ensure uninterrupted and safe care. C

MOM.2 : The organisation develops, updates and implements a hospital formulary.

Elements

(a) **A list of medications appropriate for the patients and as per the scope of the organisation's clinical services is developed collaboratively by the multidisciplinary committee.** Core

(b) The list is reviewed and updated collaboratively by the multidisciplinary committee at least annually. C

(c) The current formulary is available for clinicians to refer to. C

(d) The clinicians adhere to the current formulary. E

(e) The organisation adheres to the procedure for the acquisition of formulary medications. C

(f) The organisation adheres to the procedure to obtain medications not listed in the formulary. C

MOM.3 : Medications are stored appropriately and are available where required

Elements

(a) **Medications are stored in a clean, safe and secure environment; and incorporating the manufacturer's recommendation(s).** Core

(b) Sound inventory control practices guide storage of the medications throughout the organization. C

(c) **The organisation defines a list of high-risk medication(s).** Core

(d) High-risk medications are stored in areas of the organisation where it is clinically necessary. A

(e) **High-risk medications including look-alike, sound-alike medications and different concentrations of the same medication are stored physically apart from each other.** Core

(f) The list of emergency medications is defined and is stored uniformly. C

(g) **Emergency medications are available all the time and are replenished promptly when used.** Core

MOM. 4 : Medications are prescribed safely and rationally.

Elements

(a) Medication prescription is in consonance with good practices/ guidelines for the rational prescription of medications. C

(b) **The organisation adheres to the determined minimum requirements of a prescription.** Core

(c) Drug allergies and previous adverse drug reactions are ascertained before prescribing. C

(d) The organisation has a mechanism to assist the clinician in prescribing appropriate medication. E

(e) **Implementation of verbal orders ensures safe medication management practices.** Core

(f) Audit of medication orders/prescription is carried out to check for safe and rational prescription of medications. A

(g) Corrective and/or preventive action(s) is taken based on the audit, where appropriate. A

(h) **Reconciliation of medications occurs at transition points of patient care.** Core

MOM. 5 : Medications orders are written in a uniform manner.

Elements

(a) The organisation ensures that only authorised personnel write orders. C

(b) Medication orders are written in a uniform location in the medical records, which also reflects the patient's name and unique identification number. C

(c) Medication orders are legible, dated, timed and signed. C

(d) Medication orders contain the name of the medicine, route of administration, strength to be administered and frequency/ time of administration. C

MOM.6 : Medications are dispensed in a safe manner.

Elements

(a) Dispensing of medications is done safely. C

(b) Medication recalls are handled effectively. C

(c) Near-expiry medications are handled effectively. C

(d) **Dispensed medications are labelled.** Core

(e) **High-risk medication orders are verified before dispensing.** Core

(f) Return of medications to the pharmacy is addressed. C

MOM.7 : Medications are administered safely.

Elements

(a) Medications are administered by those who are permitted by law to do so. C

(b) Prepared medication is labelled before preparation of a second drug. C

(c) The patient is identified before administration . C

(d) **Medication is verified from the medication order and physically inspected before administration.** Core

(e) Strength is verified from the order before administration. C

(f) The route is verified from the order before administration. C

(g) Timing is verified from the order before administration. C

(h) **Measures to avoid catheter and tubing mis-connections during medication administration are implemented.** Core

(i) Medication administration is documented. C

(j) Measures to govern patient's self-administration of medications are implemented. C

(k) Measures to govern patient's medications brought from outside the organisation are implemented. C

MOM. 8 : Patients are monitored after medication administration.

Elements

(a) Patients are monitored after medication administration. C

(b) Medications are changed where appropriate based on the monitoring. C

(c) **The organization captures near miss ,medication error and adverse drug reaction.** Core

(d) Near miss, medication error and adverse drug reaction are reported within a specified time frame. C

(e) Near miss, medication error and adverse drug reaction are collected and analysed. C

(f) Corrective and/or preventive action(s) are taken based on the analysis. C

MOM.9 : Narcotic drugs and psychotropic substances, chemotherapeutic agents and radioactive agents are used in a safe manner.

Elements

(a) Narcotic drugs and psychotropic substances, chemotherapeutic agents and radioactive agents are used safely. C

(b) Narcotic drugs and psychotropic substances, chemotherapeutic agents and radioactive agents are prescribed by appropriate caregivers. C

(c) Narcotic drugs and psychotropic substances, chemotherapeutic agents and radioactive agents drugs are stored securely. C

(d) Chemotherapy and radioactive agents are prepared properly and safely and administered by qualified personnel. C

(e) A proper record is kept of the usage, administration and disposal of narcotic drugs and psychotropic substances, chemotherapeutic agents and radioactive agents. C

MOM.10 : Implantable prosthesis and medical devices are used in accordance with laid down criteria.

Elements

(a) Usage of the implantable prosthesis and medical devices is guided by scientific criteria for each item and national/ international recognised guidelines/ approvals for such specific item(s). C

(b) The organisation implements a mechanism for the usage of the implantable prosthesis and medical devices. C

(c) Patient and his/her family are counselled for the usage of the implantable prosthesis and medical device, including precautions if any. C

(d) The batch and the serial number of the implantable prosthesis and medical devices are recorded in the patient's medical record, the master logbook and the discharge summary. C

(e) Recall of implantable prosthesis and medical devices are handled effectively. A

MOM.11: Medical supplies and consumables are stored appropriately and are available where required.

Elements

(a) The organisation adheres to the defined process for the acquisition of medical supplies and consumables. C

(b) Medical supplies and consumables are used in a safe manner, where appropriate. C

(c) Medical supplies and consumables are stored in a clean, safe and secure environment; and incorporating the manufacturer's recommendation(s). C

(d) Sound inventory control practices guide storage of medical supplies and consumables. C

(e) There is a mechanism in place to verify the condition of medical supplies and consumables . C

Chapter 4: Patients Rights and Education (PRE)

Elements

PRE.1 : The organisation protects and promotes patient and family rights and informs them about their responsibilities during care.

(a) Patient and family rights and responsibilities are documented, displayed and they are made aware of the same. C

(b) Patient and family rights and responsibilities are actively promoted. A

(c) **The organisation protects patient and family rights**. Core

(d) **The organization has a mechanism to report a violation of patient and family rights**. Core

(e) **Violation of patient and family rights are monitored, analysed, and corrective/preventive action taken by the top leadership of the organisation.** Core

PRE.2. : Patient and family rights support individual beliefs, values and involve the patient and family in decision-making processes.

Elements

(a) Patients and family rights include respecting values and beliefs, any special preferences, cultural needs, and responding to requests for spiritual needs. C

(b) Patient and family rights include respect for personal dignity and privacy during examination, procedures and treatment. C

(c) Patient and family rights include protection from neglect or abuse. C

(d) **Patient and family rights include treating patient information as confidential**. Core

(e) Patient and family rights include the refusal of treatment. C

(f) Patient and family rights include a right to seek an additional opinion regarding clinical care. C

(g) **Patient and family rights include informed consent before the transfusion of blood and blood components, anaesthesia, surgery, initiation of any research protocol and any other invasive/high-risk procedures/treatment**. Core

(h) Patient and family rights include a right to complain and information on how to voice a complaint. C

(i) Patient and family rights include information on the expected cost of the treatment. A

(j) Patient and family rights include access to their clinical records. C

(k) Patient and family rights include information on the name of the treating doctor, care plan, progress and information on their health care needs. C

(l) l. Patient rights include determining what information regarding their care would be provided to self and family. C

PRE.3: The patient and/or family members are educated to make informed decisions and are involved in the care planning and delivery process.

Elements

(a) **The Patient and/or family members are explained about the proposed care, including the risks, alternatives and benefits**. Core

(b) The patient and/or family members are explained about the expected results. C

(c) The patient and/or family members are explained about the possible complications. C

(d) The care plan is prepared and modified in consultation with the patient and/or family members. A

(e) The patient and/or family members are informed about the results of diagnostic tests and the diagnosis. C

(f) The patient and/or family members are explained about any change in the patient's condition in a timely manner. C

(g) The patient and/or family members are provided multi-disciplinary counselling when appropriate. A

PRE.4 : Informed consent is obtained from the patient or family about their care.

Elements

(a) **The organisation obtains informed consent from the patient or family for situations where informed consent is required**. Core

(b) Informed consent process adheres to statutory norms. C

(c) **Informed consent includes information regarding the procedure; it's risks, benefits, alternatives and as to who will perform the procedure in a language that they can understand**. Core

(d) The organisation describes who can give consent when a patient is incapable of independent decision making and implements the same. C

(e) **Informed consent is taken by the person performing the procedure**. Core

PRE.5: Patient and families have a right to information and education about their healthcare needs.

Elements

(a) **Patient and/or family are educated in a language and format that they can understand**. Core

(b) Patient and/or family are educated about the safe and effective use of medication and the potential side effects of the medication, when appropriate. C

(c) Patient and/or family are educated about food-drug interaction. C

(d) Patient and/or family are educated about diet and nutrition. C

(e) Patient and/or family are educated about immunisations. C

(f) Patient and/or family are educated on various pain management techniques, when appropriate. C

(g) Patient and/or family are educated about their specific disease process, complications and prevention strategies. C

(h) Patient and/or family are educated about preventing healthcare associated infections. C

(i) The patients and/or family members' special educational needs are identified and addressed. A

PRE.6: Patients and families have a right to information on expected costs.

Elements

(a) **The patient and/or family members are made aware of the pricing policy in different settings (out-patient, emergency, ICU and inpatient)**. Core

(b) The relevant tariff list is available to patients. C

(c) The patient and/or family members are explained about the expected costs. C

(d) Patient and/or family are informed about the financial implications when there is a change in the care plan. C

PRE.7: The organisation has a mechanism to capture patient's feedback and to redress complaints.

Elements

(a) The organisation has a mechanism to capture feedback from patients, which includes patient satisfaction. C

(b) The organisation has a mechanism to capture patient experience. A

(c) **The organisation redress patient complaints as per the defined mechanism**. Core

(d) Patient and/or family members are made aware of the procedure for giving feedback and/or lodging complaints. C

(e) Feedback and complaints are reviewed and/or analysed within a defined time frame. C

(f) Corrective and/or preventive action(s) are taken based on the analysis where appropriate. C

PRE.8: The organisation has a system for effective communication with patients and/or families.

Elements

(a) Communication with the patients and/or families is done effectively. C

(b) The organisation shall identify special situations where enhanced communication with patients and/or families would be required. C

(c) Enhanced communication with the patients and/or families is done effectively. C

(d) The organisation ensures that there is no unacceptable communication. C

(e) The organisation has a system to monitor and review the implementation of effective communication. A

Chapter 5 : Hospital Infection Control (HIC)

HIC.1 : The organisation has a comprehensive and coordinated Hospital Infection Prevention and Control (HIC) programme aimed at reducing/ eliminating risks to patients, visitors, providers of care and community.

Elements

(a) **The hospital infection prevention and control programme is documented, which aims at preventing and reducing the risk of healthcare associated infections in the hospital.** Core

(b) The hospital infection prevention and control programme identifies high-risk activities, and has written guidance to prevent and manage infections for these activities. C

(c) The infection prevention and control programme is reviewed and updated at least once a year. C

(d) The infection prevention and control programme is reviewed based on infection control assessment tool. A

(e) The organisation has a multi-disciplinary infection control committee, which co ordinates all infection prevention and control activities. C

(f) The organisation has an infection control team, which coordinates the implementation of all infection prevention and control activities. C

(g) The organisation has designated infection control officer as part of the infection control team. C

(h) The organisation has designated infection control nurse(s) as part of the infection control team. C

(i) The organisation implements information, education and communication programme for infection prevention and control activities for the community. C

(j) The organisation participates in managing community outbreaks. C

HIC.2 : The organisation provides adequate and appropriate resources for infection prevention and control.

Elements

(a) **The management makes available resources required for the infection control programme.** Core

(b) The organisation earmarks adequate funds from its annual budget in this regard. C

(c) Adequate and appropriate personal protective equipment, soaps, and disinfectants are available and used correctly. C

(d) **Adequate and appropriate facilities for hand hygiene in all patient-care areas are accessible to healthcare providers.** Core

(e) Isolation/barrier nursing facilities are available. A

HIC.3 : The organisation implements the infection prevention and control programme in clinical areas.

Elements

(a) **The organisation adheres to standard precautions at all times.** Core

(b) **The organisation adheres to hand-hygiene guidelines.** Core

(c) The organisation adheres to transmission-based precautions. C

(d) **The organisation adheres to safe injection and infusion practices.** Core

(e) Appropriate antimicrobial usage policy is established and documented. C

(f) **The organisation implements the antimicrobial usage policy and monitors the rational use of antimicrobial agents.** Core

(g) The organisation implements an antibiotic stewardship programme. E

HIC. 4 : The organisation implements the infection prevention and control programme in support services.

Elements

(a) The organisation has appropriate engineering controls to prevent infections. C

(b) The organisation designs and implements a plan to reduce the risk of infection during construction and renovation. C

(c) **The organisation adheres to housekeeping procedures.** Core

(d) **Biomedical waste (BMW) is handled appropriately and safely.** Core

(e) The organisation adheres to laundry and linen management processes. C

(f) The organisation adheres to kitchen sanitation and food-handling issues. C

HIC.5 : The organisation takes actions to prevent healthcare associated infections (HAI) in patients.

Elements

(a) The organisation takes action to prevent catheter-associated urinary tract Infections. C

(b) The organisation takes action to prevent infection-related ventilator associated complication/ventilator-associated pneumonia. C

(c) The organisation takes action to prevent catheter linked blood stream infections. C

(d) The organisation takes action to prevent surgical site infections. C

HIC.6 : The organisation performs surveillance to capture and monitor infection prevention and control data.

Elements

(a) **The scope of surveillance incorporates tracking and analysing of infection risks, rates and trends.** Core

(b) Verification of data is done regularly by the infection control team. C

(c) Surveillance is directed towards the identified high-risk activities. C

(d) **Surveillance includes monitoring compliance with hand-hygiene guidelines.** Core

(e) Surveillance includes mechanisms to capture the occurrence of multi-drug resistant organisms and highly virulent infections. C

(f) **Surveillance includes monitoring the effectiveness of housekeeping services.** Core

(g) Feedback regarding surveillance data is provided regularly to the appropriate health care provider. C

(h) The organisation identifies and takes appropriate action to control outbreaks of infections. C

(i) Surveillance data is analysed, and appropriate corrective and preventive actions are taken. C

HIC.7 : Infection prevention measures include sterilisation and/or disinfection of instruments, equipment and devices.

Elements

(a) The organisation provides adequate space and appropriate zoning for sterilisation activities. C

(b) **Cleaning, packing, disinfection and/or sterilisation, storing and the issue of items is done as per the written guidance.** Core

(c) Reprocessing of single-use instruments, equipment and devices are done as per written guidance. C

(d) Regular validation tests for sterilisation are carried out and documented. C

(e) The established recall procedure is implemented when a breakdown in the sterilisation system is identified. C

HIC.8 : The organisation takes action to prevent or reduce healthcare associated infections in its staff.

Elements

(a) The organisation implements occupational health and safety practices to reduce the risk of transmitting microorganisms among health care providers. C

(b) The organisation implements an immunisation policy for its staff. C

(c) The organisation implements work restrictions for health care providers with transmissible infections. A

(d) The organisation implements measures for blood and body fluid exposure prevention. C

(e) Appropriate post-exposure prophylaxis is provided to all staff members concerned. C

Chapter 6 : Patient Safety and Quality Improvement (PSQ)

PSQ.1: The organisation implements a structured patient-safety programme.

Elements

(a) **The patient-safety programme is developed, implemented and maintained by a multi-disciplinary safety committee.** Core

(b) The patient-safety programme is comprehensive and covers all the major elements related to patient safety. C

(c) The programme covers incidents ranging from "no harm" to "sentinel events". C

(d) Designated patient safety officer(s) coordinates implementation of the patient safety programme. C

(e) Designated clinical safety officer(s) coordinates implementation of the clinical aspects of the patient-safety programme. E

(f) The patient-safety programme identifies opportunities for improvement based on the review at pre-defined intervals. C

(g) The organisation performs proactive analysis of patient safety risks and makes improvements accordingly. E

(h) The patient-safety programme is reviewed and updated at least once a year. C

(i) **The organisation adapts and implements national/ international patient-safety goals/solutions.** Core

PSQ.2 : The organisation implements a structured quality improvement and continuous monitoring programme.

Elements

(a) **The quality improvement programme is developed, implemented and maintained by a multi-disciplinary committee.** Core

(b) The quality improvement programme is comprehensive and covers all the major elements related to quality assurance. C

(c) The quality improvement programme improves process efficiency and effectiveness. E

(d) There is a designated individual for coordinating and implementing the quality improvement programme. C

(e) The quality improvement programme identifies opportunities for improvement based on the review at pre-defined intervals. C

(f) The quality improvement programme is reviewed and updated at least once a year. C

(g) Audits are conducted at regular intervals as a means of continuous monitoring. C

(h) **There is an established process in the organisation to monitor and improve the quality of nursing care.** Core

PSQ.3 : The organisation identifies key indicators to monitor the structures, processes and outcomes, which are used as tools for continual improvement.

Elements

(a) The organisation identifies and monitors key indicators to oversee the clinical structures, processes and outcomes. C

(b) **The organisation identifies and monitors the key indicators to oversee infection control activities.** Core

(c) The organisation identifies and monitors key indicators to oversee the managerial structures, processes and outcomes. C

(d) **The organisation identifies and monitors key indicators to oversee patient safety activities.** Core

(e) The organisation has a mechanism to capture patient reported outcome measures. E

(f) Verification of data is done regularly by the quality team. C

(g) There is a mechanism for analysis of data which results in identifying opportunities for improvement. C

(h) The improvements are implemented and evaluated. C

(i) Feedback about care and service is communicated to staff. A

PSQ.4 : The organisation uses appropriate quality improvement tools for its quality improvement activities.

Elements

(a) **The organisation undertakes quality improvement projects.** Core

(b) The organisation uses appropriate analytical tools for its quality improvement activities. C

(c) The organisation uses appropriate statistical tools for its quality improvement activities. C

(d) The organisation uses appropriate managerial tools for its quality improvement activities. C

PSQ.5 : There is an established system for clinical audit.

Elements

(a) Clinical audits are performed to improve the quality of patient care. C

(b) The parameters to be audited are defined by the organisation. C

(c) Medical and nursing staff participate in clinical audit. A

(d) Patient and staff anonymity are maintained. C

(e) Clinical audits are documented. C

(f) Remedial measures are implemented. C

PSQ.6 : The patient safety and quality improvement programme are supported by the management.

Elements

(a) The management creates a culture of safety. A

(b) The leaders at all levels in the organisation are aware of the intent of the patient safety and quality improvement programme and the approach to its implementation. C

(c) Departmental leaders are involved in patient safety and quality improvement. C

(d) The management makes available adequate resources required for patient safety and quality improvement programme. C

(e) Organisation earmarks adequate funds from its annual budget in this regard. C

(f) The management identifies organisational performance improvement targets. F

(g) The management uses the feedback obtained from the workforce to improve patient safety and quality improvement programme. E

PSQ.7 : Incidents are collected and analysed to ensure continual quality improvement.

Elements

(a) **The organisation implements an incident management system.** Core

(b) The organisation has a mechanism to identify sentinel events. C

(c) The organisation has established processes for analysis of incidents. C

(d) Corrective and preventive actions are taken based on the findings of such analysis. C

(e) The organisation incorporates risks identified in the analysis of incidents into the risk management system. A

(f) The organisation shall have a process for informing various stakeholders in case of a near miss/adverse event/sentinel event. E

Chapter 7 : Responsibilities of Management (ROM)

ROM.1 : The organisation identifies those responsible for governance and their roles are defined.

Elements

(a) **Those responsible for governance are identified, and their roles and responsibilities are defined and documented.** Core

(b) Those responsible for governance lay down the organisation's vision, mission and values. C

(c) Those responsible for governance approve the strategic and operational plans and the organisation's annual budget. C

(d) Those responsible for governance monitor and measure the performance of the organisation against the stated mission. A

(e) Those responsible for governance appoint the senior leaders in the organisation. C

(f) Those responsible for governance support safety initiatives and quality improvement plans. C

(g) Those responsible for governance support the ethical management framework of the organisation. C

(h) Those responsible for governance inform the public of the quality and performance of services. E

ROM.2 : The leaders manage the organisation in an ethical manner.

Elements

(a) The leaders make public the vision, mission and values of the organisation. C

(b) **The leaders establish the organisation's ethical management framework.** Core

(c) The ethical management framework includes processes for managing issues with ethical implications, dilemmas and concerns, E

(d) The organisation discloses its ownership. C

(e) The organisation honestly portrays its affiliations and accreditations. C

ROM.3 : The organisation is headed by a leader who shall be responsible for operating the organisation on a day-to-day basis.

Elements

(a) The person heading the organisation has requisite and appropriate administrative qualifications. C

(b) The person heading the organisation has requisite and appropriate administrative experience. C

(c) **The leader is responsible for and complies with the laid-down and applicable legislations, regulations and notifications.** Core

(d) The leader appoints/participates in the recruitment of senior leadership of the organisation who will assist in the day-to-day functioning of the organisation. C

(e) The leader ensures that each organisational programme, service, site or department has effective leadership. E

(f) The performance of the organisation's leader is reviewed for effectiveness. A

ROM.4 : The organisation displays professionalism in its functioning.

Elements

(a) The organisation has strategic and operational plans, including long-term and short-term goals commensurate to the organisation's vision, mission and values in consultation with the various stakeholders. C

(b) The organisation coordinates the functioning with departments and external agencies and monitors the progress in achieving the defined goals and objectives. A

(c) The organisation plans and budgets for its activities annually. C

(d) The functioning of committees is reviewed for their effectiveness. A

(e) The organisation documents staff rights and responsibilities. C

(f) The organisation documents the service standards that are measurable and monitors them. C

(g) Systems and processes are in place for change management. E

ROM. 5 : Management ensures that patient-safety aspects and risk-management issues are an integral part of patient care and hospital management.

Elements

(a) **Management ensures proactive risk management across the organisation.** Core

(b) Management provides resources for proactive risk assessment and risk reduction activities. C

(c) Management ensures integration between quality improvement, risk management and strategic planning within the organisation. C

(d) Management ensures implementation of systems for internal and external reporting of system and process failures. A

(e) Management ensures that it has a documented agreement for all outsourced services that include service parameters. C

(f) Management monitors the quality of the outsourced services and improvements are made as required. A

Chapter 8 : Facility Management and Safety (FMS)

FMS.1 : The organisation has a system in place to provide a safe and secure environment.

(a) **Patient-safety devices and infrastructure are installed across the organisation and inspected periodically.** Core

(b) The organisation has facilities for the differently-abled. C

(c) **Facility inspection rounds to ensure safety are conducted at least once a month.** Core

(d) Inspection reports of facility rounds are documented, and corrective and preventive measures are undertaken. C

(e) Before construction, renovation and expansion of existing hospital, risk assessment are carried out. E

FMS.2: The organisation's environment and facilities operate in a planned manner and promotes environment-friendly measures.

(a) Facilities and space provisions are appropriate to the scope of services. C

(b) As-built and updated drawings are maintained as per statutory requirements. C

(c) **There are internal and external sign postings in the organisation in a manner understood by the patient, families and community.** Core

(d) **Potable water and electricity are available round the clock.** Core

(e) Alternate sources for electricity and water are provided as a backup for any failure/shortage. C

(f) The organisation tests the functioning of these alternate sources at a predefined frequency. C

(g) The organisation takes initiatives towards an energy-efficient and environmentally friendly hospital. E

FMS.3 : The organisation's environment and facilities operate to ensure the safety of patients, their families, staff and visitors.

(a) Patient safety aspects in terms of structural safety of hospitals especially of critical areas are considered while planning, design and construction of new hospitals and re-planning, assessment, and retrofitting of existing hospitals. E

(b) Operational planning identifies areas which need to have extra security and describes access to different areas in the hospital by staff, patients, and visitors. C

(c) The organisation conducts electrical safety audits for the facility. A

(d) There is a procedure which addresses the identification and disposal of material(s) not in use in the organisation. C

(e) **Hazardous materials are identified and used safely within the organisation.** Core

(f) The plan for managing spills of hazardous materials is implemented. C

FMS.4 : The organisation has a programme for the facility, engineering support services and utility system.

(a) The organisation plans for utility and engineering equipment in accordance with its services and strategic plan. C

(b) Equipment is inventoried, and proper logs are maintained as required. C

(c) **The documented operational and maintenance (preventive and breakdown) plan is implemented.** Core

(d) Utility equipment, are periodically inspected and calibrated (wherever applicable) for their proper functioning. C

(e) Competent personnel operate, inspect, test and maintain equipment and utility systems. C

(f) Maintenance staff is contactable round the clock for emergency repairs. C

(g) Downtime for critical equipment breakdowns is monitored from reporting to inspection and implementation of corrective actions. A

(h) Written guidance supports equipment replacement, identification of unwanted material and disposal. C

FMS.5 : The organisation has a programme for medical equipment management.

(a) The organisation plans for medical equipment in accordance with its services and strategic plan. C

(b) Medical equipment is inventoried, and proper logs are maintained as required. C

(c) **The documented operational and maintenance (preventive and breakdown) plan for medical equipment is implemented.** Core

(d) Medical equipment is periodically inspected and calibrated for their proper functioning. C

(e) Qualified and trained personnel operate and maintain medical equipment. C

(f) Written guidance supports medical equipment replacement and disposal. C

(g) There is a monitoring of medical equipment and medical devices related to adverse events, and compliance hazard notices on recalls. C

(h) Downtime for critical equipment breakdown is monitored from reporting to inspection and implementation of corrective actions. A

FMS.6 : The organisation has a programme for medical gases, vacuum and compressed air.

(a) Written guidance governs the implementation of procurement, handling, storage, distribution, usage and replenishment of medical gases. C

(b) **Medical gases are handled, stored, distributed and used in a safe manner.** Core

(c) The procedures for medical gases address the safety issues at all levels. C

(d) **Alternate sources for medical gases, vacuum and compressed air are provided for, in case of failure.** Core

(e) The organisation regularly tests the functioning of these alternate sources. C

(f) There is an operational, inspection, testing and maintenance plan for piped medical gas, compressed air and vacuum installation. C

FMS.7 : The organisation has plans for fire and non-fire emergencies within the facilities.

(a) The organisation has plans and provisions for early detection, abatement and containment of the fire, and non-fire emergencies. Core

(b) The organisation has a documented and displayed exit plan in case of fire and non-fire emergencies . C

(c) Mock drills are held at least twice a year. C

(d) There is a maintenance plan for fire-related equipment and infrastructure. C

(e) The organisation has a service continuity plan in case of fire and non-fire emergencies. A

Chapter 9 : Human Resource Management (HRM)

HRM.1 : The organisation has a documented system of human resource planning.

(a) Human resource planning supports the organisation's current and future ability to meet the care, treatment and service needs of the patient. E

(b) **The organisation maintains an adequate number and mix of staff to meet the care, treatment and service needs of the patient.** Core

(c) The organisation has contingency plans to manage long- and short-term workforce shortages, including unplanned shortages. A

(d) The job specification and job description are defined for each category of staff. C

(e) The organisation performs a background check of new staff. C

(f) Reporting relationships are defined for each category of staff. C

(g) Exit interviews are conducted and used as a tool to improve human resource practices. A

HRM.2 : The organisation implements a defined process for staff recruitment.

(a) **Written guidance governs the process of recruitment.** Core

(b) A pre-employment medical examination is conducted on the staff. C

(c) **The organisation defines and implements a code of conduct for its staff.** Core

(d) Administrative procedures for human resource management are documented . C

HRM.3: Staff are provided induction training at the time of joining the organisation.

(a) **Staff are provided with induction training.** Core

(b) The induction training includes orientation to the organisation's vision, mission and values. C

(c) The induction training includes awareness on staff rights and responsibilities and patient rights and responsibilities. C

(d) The induction training includes training on safety. C

(e) The induction training includes training on cardio-pulmonary resuscitation for staff providing direct patient care. C

(f) The induction training includes training in hospital infection prevention and control. C

(g) The induction training includes orientation to the service standards of the organization. C

(h) The induction training includes an orientation on administrative procedures. C

(i) The induction training includes an orientation on relevant department/unit/ service/programme's policies and procedures. C

HRM.4 : There is an on-going programme for professional training and development of the staff.

(a) **Written guidance governs training and development policy for the staff.** Core

(b) The organisation maintains the training record. C

(c) Training also occurs when job responsibilities change/new equipment is introduced. C

(d) Feedback mechanisms are in place for improvement of training and development programme. C

(e) Evaluation of training effectiveness is done by the organisation. C

(f) The organisation supports continuing professional development and learning. A

HRM.5 : Staff are appropriately trained based on their specific job description.

(a) Staff involved in blood transfusion services are trained on the handling of blood and blood products. C

(b) Staff are trained in handling vulnerable patients. C

(c) Staff are trained in control and restraint techniques. C

(d) Staff are trained in healthcare communication techniques. C

(e) **Staff involved in direct patient care are provided training on cardiopulmonary resuscitation periodically.** Core

(f) Staff are provided training on infection prevention and control. C

HRM.6 : Staff are trained in safety and quality-related aspects.

(a) Staff are trained on the organisation's safety programme. C

(b) Staff are provided training on the detection, handling, minimisation and elimination of identified risks within the organisation's environment. C

(c) Staff members are made aware of procedures to follow in the event of an incident. C

(d) Staff are trained in occupational safety aspects. C

(e) **Staff are trained in the organisation's disaster management plan.** Core

(f) **Staff are trained in handling fire and non-fire emergencies.** Core

(g) Staff are trained on the organisation's quality improvement programme. C

HRM.7 : An appraisal system for evaluating the performance of staff exists as an integral part of the human resource management process.

(a) Performance appraisal is done for staff within the organisation. C

(b) The staff are made aware of the system of appraisal at the time of induction. C

(c) Performance is evaluated based on the pre-determined criteria. C

(d) The appraisal system is used as a tool for further development. A

(e) Performance appraisal is carried out at defined intervals and is documented. C

HRM.8 : Process for disciplinary and grievance handling is defined and implemented in the organisation.

(a) Written guidance governs disciplinary and grievance handling mechanisms. C

(b) The disciplinary and grievance handling mechanism is known to all categories of staff of the organisation. C

(c) The disciplinary policy and procedure are based on the principles of natural justice. C

(d) **The disciplinary and grievance procedure is in consonance with the prevailing laws.** Core

(e) There is a provision for appeals in all disciplinary cases. C

(f) Actions are taken to redress the grievance. C

HRM.9 : The organisation promotes staff well-being and addresses their health and safety needs.

(a) Staff well-being is promoted. A

(b) Health problems of the staff, including occupational health hazards, are taken care of in accordance with the organisation's policy. C

(c) Health checks of staff dealing with direct patient care are done at least once a year and the findings/results are documented. C

(d) Organisation provides treatment to staff who sustain workplace-related injuries. C

(e) **The organisation has measures in place for prevention and handling workplace violence.** Core

HRM.10: There is documented personal information for each staff member.

(a) Personal files are maintained with respect to all staff, and their confidentiality is ensured. C

(b) The personal files contain personal information regarding the staff's qualification, job description, verification of credentials and health status. C

(c) Records of in-service training and education are contained in the personal files. C

(d) Personal files contain results of all evaluations and remarks. C

HRM.11 : There is a process for credentialing and privileging of medical professionals, permitted to provide patient care without supervision.

(a) **Medical professionals permitted by law, regulation and the organisation to provide patient care without supervision are identified.** Core

(b) The education, registration, training and experience of the identified medical professionals are documented and updated periodically. C

(c) The information about medical professionals is appropriately verified when possible. C

(d) **Medical professionals are granted privileges to admit and care for patients in consonance with their qualification, training, experience and registration.** Core

(e) The requisite services to be provided by the medical professionals are known to them as well as the various departments/units of the organisation. C

(f) Medical professionals admit and care for patients as per their privileging. C

HRM.12: There is a process for credentialing and privileging of nursing professionals, permitted to provide patient care without supervision.

(a) **Nursing staff permitted by law, regulation and the organisation to provide patient care without supervision are identified.** Core

(b) The education, registration, training and experience of nursing staff are appropriately verified, documented and updated periodically. C

(c) The information about the nursing staff is appropriately verified when possible. C

(d) **Nursing staff are granted privileges in consonance with their qualification, training, experience and registration.** Core

(e) The requisite services to be provided by the nursing staff are known to them as well as the various departments/units of the organisation. C

(f) Nursing professionals care for patients as per their privileging. C

HRM.13: There is a process for credentialing and privileging of para-clinical professionals, permitted to provide patient care without supervision.

(a) **Para-clinical professionals permitted by law, regulation and the organisation to provide patient care without supervision are identified.** Core

(b) The education, registration, training and experience of para clinical professionals are appropriately verified, documented and updated periodically . C

(c) **Para-clinical professionals are granted privileges in consonance with their qualification, training, experience and registration.** Core

(d) The requisite services to be provided by the para-clinical professionals are known to them as well as the various departments/units of the organisation. C

(e) Para-clinical professionals care for patients as per their privileging. C

Chapter 10 : Information Management System (IMS)

IMS.1 : Information needs of the patients, visitors, staff, management and external agencies are met.

(a) **The organisation identifies the information needs of the patients, visitors, staff, management external agencies and community.** Core

(b) Identified information needs are captured and/or disseminated. C

(c) Information management and technology acquisitions are commensurate with the identified information needs. C

(d) A maintenance plan for information technology and communication network is implemented. C

(e) Contingency plan ensures continuity of information capture, integration and dissemination. A

(f) The organisation ensures that information resources are accurate and meet stakeholder requirements. E

(g) The organisation contributes to external databases in accordance with the law and regulations. C

IMS.2 : The organisation has processes in place for management and control of data and information.

(a) Processes for data collection are standardised. C

(b) Data is analysed to meet the information needs. C

(c) The organisation disseminates the information in a timely and accurate manner. C

(d) The organisation stores and retrieves data according to its information needs. C

(e) Clinical and managerial staff participate in selecting, integrating and using data for meeting the information needs. C

IMS.3 : The patients cared for by the organisation have a complete and accurate medical record.

(a) The unique identifier is assigned to the medical record. C

(b) The contents of the medical record are identified and documented. C

(c) **The medical record provides a complete, up-to-date and chronological account of patient care.** Core

(d) Authorised staff make the entry in the medical record. C

(e) Entry in the medical record is signed, dated and timed. C

(f) The author of the entry can be identified. C

(g) The medical record has only authorised abbreviations. C

IMS.4 : The medical record reflects the continuity of care.

(a) The medical record contains information regarding reasons for admission, diagnosis and care plan. C

(b) The medical record contains the details of assessments, re-assessments and consultations. C

(c) The medical record contains the results of investigations and the details of the care provided. C

(d) Operative and other procedures performed are incorporated in the medical record. C

(e) When a patient is transferred to another organisation, the medical record contains the details of the transfer. C

(f) The medical record contains a copy of the discharge summary. C

(g) In case of death, the medical record contains a copy of the cause of death report. C

(h) Care providers have access to current and past medical record. C

IMS.5 : The organisation maintains confidentiality, integrity and security of records, data and information.

(a) **The organisation maintains the confidentiality of records, data and information.** Core

(b) **The organisation maintains the integrity of records, data and information.** Core

(c) **The organisation maintains the security of records, data and information.** Core

(d) The organisation uses developments in appropriate technology for improving confidentiality, integrity and security. A

(e) The organisation discloses privileged health information as authorised by the patient and/or as required by law. C

(f) Request for access to information in the medical records by patients/physicians and other public agencies are addressed consistently. C

IMS.6: The organisation ensures availability of current and relevant documents, records, data and information and provides for retention of the same.

(a) **The organisation has an effective process for document control.** Core

(b) **The organisation retains patient's clinical records, data and information according to its requirements.** Core

(c) The retention process provides expected confidentiality and security. C

(d) The destruction of medical records, data and information are in accordance with the written guidance. C

IMS.7: The organisation carries out a review of medical records.

(a) **The medical records are reviewed periodically**. Core

(b) The review uses a representative sample based on statistical principles. C

(c) The review is conducted by identified individuals. C

(d) The review of records is based on identified parameters. C

(e) The review process includes records of both active and discharged patients. C

(f) The review points out and documents any deficiencies in records. C

(g) Appropriate corrective and preventive measures are undertaken. C

Accreditation Process.

- Applications are received
- Screening of applications is done.
- Pre-assessment survey.
- Assessment survey.
- Review of the recommendations of the assessing body by the accreditation committee.
- Recommendations to the Board.
- Accreditation decision.

Who can apply?

- Currently in operation as a health care organization.
- Preferably registered.
- Willing to assume responsibility for improving quality of care.
- Should be able to meet the prescribed standards of the accrediting organization.

Steps to accreditation

1. Obtain copy of NABH standards.
2. Carry out self assessment on status of compliance with the NABH standards.
3. Indentify gap areas and prepare action plan to bridge the gaps.
4. Ensure that NABH standards are implemented and integrated with hospital functioning.
5. Obtain copy and submit application form for assessment.
6. Pay the accreditation fee.
7. Receive the assessment program
8. Facilitate the assessment.

9. Receive recommendation on accreditation
10. Maintain quality improvement programme based on continuous monitoring of patient care services.

Initial presentation by the Hospital

- Organogram.
- Quality management team.
- Methodology followed for quality improvement.
- Facilities provided.
- Inputs on resources provided for quality improvement.
- Identified high risk area for patient care and safety.
- Sentinel events being monitored
- Key monitoring indicators.
- Resource
- Volume
- Utilization
- Performance
- Control charts
- Problems faced and remedial measures undertaken.

Document review

- Quality manual.
- Various policies and procedures.
- Minutes of meetings of various committees.
- Medical records.
- Medical/Nursing audit.
- Adverse events.
- Action taken reports.
- Personal records of staff.

Observations

- Facility safety
- Level of compliance with laid down procedures and policies.
- Bio-Medical Waste (BMW) management.
- Standard precautions.

- Patient care.
- Fire safety
- Equipment management.

Patient and staff interviews

Scoring pattern

NABH has laid down the following Pattern.

- Non compliance – 0
- Partial compliance-5
- Full compliance -10

Duration of Accreditation Awards.

Generally three years with one reassessment survey to ensure continued compliance and to assess the CQI programme. If during accreditation the Accreditation Organization receives inputs that the organization is substantially out of compliance with the current standard then resurvey or withdrawal of accreditation decision may be resorted to.

References

- Sheth Sudha. Accreditation of hospitals Health care Management: October 2001.
- Chatterjee . B. Chandrima. Accreditation of hospitals. An overview. Health Care Management September 2005.
- Sharma D.k. Hospital Accreditation. Why and where fore. Symposium on quality assurance and medical audit in hospitals July 1992.
- Francis. P.A. Regulating hospitals and Nursing homes. Editorial pharma biz: September 2005
- Standards for Hospitals. First edition Joint commission International Accreditation 2000. www.jcwc.com
- B.k Rana. National Accreditation Board for Hospitals and Health care providers. Ind Medica. Cyber lectures 2006. www.indmedica.com
- JK Das. National Accreditation for Hospitals and Health care providers. NIHFW. New Delhi. www.NIHFW.org.
- K.R. Singhal. Awareness on "NABH standards for Hospitals". National Centre for quality Management. AJMER Centre 2006.
- Accreditation Standards for Hospitals. 5th Edition. National Accreditation Board for Hospitals and Health care Providers (NABH). IEEA.

7

Rights of the Patients

Health is a wide ranging concept and it is duty of State to protect and promote health of its citizens. When a patient is being treated by a medical team both the partners have rights and responsibilities towards each other. Patient means a person who is admitted to an acute care inpatient facility for a continuous period longer than 24 hours, for the purpose of diagnosis or treatment bearing on the physical and mental health of that person. Patient also means any person who is receiving treatment on an out patient basis or in a community support program or other community based program. Patient has also been defined as any person suffering from illness or using health services.

Patients shall at admission be told that there are legal rights for their protection during their stay at the facility or throughout their course of treatment and maintenance in the community. Explanation of the written statement of rights shall be available to patients, their guardians or their chosen representatives upon reasonable request to the administrator. Sufficient information about medical services and the best way to use them shall be made available to the public. Patients shall be given by their physicians complete and current information concerning their diagnosis, treatment, alternatives, risks and prognosis as required by the physician's legal duty to disclose. This information shall be in terms and languages the patients can reasonably be expected to understand. This information shall include the likely medical or major psychological results of the treatment and its alternatives. In case where it is medically inadvisable, doctor can use therapeutic privileges and not disclose information because it would be harmful to the patient. This privilege is less used these days because of the decreasing paternalistic attitudes of doctors. One should also consider the moral and legal implications of not disclosing information. A high degree of respect for the patient is needed to make this Judgment. This is where virtues in the doctor's personality are important. The patient shall have the right not to be informed if he so requests. The patient shall have the right to choose if and who will be informed on his behalf. The patient has the right to know about the identity and status of all those who provide health care as well as regulations concerning the terms and the procedures of stay and the medical care offered by the establishment. Patient has right to refuse treatment. Patients who receive services from an outside provider are entitled upon request to be told the identity of the provider. Information shall include the name of the outside provider, the address and description of the service which may be rendered. A patient who no longer has a medical reason to stay in a medical institution shall have the right to full explanation before he is transferred to another institute or be discharged. The transfer can take place only if another institution has agreed to accept the patient. When a patient is discharged he should be offered out- patient services. For every procedure which is to be performed on a patient, consent has to be taken. All the relevant information has to be given to the patient regarding the procedure, its risks and the alternatives available. The patient should have thorough understanding of the procedure and should volunteer for it. He should know the competence of the person who is performing the procedure. Five conditions for informed consent are: disclosures of information, understanding, voluntariness, competence and consent. Should the patient not be in a position to express his wishes and should emergency treatment or other procedure be necessary his consent shall be considered as given unless it is obvious that under the circumstances he would have reasonably objected. In case when due to the condition of the patient a person is appointed or should have been appointed to give consent and treatment is urgent, then this can take place if the consent cannot be obtained in time, unless it is obvious that under the circumstances he would have reasonably objected. When consent is to be taken from person appointed by law for a particular patient he should be thoroughly informed about the procedure to be performed. If a person who is appointed by law to give consent for a patient refuses to give consent and doctor thinks that treatment is necessary to save life of the patient, the case then is to be labeled as medico-legal and referred to law enforcing agency for decision.

Confidentiality is the corner stone of the doctor patient relationship. Patients have to be assured confidential treatment of their personal and medical records. The patient can review his medical record without charge. Patient can obtain a copy of medical record for which hospital can charge a reasonable fee, however copy cannot be denied if patient cannot afford to pay. The patient has to be provided a written discharge plan and written description of how he can approach the hospital when needed. Information which is put on the person's file is not merely something which needs to be explained in terms the patient can understand and act upon, but is in fact owned by the patient. Although the medical record is owned by the hospital but the information contained is owned by the patient and is to be respected as such and may refuse its release to any individual outside the facility. Confidential information shall be disclosed when consent has been obtained from patient or if the law permits it in exceptional cases. The consent is considered to have been given when information is given to a person who is involved in treatment of the patient. Doctors have dual role when working as occupational physicians for companies. Doctor in such case must explain his duty to the third party and patient as well. First duty of the doctor in such a case is toward the patient and any information cannot be revealed without consent of the patient. Doctor may however feel obliged to warn a person who is going to be affected by disease of the patient. This is what is called as "Double effects" but are difficult to answer. Data protection Acts oblige doctor to protect information and are responsible for it not being divulged or used for means other than patient has consented for. Patients shall have the right to respectfulness and privacy as it relates to their medical and personal care program. Patient has the right to correction of his medical record which is inaccurate, incomplete or unclear.

Whenever circumstances call for a selection among patients for specific medial care, this shall be made without discrimination, in a fair manner and shall be based on medical criteria. Upon admission to a facility a patient or his legal guardian shall be given opportunity to authorize disclosure of the patient's presence in the facility to callers or visitors who may seek to communicate with the patient. Patient has the right to complain about the care and services he is receiving and to have hospital to respond to it. Patient has a right to an itemized bill and explanation of all charges. Patient has the right to make known his wishes in regard to anatomical gifts to appropriate authority.

References

1. Pierre Mallia. Biomedical ethics- Patients rights. Student BMJ 2003; 11:175-218.
2. Charter of patients rights. Patients rights movement and working group for the construction of the charter Cyprus – 2001. (www.active citizenship.net/ documents)
3. Statutory bill of rights. Public health law (PHL) 2803 (1) (g) patients rights, IONYCRR, 405.7, 406.7 (a) (1), 405.7 (c)

8

Quality in Laboratories

The aim of quality control in laboratories is to produce accurate results every time. Two yard sticks used are accuracy and precision. Accuracy is concerned with the relationship of a set of results to the true value. This can be done by relating the mean of the replicate analysis to the true value. Precision measurements are concerned with agreement between replicate analyses. Rarely are the results same when a certain test is performed on a same sample repeatedly under ordinary working conditions, instead a scatter of results is obtained. The distribution of the results of such measurements is a measure of the precision of a method.

The functioning of a laboratory can be divided into three components.

1. Pre-Analytical activities
2. Analytical activities
3. Post analytical activities.

Each laboratory quality programme defines requirements for a lab in terms of physical facilities, policy, procedures etc.

- Ventilation in the facility should be adequate.
- Temperature and humidity must be regularly monitored.
- Proper layout .
- Equipment manufactures quality control recommendations should be strictly followed.

- Daily equipment function checks be performed before sample testing.
- Quality control procedures for equipment to be performed at least each day of the use.
- Quality manual ,SOPs manual (Standard operating procedures manual) should be available in the laboratory and all staff members should have access to the same.
- All health and safety measures should be followed.
- Proper qualified personnel should be available.
- Job description of all categories of workers should be available.
- Organogram of the laboratory as part of the health organization and also internal laboratory organization should be available.
- Staff appraisals should be done.
- CMEs should be regularly done.
- Internal and external audits should be regularly carried out.

Quality Assurance Activities

Pre- analytical Activities

Quality control starts right from the ordering of investigation.

Test ordering process: Test requisition should be complete and should include name of patient, hospital number, sex, age, and clinical information. Date & time of ordering should be mentioned. The person requesting for investigation should identify himself.

Specimen collection procedures: - Samples should be taken by trained staff. Standard precautions should be observed while drawing samples. Labeling instructions of samples should be laid down and communicated to personnel concerned.

Transportation to the laboratory: - After collecting the samples in well defined condition they should be transported to lab in such a way and within such time that no changes occur. The specimens taken should be placed in adequate containers for transport to the laboratory. Request forms should be placed in separate water proof bags or envelops.

Automated computer systems in the form of LAN (Local Area Network) are used for ordering tests which reduce the chances of error. If the patient is not prepared properly for investigation or any clinical information not provided, the whole process of quality control is undermined.

Analytical Activities

Well established and scientifically recognized methods should be used and method used should be documented. There should be calibration of equipment and devices and maintenance schemes as advised by manufacturer should be strictly followed. Control samples should be tested in same manner as patient samples. Once the specimen reaches the laboratory worker should have control over the specimen handling techniques . There should be early separations of blood serum. The time required to mix a specimen where deposits occur is frequently under-estimated. The temperature change that occurs in a biologic fluid during centrifugation should be known and monitored. Procedures which can be automated, should be automated to reduce human error. Many test methods use automated analyzers. Most instruments have internal control systems to detect error. External control systems also bring abnormal results to the operator's attention. Internal quality control measures by using control replications and random sample check determine the drifts occurring in the daily tests. Appropriate remedies to correct any deviations should be implemented immediately. External quality control by periodic analysis of samples from reputed quality control programmers can be done. The variance index scores are measures of performance. Performance comparisons with other laboratories are provided. These measures help to assess the quality of work in comparison with international laboratories and also to implement corrective procedures if the performance is not upto standard. Good quality reagents should be used.

Post- Analytic Activities

As test results are made available to the heath care provider, quality continues to be monitored. The test results have to be sent to appropriate party and should be reported timely. Reference ranges should be included. There should be immediate notification of results exceeding critical limits. Results can be reported electronically through LAN. There has to be proper handling of hazardous waste both chemical and biological, as per Bio-Medical Waste Management and handling rules.

Quality Control officer

In large laboratories there should be a Quality Control Officer who should have complete knowledge of laboratory procedures but should not be part of those who actually perform the tests nor should he be identified with Head of the laboratory. He should be in direct contact and access to the Head of the laboratory. He should ideally be appointed from the hospital staff itself and not from outside. He should be responsible for monitoring the quality control activities by using quality control techniques. He should identify the problems and find solutions thereof.

Safety in laboratories

The good laboratory safety practices is a step toward the achievement of a safe and healthful work environment. One cannot remove all the dangers and hazards from a laboratory but can make a laboratory reasonably safe. A Laboratory Safety Coordinator is appointed by Laboratory Head and is responsible for overall safety in laboratories including chemical safety, explosion hazards, electrical hazards, emergency contingency plans and hazardous waste disposal.

General principles of safety in laboratories

- Wear lab coat, gloves and safety glasses with side shields to protect from unintended splashes and explosions.
- Use safety shields to protect against explosion hazards.
- Never pipette by mouth. Use pipette pump or bulb.
- Wash your hands properly before leaving the laboratory.
- If there has been a spill take care of people first and then clear the spill.
- In case of chemical spills MSDS (Material safety data sheet) is a valuable document that should be consulted before medical attention is sought.
- MSDS provides information on physical and chemical properties, toxicity, health hazards, fire and explosion limits,

reactivity, spill and clean up, handling and storage. MSDS should be used wisely.

- It is the responsibility of the Laboratory Director to ensure the development and adoption of a biosafety management plan and a safety or operations manual, SOPs (Standard operating procedures) manual.
- Laboratory Safety Officer should ensure that regular training in laboratory safety is provided.
- Personnel should be advised of special hazards and required to read the safety or operations manual and follow standard practices and procedures. The laboratory safety officer should ensure that all personnel understand these. A copy of the safety manual should be available in the laboratory.
- Understand the chemistry and predict potential hazards.
- Proper chemical storage.
- Never work in the lab alone.
- Keep emergency number handy.
- Make chemical hygiene plan specific to each laboratory.
- Know your hazards and steps to be taken to ensure your own safety.
- Use common sense in emergency situations.
- When working with unknown assume the worst and take extreme precautions to protect yourself and the environment.
- Know position of first aid kits.
- Familiarize yourself with escape route.
- Every body should know about Safety Officer and his number.
- Take special precautions when working with radioactive materials, lasers, ultraviolet radiations, recombinant DNA molecules, chemical carcinogens, biohazardous agents, compressed gas cylinders and cryogenic liquids.
- Avoid underestimating the risk.

References

1. Quality assurance and quality control Monitored at each step. How reliable is laboratory testing. American Association for clinical Chemistry 2001-2007.

2. C. Snehlasha. Quality control and quality assurance in laboratory research. International Journal Diabetes Dev Countries. 1998. Vol. 18: p. 44-45.
3. Basic laboratories - Biosafety levels 1 and 2. Laboratory biosafety manual 3rd edition WHO 2004. p. 9-19.
4. Laboratory safety policies in Policies and procedure Manual. Kansas State University Chapter 3730: 2002.
5. G. Sudhakar Reddy. Occupational safety and environmental Health. University of Michigan Ann Arbor, Michigan, USA.

9

Techniques of Management

Health is a complex organization with number of subsystems and players. Public hospitals, private sector and community health services come together to provide best patient care possible. Even in a single hospital there are number of subsystems which influence the outcome. In a developing country like ours where resources are meagre it becomes important that these resources are utilized properly and scientifically. In this scenario of meagre resources and number of options how to utilize them it is important that modern techniques of management are used in decision making. These management techniques make use of mathematical and statistical models . These techniques are quantitative and semi-quantitative and are useful in increasing efficiency by reducing costs and ensuring better health care.

Modern Management Techniques

Statistical Techniques

- Time trends & forecasting
- Decision theory and tree

Activity Analysis

- Time motion studies
- Work sampling and activity analysis
- Queuing theory
- Gantt chart & work schedule

Mathematical techniques

- Simulation study/models
- Systems analysis
- Linear programming
- Inventory control
- Network analysis
- PERT
- CPM

Financial Techniques

- Investment Analysis
- Break Even Analysis.
- Cost accounting & costing of service.
- Cost benefit analysis
- Cost effectiveness analysis
- Budgeting.

Miscellaneous

- Situational analysis
- SWOT analysis

Time trends & forecasting

Trend analysis is the widespread practice of collecting information and attempting to spot a pattern. Trend analysis is a mathematical technique that uses historical results to predict future outcome. This is achieved by tracking variances in cost and schedule performance. Trend analysis often refers to techniques for extracting an underlying pattern of behavior in a time series which would otherwise be partly or nearly completely hidden. If the trend can be assumed to be linear, trend analysis can be undertaken within a formal regression analysis. If the trends have other shapes than linear, trend testing can be done by non-parametric methods, e.g. smoothing. Trend analysis is the process of looking at current trends in order to predict future ones and is considered a form of comparative analysis. This can include attempting to determine whether a current market trend, such as gains in a particular market sector, is likely to continue, as well as whether a trend in one market area could result in a trend in another.

Forecasting is one of the first steps in planning; the success of the plans depends on the accuracy of the forecasts. In the service industries like the hospitals, there are many plans that depend on the forecast, from capacity planning to aggregate planning, from layout decisions to the daily schedules. There are number of situations in hospitals where trend analysis is needed for forecasting . The examples are forecasting demand of supplies, load of patients in out patient department, requirement of hospital beds, requirement of staff etc. Forecasting analysts try to minimize the effects of bias and random errors by selecting the appropriate forecasting models but eliminating all forms of errors is impossible. The methods used are: Moving averages, exponential smoothing method with an alpha 0.1, exponential smoothing method with an alpha 0.5, Double exponential smoothing method with an alpha 0.2, gamma 0.3, Trend analysis method with linear trend, trend analysis method with quadratic trend, Trend analysis method with growth curve, Winters Method with alpha 0.2, gamma 0.2, delta 0.2. The overall accuracy of a forecasting model can be determined by comparing the forecasted values for the past known period with the actual or deserved demand for these periods. Simple moving average (SMA) is a calculation that takes the arithmetic mean of a given set of prices over the specific number of days in the past; for example, over the previous 15, 30, 100, or 200 days. Exponential moving averages (EMA) is a weighted average that gives greater importance to the price of a stock on more recent days, making it an indicator that is more responsive to new information. The simplest form of a moving average, known as a simple moving average (SMA), is calculated by taking the arithmetic mean of a given set of values over a specified period of time. In other words, a set of numbers or prices in the case of financial instruments are added together and then divided by the number of prices in the set. The simple moving average method is highly dependent on n, the number of terms selected for constructing the average. The equation is shown as Equation 1 as follows:

$$Ft+1 = (Yt + Yt-1 + Yt-2 + \ldots\ldots + Yt-n+1)/n \quad (1)$$

Where: Ft+1 = the forecast value for the next period, Yt = the actual value at period, and t n = the number of term in the moving average.

For the double weighted moving average method, it requires determining two averages. The first moving average is computed; a second moving average is calculated. In addition, Five equations are used in the double moving average which are stated as follows:

Mt = Ft+1 = (Yt +Yt-1 +Yt-2 + ...+Yt-n+1)/n (2)

M’t = (Mt + Mt-1 +Mt-2 + ...+Mt-n+1)/n (3)

At = 2Mt - M ’ t (4)

Bt=1 2n(Mt - M’t) (5)

Ft+p = At + Bt p (6)

Where: n = the number of period in the double moving average. Yt = the actual series value at time period, p = the number of period ahead to be forecast. For the simple exponential smoothing method, it uses a weighted moving average of past data as the basis for a forecast. This method keeps a running average of demand and adjusts it for each period in proportion to the difference between the latest actual demand figure and the latest value of the average. The equation for the simple exponential smoothing method is shown as follows :

Ft+1 = α Yt + (1-α) Ft-1 (7)

where Ft+1 = the new smoothing value or the forecast value for the next period, α= the smoothing constant (0 < α The exponential moving average is a type of moving average that gives more weight to recent prices in an attempt to make it more responsive to new information. To calculate an EMA, one must first compute the simple moving average (SMA) over a particular time period. Next, one must calculate the multiplier for weighting the EMA (referred to as the “smoothing factor”), which typically follows the formula: [2/(selected time period + 1)]. So, for a 20-day moving average, the multiplier would be [2/(20+1)]= 0.0952. Then you use the smoothing factor combined with the previous EMA to arrive at the current value. The EMA thus gives a higher weighting to recent prices, while the SMA assigns equal weighting to all values.

Decision theory and Tree

According to Simons decision making Theory, decision making has following stages.

- Intelligence Activity Stage: This stage identifies the problems of an organisation and the head of the organisation has to analyse and understand the organisational environment to proceed to a resolution.
- Design Activity Stage: After problem identification, the organisation head starts to look for various suitable courses or strategies or alternatives and identifies the merits and demerits of each.
- Choice Activity Stage: Once alternatives have been developed, the administration begins the choice activity stage. It critically evaluates the different consequences of all alternatives available and a decision is taken after examining the above mentioned alternatives' merits and demerits and the most suitable course of action is selected. This stage requires skills such as judgement, creativity, quantitative analysis and experience in the decision making process.

In regard to organisational decision making Simon identified two types of decision making:

Programmed decisions: Decisions having repetitive components and where pre established examples are present.

Non Programmed decisions: Non repetitive in nature and directed towards solving problems in new environments and new variables.

Simon advocated delegating to sub-units programmed decisions whereas non-programmed decisions should be retained with the upper level strategic management.

Though there are many slight variations of the decision-making framework floating around, professionals use these seven steps.

The steps involved in the process of decision making are:-

1. Detect Problem
2. Diagnose Problem
3. Establish Decision Criteria
4. Develop Alternatives
5. Evaluate Alternatives
6. Implementation
7. Evaluate the decision.

Detect Problem: The most crucial step in good decision making is to recognise a decision needs to be made. It goes without saying that if the need for a decision is not identified then an appropriate action cannot be taken. Most decisions stem from two main causes- a need to correct a problem and a desire to exploit a new opportunity.

Diagnose Problem: Once a problem has been recognised it must be defined and the nature of the problem diagnosed. Sometimes a problem is diagnosed at a very superficial level and a decision is made to treat the symptoms of the problem rather than its real cause.

A very simple approach to problem diagnosis is to ask

(i) What is the evidence that a problem really exists?

(ii) Where does the problem appear to arise?

(iii) When does the problem appear to arise?

(iv) How urgent is the problem?

(v) Who is most involved with the problem?

(vi) What factors, people, departments, organisations, processes are related to the problem?

(vii) Why did the problem occur?

Establish Decision Criteria: Establishing the criteria which a good decision should possess is a vital part of the diagnostic phase. It is often overlooked. Many people do not develop decision criteria until after alternative solutions have been identified. This has a major disadvantage. The decision criteria may be distorted to favour one of the alternatives instead of being thought out in a logical way.

Some of the frequently used criteria are:

- Usefulness for direct patient care.
- Financial benefits
- Financial costs
- Physical resources needed
- Human resources needed
- Quantity (more production)
- Quality (better performance)
- Certainty of desired outcome (risk) etc.

The combination of criteria used to decide between alternative solutions will depend on the exact nature of the problem.

Develop Alternatives: The next stage is to develop alternative solutions. Often managers accept the first reasonable solution that occurs. This is called satisficing and it is very common. Satisficing means accepting a solution which meets minimum requirements. It is the opposite of optimising which is the acceptance of the solution that provides the best possible answer. Research suggests that most managers accept satisfactory rather than optimal solutions.

In most circumstances it is important to generate several alternative solutions which can be evaluated and the best one chosen. If the decision is important, special techniques may be employed to produce enough alternatives. The main techniques are : employee suggestions, idea quotes, brain storming, nominal group technique, delphi technique etc.

Evaluate Alternatives :

Decision Trees

A decision tree is a decision support tool that uses a structured graphical depiction of alternatives. This method creates a visual depiction of choices so decision makers can have a clearer understanding of them. Decision trees help divide larger decisions into smaller ones and are useful for uncovering all available options.

Decision trees have a starting point and then branch out, with each branch representing a different event, action, or outcome. Resource costs, benefits, and probabilities can be recorded by each option.

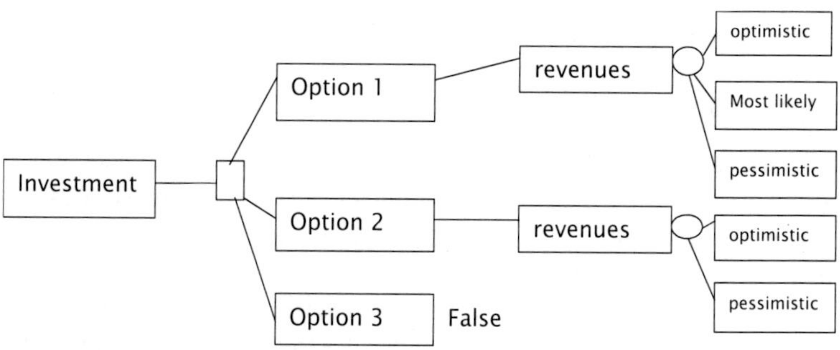

Fig 9.1: Showing Decision tree

Decision trees have three types of nodes at each part of the diagram:

- Decision nodes: these are the alternatives themselves and represent the point where a decision must be made.
- Change nodes: these are points where choices must be made; in their simplest form these may be represented by Yes/No or Go/No Go options.
- Conclusion or end nodes: these are the points that appear when there are no more alternatives or choices to be made, and they state the outcome of a particular decision branch.

When a decision maker has successfully and accurately defined the problem and generated alternatives, he or she can then conduct analysis useful to evaluating and assessing each. This typically involves analysis of quantitative data such as costs or revenues. Qualitative data is also used to be sure that considerations such as consistency with strategy, effects on relationships, or ethical implications are taken into account.

A first step in analysis is identifying all the sources of data needed to understand the various alternatives and their potential outcomes. Finding this data often involves research if relevant data does not exist. The results of data analysis are typically gathered, summarized, and synthesized as the basis for discussions and deliberations by decision makers.

There are a few approaches that can be used to help structure the analysis and assessment of potential decision alternatives. These range from simple tools such as lists of pros and cons to more complex models such as decision trees and influence diagrams, which can capture more variables and include more data.

A decision tree specifies alternatives visually and creates paths of subdecisions to be made or uncertainties to be considered in order to estimate the outcome of a given choice. It includes a value for each alternative, such as a financial outcome, and notes the probabilities that each outcome will occur. Decision trees sometime include the results of financial analysis such as net present value, which determines the present or current value of a stream of incoming cash flows that a project will bring in sometime in the future. One limitation to using decision trees is that they can become highly complicated as decisions become more complex or outcomes involve greater numbers of variables.

Another tool that decision makers can use to analyse alternatives is an influence diagram. An influence diagram is a compact graphical and mathematical representation of a decision situation. It groups sets of variables into things that are known and factors that are uncertain and links them to the choice to be made and the criteria for assessing it. Influence diagrams are directly applicable in group decisions because they allow incomplete sharing of information among team members to be modelled and for estimates to be made explicitly.

Influence diagrams are closely related to decision trees and often used in conjunction with them. An influence diagram displays a summary of the information contained in a decision tree. It involves four variable types for notation: a decision (a rectangle), chance (an oval), objective (a hexagon), and function (a rounded rectangle). Influence diagrams also use solid lines to denote influence. Their appearance is very similar to a flowchart. Influence diagrams show

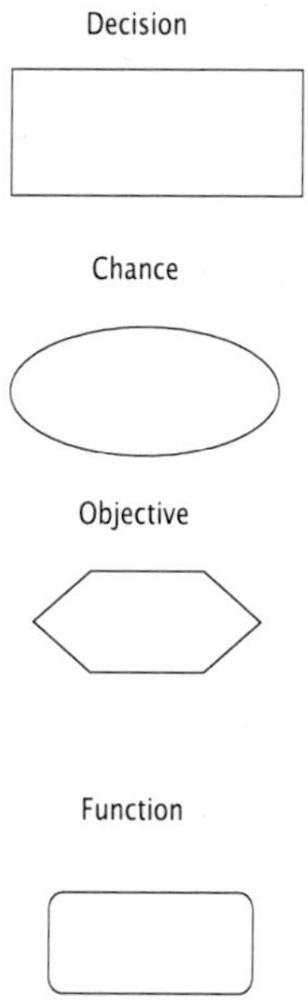

Fig : 9.2: Implementation

the dependencies among variables. This is an important distinction between influence diagrams and decision trees. Decision trees offer much more detail about each possible decision. An influence diagram involves 4 variable types for notation: a decision (a rectangle), chance (an oval), objective (a hexagon), and function (a rounded rectangle).

The implementation of a proposed solution to a problem is, in effect, the initiation of a new order of things or the introduction of change. And change must be managed. User expectations must be managed as part of change management. The definition of implementation is somewhat complicated because implementation is a long, involved process with vague boundaries. Simplistically, the implementation phase involves putting a recommended solution to work. Many generic implementation issues, such as resistance to change, degree of support of top management, and user training, are important in dealing with managerial decisions.

Finally data is collected about the alternative, alternative evaluated and impact of the decision followed.

Time and Motion Study

Time and motion study (also referred to as motion and time study, the terms are used interchangeably) is the scientific study of the conservation of human resources in the search for the most efficient method of doing a task. A fascination with the word "efficiency" began in the late 19th and early 20th centuries when it was considered one of the most important concepts. Time study began in the 1880s as a means of wage-rate setting by Frederick W. Taylor, who is regarded as the "father of scientific management." It consists of a wide variety of procedures for determining the amount of time required, under certain standard conditions of measurement, for tasks involving some human activity. Motion study was developed by Frank B. Gilbreth and Lillian M. Gilbreth and consists of a wide variety of procedures for the description, systematic analysis, and means of improving work methods. It is difficult to separate these two aspects completely. Therefore, the combined term usually refers to all three phases of the activity: method determination, time appraisal, and development of material for the application of these data. Frank and Lillian also broadened scientific management by including the human element, therefore using psychology to gain the cooperation of employees. Motion and time analysis could be used to help find a preferential way of doing the work and could assist in effectively managing or controlling the activity. This approach has been successfully applied to factories, hospitals, department stores, housework, banks, cafeteria work, libraries, music, and to many other human activities. For instance, factories have used it to reduce wasted time and improve the time to compete a task, while banks use it to help team members reach their sales goals. However, the goal of a time and motion study is not simply efficiency. These studies are done to create a baseline that can be used in the future when evaluating procedural, equipment, or personnel changes. The goal can be to understand the skills required to enable individuals to perform the work and, thus, to provide the correct training. Another may be to reduce the discomfort experienced, especially in the case of surgical procedures—a goal such as this, namely, to create less tissue damage, may run counter to efficiency.

Objectives of Work Study :

(i) Work study brings higher productivity

(ii) Work study improves existing method of work for which cost becomes lower

(iii) It eliminates wasteful elements

(iv) It sets standard of performance

(v) It helps to use machine and human more effectively

(vi) It improves by saving in time and loss of material also.

Steps Involved in Work Study:

The steps of work study are:

(i) It selects the jobs which are to be studied

(ii) It examines critically the recorded facts which are already done

(iii) It records from direct observations all the matters which are happened

(iv) It defines new method

(v) It also installs the new method

(vi) It also maintains the new standard

(vii) It develops most economic and appropriate methods

(viii) It measures the work content in the method, that is selected and compute a standard time.

Types of Work Study:

1. Method Study: According to ILO, method study is "the systematic recording, analysis and critical examination of existing and proposed ways of doing work and the development and application of easier and more effective method". In short, it is a systematic procedure to analyse the work to eliminate unnecessary operations.

   The objectives of method study are:

   (i) It improves the proper utilisation of manpower, machine and materials;

   (ii) It also improves the hospital layout, work place, etc.

   (iii) It also improves the process and procedure

   (iv) It develops better physical working environment

   (v) It reduces undesirable fatigue.

   The steps of method study are:

   (i) At first select the proper work which are to be studied

   (ii) Record all the facts of existing method

   (iii) Examine the facts very critically

   (iv) Develop the most practical, economic, and effective method

   (v) Install the method and the same should be maintained.

2. Time and Motion Study: According to ILO, Time Study means "a technique for determining as accurately as possible from a limited number of observations the time necessary to carry out a given activity at a different standard of performance". In other words, "time study is the art of observing and recording time required to do each detailed element of an individual operation." Practically, it studies the time taken on each element of a job.

   Motion study, on the other hand, is the study of the body motion used in performing an operation, with the thought of improving the operation by eliminating unnecessary motion and simplifying necessary motion and thus establishing the most favourable motion sequence for maximum efficiency.

So, in short, 'Time Study' means the determination of standard time that is taken by a worker of average ability under normal working conditions for performing a job. But 'Motion Study' determines the correct method of doing a job to avoid wasteful movements.

Steps

1. Time and Motion studies eliminate wasteful movements
2. They examine the proposed method critically and determine the most effective one
3. They determine for each element having a stop-watch
4. They record all the parts of a job which are done by the existing method
5. They install the method as standard one
6. They critically observe the workers who are engaged with the work
7. They assess the proper speed of the operator who is working.

Work Sampling and Activity Analysis

Work sampling also called activity sampling is the statistical technique used for determining the proportion of time spent by workers in various defined categories of activity. It is as important as all other statistical techniques because it permits quick analysis, recognition, and enhancement of job responsibilities, tasks, performance competencies, and organizational work flows.

- In a work sampling study, a large number of observations are made of the workers over an extended period of time. For statistical accuracy, the observations must be taken at random times during the period of study, and the period must be representative of the types of activities performed by the subjects. Idea is to develop standard times to perform a task. Standard times have been defined as the time required by an average skilled operator, working at normal pace to perform a specified task using a prescribed method allowing time for personal needs, fatigue and delay. The standards derived from work sampling might specify the proportion of time that should be devoted to specific activities rather than the time required to perform a task. There must be sufficient time available to perform this study say several weeks or more. Work sampling is commonly used to study the activities of multiple workers rather than one worker. The job to be studied should have relatively long cycle time. The last condition is the non-repetitive work cycles. The work is not highly repetitive. The jobs consist of various tasks rather than a single repetitive task. However, it must be possible to classify the work activities into a distinct number of categories. There are several recommended steps when starting to prepare a work sampling study.

- Define the manufacturing tasks for which the standard time is to be determined.
- Define the task elements. These are the defined broken-down steps of the task that will be observed during the study. These are actual direct work, idle, waiting for work etc.
- Design the study. This includes designing the forms that will be used to record the observations, determining how many observations will be required, deciding on the number of days or shifts to be included in the study, scheduling the observations, and finally determining the number of observers needed.
- Identify the observers who will do the sampling.
- Start the study. All those who are affected by the study should be informed about it.
- Make random visits and collect the observations.
- Analyze and present the results.

The number of observations to be made for desired accuracy for desired confidence level is determined by following formula.

$$\sigma_P = \sqrt{\frac{pq}{n}}$$

$$n = \frac{pq}{\sigma_P{}^2}$$

Where

σP standard error of proportion.

P = percentage of working time.

q = percentage of idle time.

n = number of observations.

Example of work sampling can be studying nursing activities. Nurses perform direct nursing care activities as well as participate in other "indirect" nursing care activities such as ward administration, management and continued professional development activities which form part of the nursing work load in medical ward. Thus it is necessary to understand the proportion of nursing work load assigned to other activities and trends of variation in nursing activities throughout the day in order to estimate the actual staffing requirements. A work sampling method is used and a snapshot of nursing activity can be recorded at 10 minute intervals from 7.00am to 7.00 pm for a week.

Queuing Theory

The queuing theory also called the *waiting line theory*, owes its development to A K Erlang's efforts to analyze telephone traffic congestion for services of the Copenhagen automatic telephone system. The waiting lines develop because the service to a patient/customer may not be rendered immediately as the patient/customer reaches the service facility. Thus lack of adequate service facility would cause waiting lines of patients/customers to be formed. The only way that the service demand can be met is to increase the capacity to such high level as can always meet the peak demand with no queues. But adding to the capacity may be a costly affair and uneconomic after a stage because then it shall remain idle to varying degree when there are no or few patients/customers. Providing too low service would cause excessive waiting which has a cost in terms of patient/customer frustration, loss of goodwill . The goal of queuing modelling is the achievement of an economic balance between the cost of providing service and the cost associated with the wait required for that service.

The elements of a system are :

Arrival Process : finite or infinite, single arrivals or group arrivals, regular arrivals or arrivals in random way, deterministic arrivals or probabilistic arrivals.

Service system : (a) structure of service system b) speed of a service

Structure of the service system:

(1) Single Service facility.

(2) Multiple parallel facilities with single queue.

(3) Multiple parallel facilities with multiple queues.

(4) Service facilities in series.

Speed of service:

The speed with which service is provided can be expressed as service rate and as service time. The service rate describes the number of customers serviced during a particular period. The service time indicates the amount of time needed to service a customer. Generally, the queuing models are based on the assumption that service times are exponentially distributed about some average service time.

Queue structure

For the queuing models we shall consider the assumption that the customers are serviced on the first-come -first -served basis.

Another thing to consider in the queuing structure is the behavior or attitude of the patients entering the queuing system. The patients may not select queues randomly and look for the shortest queue. There may be *Jockeying* among the many queues that is patients may switch to other queues which are moving fast. There could be *reneging* ie patients stand in the queue for sometime and then leave the system because it is moving slowly. Sometimes patients upon arrival do not join the queue and decide to return for service at a later time or may abandon the system. This is known as *balking*. For the queuing models we assume that no jockeying, reneging or balking takes place.

The queuing models can be categorized as being deterministic or probabilistic. If each patient arrives at known intervals and the service time is known with certainty, the queuing model shall be deterministic in nature. The vast majority of the queuing models are based on the assumption that one or more elements of the queuing system can be expressed only in probabilistic terms. Hence all of the queuing models are of probabilistic type.

If arrival rate of patients is λ and service time μ patients per unit time two situations are possible

If $\lambda > \mu$ the waiting line shall be formed which will increase indefinitely; the service facility would always be busy; and the service system will eventually fail.

If $\lambda \leq \mu$ there shall be no waiting time; the proportion of time the service facility would be idle is $1 - \lambda/\mu$.

The ratio $\lambda/\mu = \rho$ is called the average utilization or the traffic intensity or the clearing ratio.

So if $\rho > 1$, the system would ultimately fail and

If $\rho \leq 1$, the system works and ρ is the proportion of time it is busy.

However conditions of uniform arrivals and uniform service rates has very limited practicability. Thus variable arrival rates and servicing times are more realistic assumptions.

Some of the numerous queuing models few are:

Poisson exponential single server model- infinite population.

Poisson exponential single server model- finite population.

Poisson exponential multiple server model – infinite population.

Poisson – Exponential Single Server model – infinite population

For a workable system it is necessary that $\lambda < \mu$. Even if $\lambda = \mu$, the system shall not work.

Probability that the system is idle, that is there are no customers in the system, equals $P_0 = 1 - \rho$.

The probability of having exactly n customers in the system shall be :

$$P_n = \rho^n p_0 = \rho^n(1-\rho)$$

Expected number of customers in the system :

$L_s = \lambda/\mu-\lambda$ or $\rho/1-\rho$.

Expected number of customers in the queue:

$L_q = L_s - \lambda/\mu = \lambda/\mu-\lambda - \lambda/\mu$.

With an average arrival rate of λ, the average time between the arrivals is 1/λ. Thus the mean waiting time in queue is

$$W_q = 1/\lambda .\ L_{q.}$$

Poisson – Exponential Single Server Model-Finite Population

This queuing model is based on similar assumptions as the earlier model except that the input population is finite. For this model system structure is such that we have a total of M patients in the system, consisting of queue and a single service station or in arriving state. When a patient is in arriving condition then the time it takes him to arrive is a random variable having an exponential distribution with mean =1/λ. As a result when there are n patients in the system then there are M-n patients in the arriving state and therefore the total average rate of arrivals in the system is λ(M-n). With M as the number of patients in the system and 1/λ as the average inter-arrival between successive arrivals and μ as the service rate probability that system will be idle is given by formula

$$P_0 = [\sum_{I=0}^{M} \{ M/(M-i)\ (\lambda/\mu)^i \}^{-1}$$

Expected length of queue

$$L_q = M - \lambda + \mu/\lambda\ (1-p_0)$$

Expected waiting time of patient in queue

$$W_{q =} L_q/\mu(1-p_0)$$

Poisson – Exponential Multiple Server Model – Infinite Population

This model applies when there are multiple service stations which are giving parallel identical service. It occurs in situations when there may be more than one doctor in a hospital whom the patient can visit. In cases where multiple servers are involved an important point to consider is whether there is a separate, independent queue for each server or the patients form a single queue from which they are picked up for service. Indeed if there are as many queues as the service stations, equal to, say K, the system can be thought of and analysed as one composed of K different single server queuing systems. We shall presume that the patients form a single queue. The model is based on the assumptions that; the arrival of patients follows Poisson probability law, the average arrival rate being λ, the service time has an exponential distribution and that there are K service stations, each of which provides identical service.

Using following expressions:

λ = average rate of arrivals.

μ = mean service rate of each server.

K = number of servers.

K_{μ} = mean combined service rate of all the servers.

Utilization rate of the entire system $\rho = \lambda/K\mu$.

Probability that the system shall be idle:

$$P_0 = [\sum_{i=0}^{k-1} (\lambda/\mu)^i/i + (\lambda/\mu)^k/K(1-\rho)]^{-1}$$

The expected number of patients in the waiting line:

$$L_q = (\lambda/\mu)^k \rho/K(1-\rho)^2 X (P_o)$$

Expected number of patients in the system :

$$L_s = L_q + \lambda/\mu$$

Expected waiting time in the queue :

$$W_q = L_q/\lambda$$

Expected time a patient spends in the System

$$W_s = W_q + 1/\mu$$

Gantt Chart

A Gantt chart is a commonly used graphical depiction of a project schedule. It's a type of bar chart showing the start and finish dates of a project's elements such as resources, planning and dependencies.

Henry Gantt (1861-1919), an American mechanical engineer, designed the Gantt chart.

- A Gantt chart is a visualization that helps in scheduling, managing, and monitoring specific tasks and resources in a project.

- It consists of a list of tasks and bars depicting each task's progress.
- It's the most widely used chart in project management.
- Gantt charts are used in heavy industries for projects like building dams, bridges, and highways, as well as software development and building out of other goods and services.

The Gantt chart is the most widely used chart in project management. These charts are useful in planning a project and defining the sequence of tasks that require completion. In most instances, the chart is displayed as a horizontal bar chart. Horizontal bars of different lengths represent the project timeline, which can include task sequences, duration, and the start and end dates for each task. The horizontal bar also shows how much of a task requires completion. A Gantt chart helps in scheduling, managing, and monitoring specific tasks and resources in a project. The chart shows the project timeline, which includes scheduled and completed work over a period. The Gantt chart aids project managers in communicating project status or plans and also helps ensure the project remains on track. The length of the bar is proportional to the time necessary for a task's completion. The project tasks are represented on the vertical axis. The chart identifies tasks that may be executed in parallel and those that can't be started or finished until others are complete. It can help detect potential bottlenecks and identify tasks that may have been excluded from the project timeline. The chart depicts things like: task slack time or additional time for completion of a task that shouldn't delay the project; noncritical activities that may be delayed; and critical activities that must be executed on time.

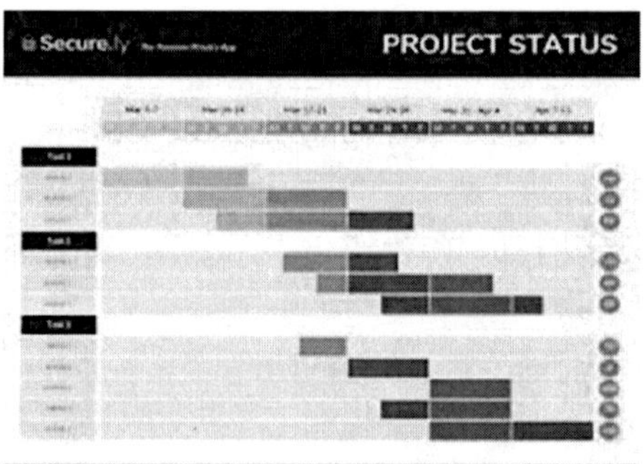

Fig. 9.3: Gantt Chart

Gantt charts can be used in managing projects of all sizes and types. These may include building infrastructure like dams, bridges, and highways.

Simulation Models

Simulation modeling is the process of creating and analyzing a digital prototype of a physical model to predict its performance in the real world. Simulation modeling is used to help designers and engineers understand whether, under what conditions, and in which ways a part could fail and what loads it can withstand. It analyses the approximate working conditions by applying the simulation software. Simulation modelling in healthcare have mainly focused on staff scheduling, resource allocation and patient waiting-time management. Simulation systems that have been designed and implemented in healthcare were attracting different operational problems such as management of patient flow inside emergency rooms, allocation of human resources around the hospital, patient admission, hospital bed utilization . It has also expanded to study the epidemiology, and consequently systems were developed to simulate populations with a specific chronic disease, or with a particular disease of a network that provides healthcare services, or during an epidemic crisis.

Systems Analysis

Systems analysis, more correctly referred to as information systems analysis, is the process by which an individual(s) studies a system such that an information system can be analyzed, modeled, and a logical alternative (independent of technology) can be chosen. The basic systems analysis project consists of two basic steps: (1) analysis (study of the system) and (2) modeling the system and choosing the logical alternative. The best way to fully describe systems analysis is to define the terminology used in the process. First, a system is a set of components that work together to achieve a particular goal or objective. Therefore, an information system is a set of components that work together to provide information for an organization. This information may be used to plan, make decisions, and/or manage an organization. The components of the information system are software, hardware, people, procedures, data/information, and communication networks. The key is that the system provides information and not data. Data are simply a list of facts, while information is a group of facts organized in such a way that the facts can be used in their present format to plan, make decisions, and and/or manage an organization. Systems analysis describes a specific set of steps (methodology) for analyzing, modeling, and choosing a logical alternative for an information system, which ultimately identifies the logical (human) requirements of an information system (software specifications, people's duties, logical procedures, data required, and information produced).

Linear Programming

Linear programming (LP, also called linear optimization) is a method to achieve the best outcome (such as maximum profit or lowest cost) in a mathematical model whose requirements are represented by linear relationships. Linear programming is a special case of mathematical programming (also known as mathematical optimization). For linear programming method to be implemented there has to be an objective, the activities to be included should be distinctly identifiable and measurable in quantitative terms, resources should be identifiable and measurable . They should be in limited supply. There should be a series of feasible alternative courses of action available to the decision maker.

Maximisation case : A laboratory is carrying out two investigations, A and B. Each unit of investigation "A" requires two units of reagents and four manpower hours for processing whereas each unit of investigation "B" requires three units of same reagent and three hours of manpower. Each week laboratory has availability of 60 units of reagents and 96 manhours. Hospital charges Rs 40 for investigation A and Rs 35 for investigation B. The objective of our Linear Programming Problem is maximisation of profit by carrying out investigations A and B. If x_1 and x_2 represent the number of investigations A and B carried out then the total profit Z is equal to $40x_1+35x_2$. Since the problem calls for a decision about the optimal values of x_1 and x_2 these are known as the decision variables. Another requirement of linear Programming is that the resources must be in limited supply which is known as constraint. As each unit of investigation A requires 2 units of reagents and each unit of investigation B requires 3 units of reagents; total consumption of reagents would be $2x_1+ 3x_2$ which cannot exceed total availability of 60 units every week. This constraint can be expressed as $2x_1+ 3x_2$

≤ 60. Similarly each unit of A requires 4 manhours and each unit of B requires 3 manhours. With the availability of 96 manhours per week the constraint is $4x_1 + 3x_2 \leq 96$. Quite obviously x_1 and x_2, being number of units produced cannot have negative values. Thus both of them can have values only greater than or equal to zero. This is non- negativity condition, expressed as $x_1 \geq 0$ and $x_2 \geq 0$.

Thus the problem is expressed as

$Z = 40x_1 + 35x_2$	Profit
$2x_1 + 3x_2 \leq 60$	Raw Material Constraint
$4x_1 + 3x_2 \leq 96$	Manpower Constraint.
$x1, x2 \geq 0$	Non-Negativity Restriction.

Minimisation case : Hospital Infection Control committee recommends 4800 litres of Hydrogen Peroxide and no less than 7200 litres of Peracetic Acid for surface disinfection of Hospital. There are two sources for obtaining these – mixtures A and B . Both of these are available in cans of 100 litres and they cost Rs 40 and Rs 24 respectively. Mixture A contains 20 litres of Hydrogen Peroxide and 80 litres of Peracetic acid while mixture B contains these in ratio of 50% each. Question is how many cans of each type should the hospital buy to achieve disinfection at minimum cost. If x_1 and x_2 are taken to represent number of cans of mixtures A and B respectively

$$Z = 40x_1 + 24x_2 \text{ ie cost.}$$

Hydrogen peroxide requirement can be expressed as $20x_1 + 50x_2 \geq 4800$. Peracetic acid requirement can be expressed as $80x_1 + 50x_2 \geq 7200$. Again decision variables representing number of cans of mixtures A and B would be non – negative. Thus $x_1 \geq 0$ and $x_2 \geq 0$.

Thus the problem is expressed as

$Z = 40x_1 + 24x_2$	Cost.
$20x_1 + 50x_2 \geq 4800$	Hydrogen Peroxide Constraint
$80x_1 + 50x_2 \geq 7200$	Peracetic acid Constraint.
$x_1, x_2 \geq 0$	Non-Negativity Restriction.

Linear programming model is based on the assumptions of Proportionality, additivity, continuity, certainty and finite choices. Proportionality means there are constant returns to scale, Additivity implies for example that total profit in the objective function is determined by the sum of the profit contributed by each of the products separately. Continuity is an assumption that the decision variables are continuous. Certainty is an assumption that, the objective function coefficients and constraint values are known with certainty. A linear programming model also assumes that a limited number of choices are available and that the decision variables do not assume negative values.

Linear programming problems can be solved by using Graphic Method or by applying algebraic method called the Simplex Method.

Maximisation Case : We consider above mentioned case, the decision variables are x_1 and x_2, the number of units of the investigations A and B respectively.

$Z = 40x_1+35x_2$	Profit
$2x_1+ 3x_2 \leq 60$	Raw Material Constraint
$4x_1+ 3x_2 \leq 96$	Manpower Constraint.
$x1,x2 \geq 0$	Non-Negativity Restriction.

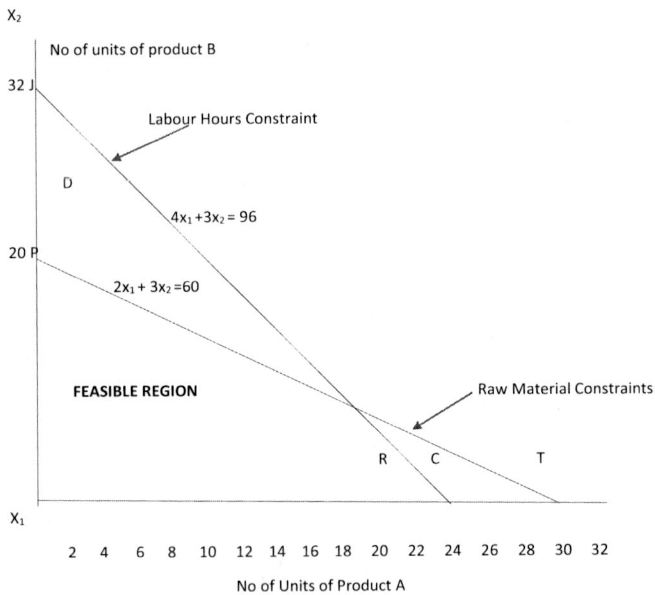

Fig: 9.4. Showing Graphic solution to Linear Programming Problem.

Minimisation Case:

Minimise $Z = 40x_1 + 24x_2$ Total Cost.

Subject to

$20x_1 + 50x_2 \geq 4800$ Phosphate Requirement.

$80x_1 + 50x_2 \geq 7200$ Nitrogen Requirement.

$x_1\ x_2 \geq 0$

Here the decision variables x_1 and x_2 represent, respectively the number of bags of mixture A and of mixture B, to be bought.

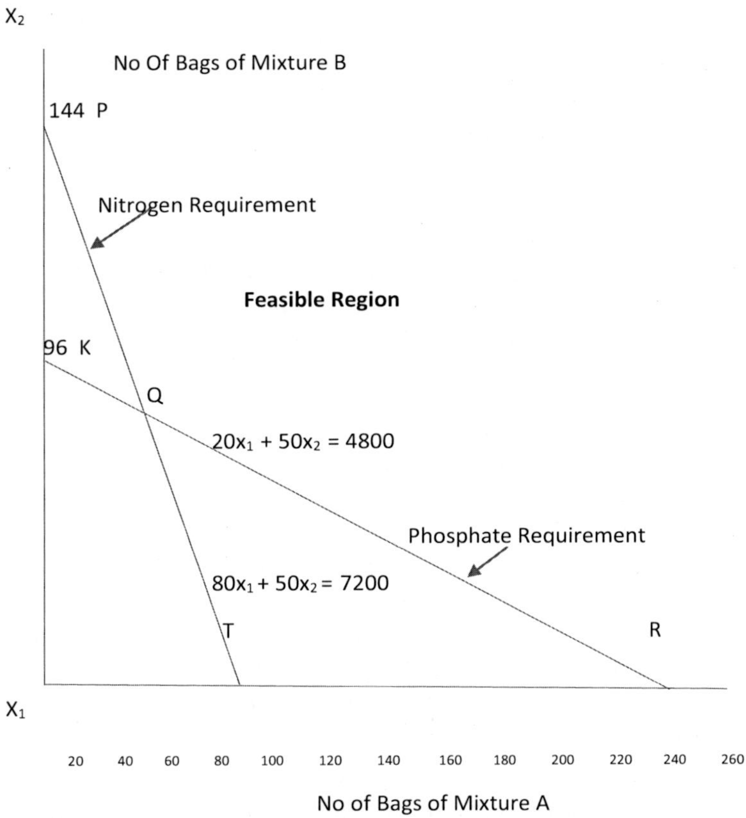

Fig. 9.5: Showing Graphic solution to Linear Programming Problem.

Inventory Control

Stock in hand is called Inventory. There has to be a balance between stock in hand and the reordering levels so that there are no stock outs and also that not much money is parked in stock. There are two inventory management systems a) Fixed Order Quantity system or re-order point system in which reorder level is determined. b) Periodic Review System where the inventories are replenished at fixed intervals of time. Here we will be discussing fixed order quantity system which is also called as the Q-system. There are various models of fixed order quantity system which are : The classical EOQ Model, EOQ with price breaks, Build Up Model/EOQ for Production Runs, Inventory model with planned Shortages. Here we will be discussing the *Classical EOQ Model.*

The Classic Economic Order Quantity model also known as Wilson Formulation is based on following basic assumptions: the demand for the item is certain, continuous and constant over time, the Lead Time ie time between placing an order and the delivery is known and fixed, per unit holding cost and the ordering cost are constant, purchase price of the item is constant and the inventory is replenished immediately as the stock level reaches equal to zero ie there are no stock overages or shortages. Suppose we begin with a stock of Q on the time 0. This will be consumed at the rate of d units per day. If the stock can be replenished instantaneously that is lead time is zero then a fresh order would be made and the inventory obtained at point T_1. Similarly when the stock is consumed an order would be made at point T_2. If the lead time is positive equal to L, we would place an order at a point when we have in stock an amount equal to the demand during the lead time so that we would have consumed it by the time fresh delivery is due to arrive. This is called the re-order level or the reorder point, R. The interval between two successive points when orders are placed or the time elapsed in consuming the entire lot of items is called inventory cycle.

For determining the optimum order quantity, we have to consider two types of costs ie ordering cost and the holding cost. Cost model would be

$$T(Q) = O(Q) + H(Q)$$

Where Q = the ordering quantity.

$T(Q)$ = total annual inventory cost.

$O(Q)$ = total annual ordering cost.

$H(Q)$ = total annual holding cost.

Total annual Ordering cost is given by the number of times an order is placed N multiplied by ordering cost per order A. Thus

$$O(Q) = N \text{ X } A$$

The value of N itself is dependant on the order quantity Q and the annual demand D. N is equal to D/Q.

$$O(Q) = D/Q \text{ X } A.$$

Total annual holding cost is obtained by multiplying the unit holding cost (measured as rupees per unit per annum) h by the average number of units held in the inventory. Average inventory held equals Q/2. The total cost of holding inventory per annum is given by formula:

$$H(Q) = Q/2 \text{ X } h$$

Total (Variable) Annual Inventory Cost is got by adding cost of both components.

Economic Order Quantity = $\sqrt{2AD/h}$

Reorder level of stock R is given by formula : Minimum Stock + Average consumption during normal delivery time.

The classic EOQ model is based on the assumption of constant and known demand for the item and the lead time. EOQ is in other words a deterministic model. What about the random variables ? When the demand is variable and so is the lead time there is a need to provide the safety or buffer stocks. Safety stock acts as a cushion against stockouts caused by random increase in demand or delay in receiving supplies. Safety stock is an important constituent of the re-order point. Re-order level would therefore be determined as the expected demand of the item during lead time plus the safety stock. Reorder level thus is given by formula :

$$R = L_d + SS$$

Where L_d is demand during lead time and SS is safety stock.

Selective approaches to inventory control: These are ABC, VED, HML, SDE, FSN .

ABC Analysis : In this the inventory items are classified on the basis of their usage in monetary terms. It is observed that usually a small number of items account for a large share of the total cost of the materials and a comparatively large number of items involves an insignificant share. In this list of the items is obtained along with their unit cost and annual consumption cost. The items are then arranged in descending order on the basis of their respective usage values. Then express the value for each item as a percentage of the aggregate usage value. Now cumulate the per cent of annual usage values. Obtain the percentage value of each of the items. For n items, each item shall represent 100/n percent. Thus if there are 20 items involved in classification then each item would represent 100/20 = 5 percent of the materials. Now cumulate these percentage values as well. Using the data on cumulated values of items and the cumulated percentage usage values, plot the curve by showing these respectively on X and Y axes.

Table 9.1: ABC Classification of items

Item	% value	Cum Value	% Number	Cum Value
11	23	23	8.3	8.3
2	20.2	43.2	8.3	16.6
5	16	59.2	8.4	25
1	9.8	69	8.3	33.3
12	7.1	76.1	8.3	41.6
6	5.6	81.7	8.4	50
3	4.2	85.9	8.3	58.3
4	3.7	89.6	8.3	66.3
7	3.4	93	8.4	75
10	3.3	96.3	8.3	83.3
8	3	99.3	8.3	91.6
9	0.7	100	8.4	100

Note: Items 11,2,& 5 are type A items, 1,12,6 are type B items. Rest are C type items. *(Adapted from Inventory Management : Quantitative Techniques in Management by N D Nohra)*

Determine appropriate divisions for A, B and C categories. The curve would rise steeply upto a point. This point is marked and the items upto that point constitute the A type items. The Curve would be Moderately slopped towards right. The point beyond which the slope is negligible is marked and the items covered beyond that point are classified as C type items because they cause only a negligible increase in cost. The other items are the B type items for which the curve depicts a gradual upward rise. After the items are classified, the inventory decisions are made on basis of this classification. "A" items would call for a strict control. "C" items can be kept in open storage and may be issued without much formalities. With regard to "B" items the policy would be fairly tight though not as tight as "A".

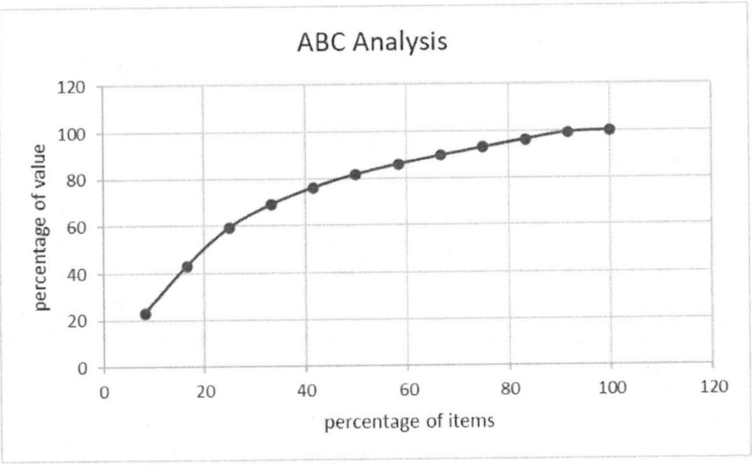

Fig 9.6: ABC Classification of items

It is seen that first 10% of items in descending order consume 70 % of money, next 20% of items consume 20% of money and next 70% of items consume 10% of money.

VED Analysis: VED analysis is classification of items on the basis of their criticality for running of hospital . Vital items (V) are those items without which functioning of hospital will come to a standstill eg Cotton, gauze, bandage, syringes, I/V fluids, defibrillator etc. Essential Items are those items absence of which will adversely affect functioning of hospital eg X-ray machine, Wheel Chair, Needle Destroyer, I/V antibiotics etc. Desirable items are required but do not stop functioning of hospital eg thermometer, Pneumatic tube system, PET CT, Creamer wire, I/V Immunoglobins etc.

HML Analysis: This is similar to ABC analysis except that here the items are classified on the basis of unit cost rather than their usage cost. The items are classified accordingly as their cost per unit as H-cost, M-cost or L-cost.

SDE Analysis: Here the items are classified on the basis of their availability. S stands for scarce items which are in short supply, D refers to Difficult items ie those that might be available in market but cannot be procured easily. E represents easily available from local market.

FSN Analysis: Based on the consumption of the items, the FSN analysis classifies items as Fast moving, Slow moving and Non moving.

Network Analysis

Network Analysis plays an important role in project management. Network analysis is a graphic depiction of "activities" and "events". By network analysis; planning, scheduling and control of a project becomes easy. Programme Evaluation and Review Technique (PERT) and Critical Path Method (CPM) are two well known network analysis techniques.

While both PERT and CPM have similarities in terms of concepts and methodology, a basic difference exists between the two techniques . PERT is useful for analyzing project scheduling problems in which the completion time of the different activities and therefore whole project is not certain. It therefore emphasizes uncertainties of the completion times of the activities. On the other hand CPM, is most appropriately used in projects in which the activity durations are known with certainty. Not only the amount of time needed to complete the various facets of the project but also the amounts of resources required for performing each of the activities are assumed to be known. Thus whereas variation in the project time is inherent in the projects where PERT is used, the time is systematically varied by using additional resources where CPM is used. Thus PERT is more probabilistic in nature and as such used more in developmental projects and research, the CPM is a deterministic technique and thus finds application in construction projects.

The first step in PERT/CPM project scheduling process is determination of all specific activities that comprise the project and their independence relationships. Once the activities comprising a project as also the interdependency relationships among them are clearly identified they can be portrayed graphically by a network or an arrow diagram. The network is constructed through a series of arrows and nodes thus expressing the sequential nature of the project. The circles at the beginning and at the end of the arrow represent the nodes or the events of beginning and completion respectively.

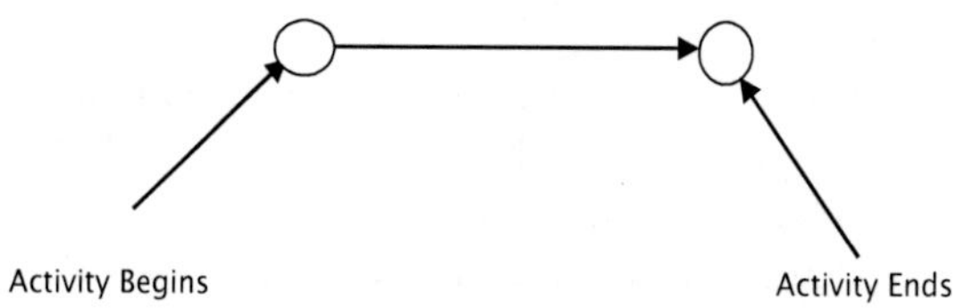

Fig 9.7: Activity And Event in Network Analysis

While formulating network certain rules are to be followed which are:

1. Each defined activity is represented by one and only one arrow in the network. No single activity can be represented more than once in the network.
2. Before an activity can be undertaken . all activities preceding it must be completed.
3. The arrows depicting various activities are indicative of the logical precedence only. The length of the arrow is not of any significance.
4. The arrow direction indicates the general progression in time. The arrow head represents the point in time at which the activity completion event takes place while tail represents the point in time activity starts. The events making the start of activities are called tail events while those marking the completion of activities are known as head events.
5. When number of activities terminate at one event, it indicates that no activity emanating from that event may start unless all activities terminating there have been completed,

6. Events are identified by numbers . Effort has to be made to have each event identified by a higher number than immediately preceding. There should be no duplication while numbering events.
7. Activities are identified by the numbers of their starting and the ending events eg 3-6, 6-7 etc.
8. An event which represents the joint completion of more than one activity is known as merge event while an event which portrays the initiation of more than one activity is called the burst event.
9. Parallel activities between two events without intervening events are prohibited. When two or more parallel activities in a project have the same head and tail events, dummy activities are needed in constructing the network.

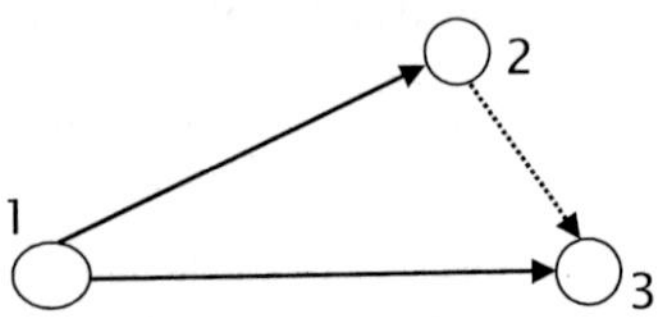

Fig 9.8: Showing Dummy activity

A dummy activity shown above which is used when two or more activities have same initial and terminal events is known as an identity dummy. Dummy activities are also used in establishing proper logical relationships when two chains of activities have a common event although they are in themselves wholly or partially independent of each other. These are known as logic dummies.

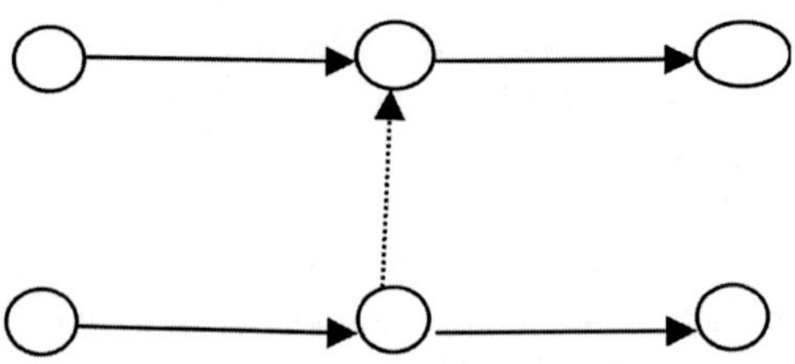

Fig 9.9: Showing Logic dummy

Looping is not permitted in a network. Thus if A precedes B, B precedes C then C cannot precede A.

Now the question is that how long the project would take to complete. This involves forward and backward pass through the network. The forward pass calculations yield the earliest start and the earliest finish times for each activity while the backward pass calculations render the least allowable start and the latest finish times for each activity. The ES time indicates the earliest that a given activity can be scheduled and EF indicates the time which the activity can be completed at the earliest. Thus each of the activities initiated from the starting node of the network are assumed to start at time 0 ie day1. The earliest finish time for each activity is obtained by adding the time duration of the activity to its earliest start time. The idea of backward pass is to compute the latest allowable times of starting and finishing, LS and LF, of each of the activities of a project. The computations in the backward pass are mirror image of forward pass calculations. The term latest allowable means that the projects terminal event is desired to occur on or before some arbitrarily scheduled time.

To know the duration of the project we have to find Critical Path. This is the path from initial node of the network to its terminal node. This is the longest path which determines the duration of project. The critical path is the bottleneck path in project network. Any delay on this path delays the whole project and needs taking corrective measures

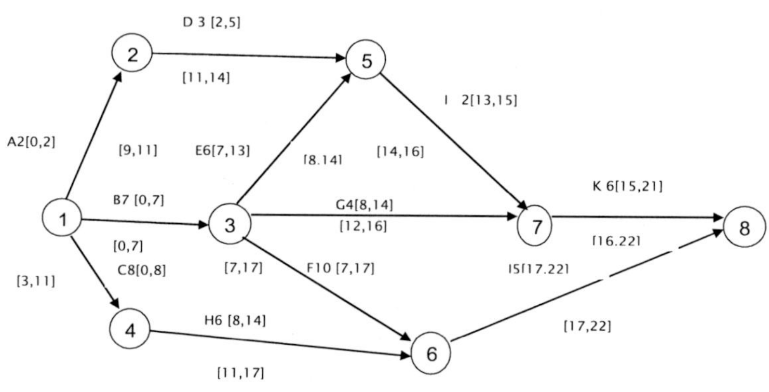

Fig 9.10: Showing activities and events for determination of ES, EF, LS and LF.

which may mean pushing more resources. There may be more than one critical paths in a given network. If for an activity, the ES time equals the LF time at the head of the arrow and if ES time equals the LF time at the tail of the arrow, the activity is possibly a critical activity lying on critical path. If this condition is met and difference between the ES time at the head of the arrow and the ES time at the tail of arrow is equal to the duration of activity, then the activity is critical and lies on the critical path. This then is sufficient evidence for criticality.

In the above figure value of 0 is assigned to initial event of the project . The earliest finish time for each activity is obtained by adding the time duration of the activity to its earliest start time. The activities A, B and C are first activities of the project and therefore ES time for each one of them is equal to zero. As activity A has a duration of 2 days its earliest finish time equals 0+2 ie 2 days. Similarly EF times for B and C are 7 and 8 respectively. For a given subsequent activity, the ES would be taken as the maximum of the EF's of activities preceding this activity. Thus the ES time for an activity leaving a particular node equals the largest value of the EF times for all activities entering the node. In the example shown above the ES for activity D, 2-5 would equal 2, the EF of preceding activity 1-2 because it is the only predecessor activity while as for activity 5-7, the ES time would be taken as 13, because of two activities terminating at event 5, being 2-5 whose EF time is 5 and 3-5 which has EF time of 13. The ES and EF times for various activities are written in brackets on the top of arrows, following description and time duration of activity. The earliest the event 8 may be therefore reached is 22. The activities 7-8 and 6-8 are the terminal activities with EF times of 21 and 22 respectively. This means that we assign a time of 22 to event 8 or in other words both the above activities would be assigned their LF time equal to 22. The LS time for an activity being equal to its LF time minus its duration for 7-8 the LS would be 22-6 ie 16, while for 6-8 it would be 22-5 ie 17.

The duration of some of the activities of a project can be cut down if additional resources ; men, material and equipment are employed on them. It is however significant to note that for technical reasons, the duration of an activity cannot be reduced indefinitely. The crash time represents the fully expedited or the minimum activity duration time that is possible and any attempts to further crash would only raise the activity direct costs without reducing the time.

Investment Analysis

To make correct investment decisions one must know how much investment is needed for a project and what will be the cash returns once project is operational, what is the availability of funds. In selecting a suitable criterion two principles are important to be kept in mind. One is that early benefits are better than late benefits and second is that other things being equal bigger benefits are better than smaller ones. There are four methods of investment analysis ie payback method, average rate of return, net present value and internal rate of return.

Payback period : The payback period of any project indicates the time period required to recover original cash investment. The investment where payback period is less is a better investment. Payback occurs when cumulative cash inflows from a project minus initial investment is equal. If C_0 is the initial investment and C_t is the cash flow in tth year then payback period would be the value of k such that

$$\sum_{T=1}^{k} C_t - C_0 = 0$$

Average rate of return Method : Here rate of return is calculated as the ratio of the average annual profits after taxes to the average investment in the project.

It is given by formula

$$\text{Average rate of Return} = \frac{\text{Average annual net earnings after taxes}}{\text{Initial Investment}} \times 100$$

OR

$$\frac{\text{Average annual net earnings after taxes}}{\text{Average investment over the life of the project}} \times 100$$

Payback period ignores the bigger the better principle and also bird in hand principle to a large extend. It over emphasizes liquidity and ignores dimensions of profitability. The average rate of return also has a limitation that it does take into account timing of cash flows . Net present value and internal rate of return takes into account timing of cash flows and are called discounted cash flow measures.

Net Present value method : The NPV of an investment proposal is determined by discounting the cash inflows back to the present at the required rate of return I and then subtracting initial investment .

$$NPV = \sum_{t=1}^{n} \frac{C_t}{(1 + i)} - C_0$$

Internal Rate of Return method : Internal rate of return is the rate at which an investment is repaid from the project. It is represented by that rate IRR so that

$$\sum_{T=0}^{n} C_i (1 + IRR)^{-1} = 0$$

Both NPV and IRR serve the same purpose however are not in complete correspondence with each other in that in some cases the two may provide different rankings. Thus a choice has to be made which method gives more accurate ranking of project.

Break Even Analysis : It is systematic analysis of costs and revenues and the resultant profit/loss to a hospital. This relationship is called cost – volume -profit relationship and the analysis is called break even analysis. This analysis is important to know the level of activity at which the hospital has just enough revenue to recover all costs. This level is a no profit no loss activity. One can also find out the level of activity at which target profit will be attained. The costs are classified as fixed and variable costs. Fixed costs are those costs for which the total amount remains constant within a specified range regardless of the variations in the activity levels. Salaries of employees, depreciation costs are examples of fixed costs. Variable costs are those costs for which the total amount varies in direct proportion to the changes in level of activity. Raw materials and labour cost of workers are examples of variable costs.

Another important parameter in CVP analysis is contribution margin which is defined as excess of selling price over the variable price. The selling price and the variable cost being constant per unit of output, the contribution margin per unit is also a constant amount.

Contribution margin = Total Sales – Total variable cost.

Also Contribution margin = Fixed Cost + Profit.

P/V ratio (profit / volume ratio) also called contribution margin ratio is an indicator of profitability of the product and is given by formula :

$$\text{P/V Ratio} = \frac{\text{Contribution margin per unit}}{\text{Selling Price}} \times 100.$$

Break Even Point = F/CM

Break even point when expressed in monetary terms is called Break Even Sales which is given by formula:

BE Sales = F/CM x S

Or

BES = F/P/v ratio.

Where F is Fixed cost per period.

V is Variable cost per unit

S is selling price per Unit.

CM is contribution margin.

There is a term called Margin of Safety which is the excess of actual sales over the break even sales. This is expressed as

Margin of safety = Actual sales – Break even sales.

Margin of safety can also be expressed as a percentage of the actual sales ie

$$\text{Margin of safety ratio} = \frac{\text{Actual Sales} - \text{Break Even sales}}{\text{Actual Sales}} \times 100.$$

The determination of break even point can also be depicted graphically. In this the level of activity ie number of units sold, sales volume in rupees is shown on X-axis and costs and revenues is shown on Y axis. Fixed cost is shown by means of a straight line parallel to the horizontal axis at a height given by amount of fixed cost. Variable cost is then added to it to get the total cost line. Then sales and revenue is plotted on the graph. This graph which is called break-even chart or cost volume profit graph gives us more information than the break even point and the margin of safety as shown in graph below.

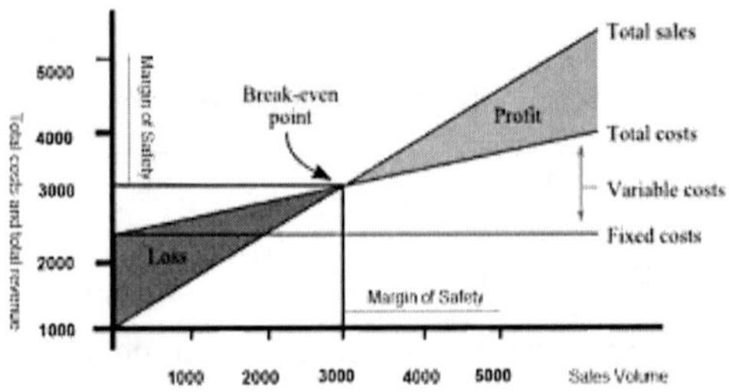

Cost accounting and costing of service

Cost accounting is the process of recognizing the cost of a product or service whereas cost accounting is a mechanism of analysing expenditure for a business. Costing is essentially the process of asserting the prices and costs of products. It is a system of determining internal financial functioning. Cost accounting on the other hand is a branch of accounting that determines the expenses incurred within a venture, through recording, analysing and predicting cost data and issues statements for the same. While costing is a process or technique cost accounting is branch of accounting. While costing is used for decision making cost accounting is a tool for management to determine future planning and budgets.

Cost accounting systems' main aim is to assist the management in their key tasks, like properly planning, evaluating, and controlling the organization's activities. Cost accounting helps in recording, summarizing, and analyzing different types of costs in an organization. These costs can be fixed costs. variable or semi-variable costs. These costs may be for a process, a product or a service. The main goal is to spend in a planned manner, control costs, and improve the organization's cost efficiency. The managers need to evaluate processes to reduce and eliminate unnecessary movement, spending, and wastage.

One important point to note here is that the accounting system and records leading to the preparation of various financial statements are mandatory and available for outsiders and the public. However, cost accounting is the system for support, review, and facilitation, for the use and view of internal organization. These reports are not public, nor an outsider has access to these systems and records, except for a few cost accounting records and reports, as per regulatory requirements. Cost accounting involves activities that record, summarize, and analyze data about costs spent at various stages and association with the organization's cost structure. Moreover, It focuses on capturing the quantitative side of data and related details that has links with cost incurrence. The cost accounting system's core objective is to work out the actual cost of production, evaluate its various components, and look for the areas to control it wherever possible. So that with the help of all these records, data analysis, and triggers, the wastages and time loss could be avoided, and production cost minimization can happen. Here, the costs can be about a product, service, department, or process. Cost accounting reports follow specific formats, as prescribed by the regulatory financial body of the respective country. It is so because these reports are for both internal uses and outsiders and regulatory bodies. Also, a statutory audit of these reports is mandatory. There are so many types of techniques and methods available in cost accounting to generate various reports. However, techniques marginal costing, break-even analysis, standard costing, etc. remain the preferred and popular ones for preparing various reports.

Costing or cost finding is determining the cost of a service eg cost of nursing in a general ward, cost of diet or cost of a particular procedure.

The purpose of costing is

- Rate setting.
- Determining profitability of a specific revenue centre.

Fixed Cost : Fixed costs are those costs which do not change when quantity of patient care changes.

Variable cost : which change with the quantity of patient care.

For example if patient days drop by 10% one would expect lower costs of meals and laundry implying that they are variable costs.

However in short term, the fall in patient days may have no effect on total wage costs since the hospital cannot dismiss workers without notice. Over a short term wages are fixed costs . Over a longer term adjustments may be possible making wages a variable cost in long term. Thus the longer the time period, the larger the portion of cost that may become variable.

Direct Cost : Direct costs are costs incurred in running a department or service or fulfilling the primary purpose of that department or service.

Indirect Cost : Indirect costs are the costs incurred by other departments or service in support of the primary function of direct patient care.

Capital cost : are costs incurred on acquisition of assets that have an economically useful life exceeding one year and that are not acquired primarily for resale. In reality assets are being worn down by the hospitals daily activities and their depreciation is an expense.

Operating costs : Operating costs are the actual costs incurred by a department to generate patient services and other functions of the department. These include salaries, supplies, maintenance etc.

Depreciation : Depreciation is notional loss suffered by fixed asset due to wear and tear and ageing. The amount charged can be kept aside so that money is available when the present asset is completely depreciated. To calculate depreciation one should know the purchase price, inflation and useful life of the equipment.

Straight line depreciation is usually used for assets like buildings, plant, furnishings etc. In straight line depreciation, asset is depreciated by a fixed amount annually for entire life span eg if original purchase price of a equipment is Rs 744000 and its useful life is 20 years, the annual depreciation for asset would be 744000/20 = Rs 37200. This approach would underestimate the true opportunity cost of the capital being used up since it ignores inflation in the purchase price. In accelerated depreciation higher rate is charged in the initial year and percentage amount of depreciation gradually decreases with passing years. Rates are decided by administrator.

To calculate charges for patient services one has to calculate total cost of revenue producing departments for which the direct cost of all non-revenue producing departments must be proportionately reallocated. These direct costs of supportive services will be indirect costs for revenue producing departments.

Two fundamental items of financial data needed by a hospital manager are allocated costs by cost centre (a programme or department within a hospital) and the unit cost of hospital services . A unit of hospital services may be as small as one meal or as broad as an entire inpatient stay. To perform these calculations precisely, the hospital needs an accurate and comprehensive financial accounting system.

- The steps for computing unit costs are
- Define the final product.
- Define cost centres.
- Identify the full cost for each input.
- Assign inputs to cost centres.
- Allocate all costs to final cost centres (compute total allocated costs).
- Compute unit cost for each final cost centre.
- Report results.

(1) Defining the final product of the cost analysis : It will depend on (a) Comparison of certain hospital departments ie compute unit costs for each department separately. (b) Comparison of multiple hospitals with similar case loads eg compute single unit cost for all inpatient care for each hospital.

One can analyse unit cost based on data for a single month, a quarter year or a year. Sometimes important data such as utility costs eg fuel, water electricity are available only on an annual basis. In such situations it may make sense to analyse data for a whole year rather than for each quarter. If hospital manager is trying to understand a rapid recent change in costs, then quarterly or monthly analysis may be appropriate.

(2) Defining cost centres: From an administrative stand point cost centres are distinguished according to the nature of their work – patient care, intermediate clinical care and overhead centres. The aim of unit cost analysis is to allocate hospital costs (direct and indirect) to centres whose costs are to be measured. Typically one would compute unit cost mainly for patient care centres, in some instances for a laboratory test or

on occasion one would like to know unit cost of an overhead service such as dietetics.

(3) Identifying the full cost for each input: An important part of computing unit costs is to make sure that you have cost data which are as complete as possible. These will include salaries, fringe benefits, donated items, drugs, maintenance, delayed payments, capital assets.

(4) Assigning inputs to cost centres: Some inputs can be assigned directly to certain cost centres. For instance if kitchen is a cost centre, then the line item food could be assigned to that cost centre. More often inputs are used by several cost centres and the analyst must seek to assign spending for an input across these centres. Various methods have been used to assign staff time to cost centres ranging from simple using administrative data to elaborate direct measurement. The direct measurement approach has the advantage of giving direct information about the sources of inefficiency where other approaches merely identify the cost centre to which expenditures should be assigned. The disadvantage of the direct measurement approach is the high cost of implementing.

(5) Allocating all costs to final cost centres: The next step is to allocate all indirect costs to the final cost centres. Where each departments use of an indirect cost centre is unknown one must devise some rule to allocate the indirect costs across departments.

Simple methods of allocating overhead costs.

Department	Method of allocation
Heating, Lighting, Cleaning.	Square meters taken up by programme divided by square meters taken up by whole hospital multiplied by department costs.
Laundry, linen	Number of requistions from the programme divided by number of requsitions from the whole hospital multiplied by departmental

Service deparments also provide service to one another and costs of one service department should also be allocated to the one to which they are transferable although it could be insignificant. Step-down method is used for assigning costs of service departments to one another and then reallocating the accumulated cost of each service department to revenue producing department.

Resource flows in a hypothetical hospital

Department providing service	Department receiving service		
	Administration	Cleaning	Pharmacy
Administration		X	X
Cleaning			X
Pharmacy			

Where X denotes the flow of resources from the department providing the service to the department receiving them.

(6) Compute unit cost for each final cost centre: At this point the total costs that were incurred at each of the final cost centres are known. What is the output of each centre in days, discharges, laboratory tests and so on ? Finding out requires utilization data to be incorporated into the analysis.

(7) Reporting results.

Estimating costs from relative values

Sech estimates could be for example one day of inpatient carecosts three times as much as one outpatient visit, or that one surgical admission costs 10% more than the average inpatient admission. These data are called external because they have to come from outside the hospital. Possible sources for these estimates could include other hospitals in the country for which step down costing studies have been carried out; judgement of clinical experts or hospital staff on relative amount of resources used for different services, studies from other countries etc. More useful information can be generated if estimates are used for similar hospitals.

Unit cost calculation from relative values for a hypothetical hospital

Ward	Reported items			Calculated items			
	Total cost	Inpatient Days	Relative value	Relative value Units	% of relative units	cost of each service	Cost/ inpatient day
Medical		500	.81	405	32.8	32847	66
Siurgical		300	1.26	378	30.7	30657	102
Obs & gynae		450	1.00	450	36.5	36496	81
All inpatient	100000	1250	1.00	1233	100	100000	80

Strengths of this approach is its simplicity and limitation is potential for inaccuracy.

Cost Benefit Analysis

A cost-benefit analysis is the process of comparing the projected or estimated costs and benefits (or opportunities) associated with a project decision to determine whether it makes sense from a business perspective. Generally speaking, cost-benefit analysis involves tallying up all costs of a project or decision and subtracting that amount from the total projected benefits of the project or decision.

If the projected benefits outweigh the costs, you could argue that the decision is a good one to make. If, on the other hand, the costs outweigh the benefits, then a company may want to rethink the decision or project. Cost-benefit analysis is a form of data-driven decision-making most often utilized in business, both at established companies and startups.

How To Conduct A Cost-Benefit Analysis

1. Establish a Framework for Your Analysis: For your analysis to be as accurate as possible, you must first establish the framework within which you're conducting it. What, exactly, this framework looks like will depend on the specifics of your organization. Identify the goals and objectives you're trying to address with the proposal. What do you need to accomplish to consider the endeavor a success? This can help you identify and understand your costs and benefits, and will be critical in interpreting the results of your analysis.
2. Identify Your Costs and Benefits: Your next step is to sit down and compile two separate lists: One of all of the projected costs, and the other of the expected benefits of the proposed project or action. When tallying costs, you'll likely to begin with direct costs, which include expenses directly related to the production or development of a product or service (or the implementation of a project or business decision). Labor costs, manufacturing costs, materials costs, and inventory costs are all examples of direct costs.

   But it's also important to go beyond. Other cost categories you must account for include:

- Indirect Costs: These are typically fixed expenses, such as utilities and rent, that contribute to the overhead of conducting business.
- Intangible Costs: These are any costs that are difficult to measure and quantify. Examples may include decreases in productivity levels while a new business process is rolled out, or reduced customer satisfaction after a change in customer service processes that leads to fewer repeat buys.
- Opportunity Costs: This refers to lost benefits, or opportunities, that arise when a business pursues one product or strategy over another.

Similarly, benefits can be:

- Direct: For example, increased revenue and sales generated from a new product
- Indirect: Such as increased customer interest in your business or brand
- Intangible: For example, improved employee morale
- Competitive: For example, being a first-mover within an industry or vertical.

3. Assign a Dollar Amount or Value to Each Cost and Benefit: Once you've compiled exhaustive lists of all costs and benefits, you must assign a dollar amount to each one. If you don't give all the costs and benefits a value, then it will be difficult to compare them accurately.
4. Tally the Total Value of Benefits and Costs and Compare: Once every cost and benefit has a dollar amount next to it, you can tally up each list and compare the two. If total benefits outnumber total costs, then there is a business case for you to proceed with the project or decision. If total costs outnumber total benefits, then you may want to reconsider the proposal. Beyond simply looking at how the total costs and benefits compare, you should also return to the framework established in step one. Does the analysis show you reaching the goals you've identified as markers for success, or does it show you falling short?

If the costs outweigh the benefits, ask yourself if there are alternatives to the proposal you haven't considered. Additionally, you may be able to identify cost reductions that will allow you to reach your goals more affordably while still being effective.

Advantages of Cost-Benefit Analysis

- It is data-driven: Cost-benefit analysis allows an individual or organization to evaluate a decision or potential project free of opinions or personal biases. As such, it offers an agnostic and evidence-based evaluation of your options, which can help your business become more data-driven and logical in how it operates.
- It makes decisions simpler: Business decisions are often complex by nature. By reducing a decision to costs versus benefits, the cost-benefit analysis can make them less complex.
- It can uncover hidden costs and benefits: Cost-benefit analysis forces you to sit down and outline every potential cost and benefit associated with a project, which can help you uncover less-than-obvious factors, such as indirect or intangible costs.

Limitations of Cost-Benefit Analysis

- It's difficult to predict all variables: While cost-benefit analysis can help you outline the projected costs and benefits associated with a business decision, it's challenging to predict all the factors that may impact the outcome. Changes in market demand, materials costs, and global business environment can occasionally be fickle and unpredictable, especially in the long term.
- It's only as good as the data used to complete it: If you're relying on incomplete or inaccurate data to finish your cost-benefit analysis, the results of the analysis will be similarly inaccurate or incomplete.
- It's better suited to short- and mid-length projects: For projects or business decisions that involve longer timeframes, cost-benefit analysis has greater potential of missing the mark, for several reasons. It typically becomes more difficult to make accurate predictions the further out you go. It's also

possible that long-term forecasts will not accurately account for variables such as inflation, which could impact the overall accuracy of the analysis.

- It removes the human element: While a desire to make a profit drives most companies, there are other, non-monetary reasons an organization might decide to pursue a project or decision. In these cases, it can be difficult to reconcile moral or "human" perspectives with the business case.

In the end, cost-benefit analysis should not be the only tool or strategy that you use in determining how to move your business into the future. It is but a single option at your disposal.

Cost-Effectiveness Analysis

Cost-effectiveness analysis helps identify neglected opportunities by highlighting interventions that are relatively inexpensive, yet have the potential to reduce the disease burden substantially. For example, each year more than a million young children die from dehydration when they become ill with diarrhea. Oral rehydration therapy (ORT) does not diminish the incidence of diarrhea, but dramatically reduces its severity and the associated mortality rate. The scientific evidence that ORT can save lives was an important step in identifying this as a neglected opportunity for improving health. Cost-effectiveness analysis helps identify ways to redirect resources to achieve more. It demonstrates not only the utility of allocating resources from ineffective to effective interventions, but also the utility of allocating resources from less to more cost-effective interventions.

Cost-effectiveness analysis is a method for assessing the gains in health relative to the costs of different health interventions. It is not the only criterion for deciding how to allocate resources, but it is an important one, because it directly relates the financial and scientific implications of different interventions. The basic calculation involves dividing the cost of an intervention in monetary units by the expected health gain measured in natural units such as number of lives saved. For example, using volunteer paramedics and trained lay people as first responders to accidents costs about US$128 per life saved in South Asia and US$283 in the Middle East and North Africa, whereas using a community-based ambulance costs about US$1,100 and US$3,500 per life saved in the same two regions, respectively. By measuring cost-effectiveness in terms of lives saved, all lives are treated equally regardless of whether the person is an infant who might live another 80 years or a middle-aged person who can expect only another 40 years of life.

"...using volunteer paramedics and trained lay people as first responders to accidents costs about US$128 per life saved in South Asia and US$283 in the Middle East and North Africa, whereas using a community-based ambulance costs about US$1,100 and US$3,500 per life saved...respectively."

Some studies calculate cost-effectiveness using years of life lost as the natural unit for measuring the effect of interventions. This measure treats each additional year of life gained from an intervention as equal. It sums the number of years of life that would be saved by an intervention. Hence an intervention that saved an infant's life (for example, preventing dehydration from diarrhea) would count more than one aimed at saving an older person's life (for instance, preventing recurrence of a stroke).

Cost-effectiveness analysis (CEA) is an alternative to cost-benefit analysis (CBA). The technique compares the relative costs to the outcomes (effects) of two or more courses of action.

CEA is most useful when analysts face constraints which prevent them from conducting cost-benefit analysis. The most common constraint is the inability of analysts to monetise benefits. CEA is commonly used in healthcare, for example, where it is difficult to put a value on outcomes, but where outcomes themselves can be counted and compared, e.g. 'the number of lives saved'.

Budgeting

A budget is a written projection of a particular department's financial performance, a specific project, a business unit, or an organization for the period under consideration. Usually, budgets for businesses or departments are created for an accounting period, i.e., for one year. However, the period could be less or more than a year. Complete flexibility is there as the method remains the same, and the business can make or plan a budget for the period they want.

Primarily, the activity of preparing a budget is called budgeting. In many organizations, it is a separate department taking care of only the preparation and implementation of budgets. Budgeting is the projection of income and expenditures that one expects an institution to earn and incur over a given period of time, usually one year. It requires continuous evaluation and control to ensure that the company's finances are managed correctly. The importance of the budget is that it becomes a reference document and thus helps in planning the activities of the organization or individual. A company can prioritize its expenditure according to the limited financial resources it has at its command. Thus this document also helps in the proper allocation of resources as per the priorities. For an entity or business organization one budget may not suffice and it may require a number of budgets. Some of them are the annual operating budget, performance budget, rolling budget, master budget, program budget, financial budget, operating budget, etc. Also, there are four key methods that companies use to create a budget. These are the traditional budgeting method, the incremental budgeting method, the zero-based budgeting method, and the activity-based budgeting method.

Budgeting is a roadmap of expenditure that the company can make according to the available resources or capital in hand. It is therefore a means of planning and controlling expenditure, as budgeting provides clear numbers or figures about the amount of money the company has. Furthermore, budgeting helps to estimate revenue over the budget period. It can plan its expenditure accordingly and ensure that it does not overspend or make commitments to spend money that the company does not have. Budgeting directs the company's scarce resources into activities that are in alignment with the organization's strategic objectives. It ensures that the company does not run out of money during the budget period for these important activities. Budgeting also helps ensure the proper availability of resources for emergencies as well as future projects. It prepares a company well in advance for crisis situations that can come from nowhere. Budgeting is an effective tool to help a company reduce wasteful spending. It shows which expenditures are not important at the present time and can be postponed. Matching available resources with revenue sources often drives management to draw up cost-cutting plans. It pushes them to find out ways to improve cash flow, to increase profits, which ultimately lead to higher returns on investment.

Making well-defined budgets is not enough. The progress of the business also needs continuous monitoring and comparison with the budgets. The comparison of budgeted performance with actual performance throws light and indicates:

- whether the company is performing as planned,
- whether the organization is on the right track and what are the chances of achieving the budgets.
- what areas are not seeing traction as desired and what is needed to get the traction.
- whether something somewhere is going wrong that requires immediate attention or there is a need for a different strategy to contain that wrong,
- it will help the organization to do midway course correction so that deviations are minimized. The expectation or performance could be re-allocated amongst the departments. It may help the organization to achieve the budgeted targets still, making internal adjustments.

Types of Budgeting Methods / Techniques

There are various types of budgets made and planned.

1. Annual Operating Budget
2. Cash Budget
3. Rolling Budgets
4. Performance Budget
5. Master Budget
6. Operating Budget
7. Program Budget
8. Financial Budget

Listed below are the most popular **types of business budgeting methods.**

1. Traditional
2. Incremental
3. Zero-Based

4. Activity-Based
5. Participative
6. Top-Down

Traditional Budget : Traditional budgeting is a method of preparing the budget in which last year's budget is taken as the base. The current year's budget is prepared by making changes to the previous year's budget by adjusting the expenses based on the inflation rate, consumer demand, market situation, etc. Past year's revenues and costs form an integral part of the current year's budget. Only those items in traditional budgets need to be justified, which are over and above the last year's budget. Incremental budget is the traditional budgeting method whereby the budget is prepared by taking the current period's budget or actual performance as a base with incremental amounts being added for the new budget period. Traditional budget is easier to prepare and implement. Only changes are required to be made in last year's budget as per the need of the current year's budget requirements. This saves lot of time and effort of managers. The Traditional budget method gives the opportunity to consolidate various projects together into a single larger one. This helps improve the performance of those underperforming projects before they were clubbed with a good performing working project. Traditional budgets are however rigid and inflexible and as these budgets are prepared at higher lower, others are less motivated and feel ignored and less important.

Zero Based Budget : As the name indicates, zero-based budgeting is a budgeting method with zero base consideration while preparing the budget. It justifies all the expenses each time we prepare a new budget. Zero-based budgeting does not aim to consider any base. Each expense has to be drilled down and analyzed well before the actual allocation of the budget. It is known as need analysis. The preparation of the budget is on the basis of the actual need of the expenses for the forecasted period. It does not consider the fact that the previous budget was lower or higher than the current budget. Zero-based budgeting targets identifying efficient and alternative methods for the organizations that opt for optimum utilization of resources. This will not only ensure efficiency and effectiveness but also wealth and profitability. Whereas traditional budgeting considers the fact that "how much" expense shall be incurred, zero-based budgeting is on the "why" approach. It goes to the root of the expense. Zero-based budgeting aims toward achieving the objectives of the organization. Zero-based budgeting completely ignores the past years' figures. Zero-based budgeting aims at cost-benefit analysis. It does not focus on studying the changes in expenses and preparing a variance analysis (such as why the expenses increased or reduced). However, it considers the necessity of the expense and the benefit which will derive from the expense. In Zero based budget previous mistakes are not repeated and obsolete processes are removed, however this type of budget requires lot of manpower and time to formulate. Sometimes, the required skills are also not present in the staff to prepare zero-based budgets.

Activity Based Budget: Activity based budgeting is a budgeting method in which budgets are prepared using Activity Based Costing after considering the overhead costs. In simple words, activity based budgeting is a management accounting tool that does not consider the past year's budget to arrive at the current year's budget. Instead, the activities that incur the cost are deeply analyzed and researched. Based on the outcome of the study, the resources are allocated to an activity. Activity based budgeting is carried out to bring efficiency to the activities of an organization. Budgets are prepared after justifying the cost drivers. Thus, activity-based budgeting is activity-oriented and not function-oriented. Activity-based budgeting method evaluates each and every cost driver. It takes into consideration all the steps involved in an activity. The irrelevant activities are eliminated, and only the necessary activities form a part of the business. Activity-based budgeting system eliminates all sorts of unnecessary activities, which helps the business to save its costs. The saved cost results in the production of goods and services at a lower cost than that of competitors. It also helps the organization gain a competitive edge in the market. Budgets under activity-based budgeting are prepared after deep research and analysis. This study removes all the unnecessary activities of the business. By doing so, the business eliminates all sorts of bottlenecks associated with an activity, and business functions are carried out more smoothly. An activity-based budgeting system helps improve the relationship between the organization and its customers. The main aim of this budgeting method is to eliminate unnecessary activities and serve the customers with the best quality at the best price. However activity-based budgeting requires a deep understanding of various functional areas of the business. If the manager preparing the budget is incapable of understanding and evaluating business areas, it would lead to inaccurate budget preparation. The process of budgeting in this method consumes a lot of resources for an organization. It needs to employ top officials for conducting numerous analyses. It is a very time-consuming task too. Implementation of activity-based budgeting requires trained employees. An employee, who is not trained enough, cannot handle the budgeting exercise effectively. Activity-based budgeting focuses on the short-term goals of the business. It does not take into account the long-term scenario of the business. Focusing more on short-term goals rather than long-term goals can prove to be very fatal for the organization.

Participative Budget : Participative budgeting is a method of budgeting wherein both the people who implement the budget and who will be affected by the budget are involved in the process of budget creation. In this type of budgeting, the top-level managers share the responsibility of making budgetary decisions with the bottom-level managers. As a result, it gives them a sense of a better stake in the firm.

Top – Down Budgeting :Top-down budgeting is a crucial method of preparing a budget for an organization or a company. Under this method, the senior management prepares a high-level budget on the basis of the company's objectives. The top management then allocates the amounts for the individual departments, who use those numbers to prepare their budget.

Managers of the individual departments may give suggestions to the top management before preparing the budget. But, it is up to the top management to include those suggestions in the budget or not.

Steps of Budgeting : The budgeting process is the process of putting a budget in place. This process involves planning and forecasting, implementing, monitoring and controlling, and finally evaluating the performance of the budget. The first step in preparing a budget is to identify the budget goals and how they will be achieved. Factors such as the business's socio-economic surroundings, sales trends, etc., have to be taken into consideration for setting the goals. Also, these goals have to be set according to the economic resources available to the hospital. A budget will be of no use without proper funding.

The next step in a budget is to scrutinize the costing for the business. Also, evaluating factors that can affect input costs during the budget period has to be done. Revision of the compensation plans of the employees takes place every year in most private hospitals. To make the budget realistic and achievable, proper provisions should be created for variations in these costs and compensation plans.

The next important step is to prepare different types of subsidiary budgets for the organization. Proper and realistic forecasts for the different types of budgets such as sales, production, cash, purchase, labor and overheads, selling, and general and administrative expenses have to be made. A realistic plan for the sources of revenue is the need for the budget period. Planning of expenditure should be accordingly as the company cannot spend more than what it earns. Thus, the revenue target decides and dictates the expected quantum of expenses to achieve these revenue targets. Smaller departments prepare their own budget in hospitals . In such cases, their collection and integration, along with the master budget, is a prerequisite. Most corporate hospitals have the policy of declaring bonuses for their employees at the end of the financial year as per their financial results. Many may declare mid-year bonuses in case of exceptional performances. Such expenses can become significant in the case of big hospitals. Hence, due provisions have to be made in the budget for such unplanned giveaways.

After finalizing all the above steps, a review of the assumptions as per the budget model should be done. Also, a thorough review of the entire budget is essential. If there is a need for any changes in the budget, it can be done now. The budget will then go to the top management for approval. They will check if it is proper. Makers will make any changes as per need. In case everything is fine with the budget, they will give the go-ahead for implementation. The implementation of the budget is not the last step in the budgetary process. The setting of proper budgetary controls comes next. This is necessary for the comparison of the actual performance with the provisions and estimates of the budget. Continuous reporting of variances has to be done. The management can take corrective actions accordingly.

A budget helps to control wasteful expenditure in an organization.

Because resources are scarce in any hospital, hence their allocation in the best possible manner is necessary for maximum returns. The budget guides the best possible utilization and allocation of resources. Moreover, it helps to maintain harmony between various departments of the business. Each department has a pre-determined share of the budget allocated to it. And it helps to take care of any daily arguments between them because of resource allocation.

Situational Analysis

A situation analysis is a detailed examination of a hospital's market presence based on internal and external factors. It examines a business's current and potential patients and how they respond to the hospitals services. Situation analysis also explores hospitals capabilities and how the current ecosystem impacts the hospital.

An analysis can forecast what results a hospital can expect—based on the decisions made—so it can adjust its strategies to meet its goals. A situational analysis can reveal many important details about a business such as:

- The opinions and experiences of patients and stakeholders.
- Hospitals strength and weakness(es).
- How a company is capitalizing on market trends.
- How it measures up to competitors.
- What's holding a business back from its desired goal(s).
- The current strategies in place to overcome the weakness(es).

A business should run a situational analysis periodically—the market is ever-evolving as customers' needs and preferences change. A regular situation analysis provides the information a company needs to create a course of action to achieve its goals. Situation analysis reveals how your hospital is performing and helps you adapt with course corrections if your plan isn't achieving the expected results.

There are several components in a situational analysis:

The hospital: An analysis of a hospital's vision, strategy, and goals—and if it's meeting them—is a good start. Examining how the hospital is performing by reviewing patient satisfaction, business, market share, and patient retention provides a useful snapshot that reveals if the hospital is fulfilling its goals. It also helps to evaluate competitors and market share.

Services: Analysing current services as well as future facilities is a vital component of a situation analysis. Market research is needed to determine how viable a new service will be.

A market analysis conducted with potential patients who offer feedback or opinions about the product, service, or pricing can shed light on who the target market is and how to improve hospitals offerings. Examine products and services separately to identify which products best meet your clients' needs and which ones need adjusting.

Opportunities: Unmet or underserved needs represent opportunities. Knowing how to capture that market share is essential to a hospitals success. But before a hospital can successfully target an untapped market, it should understand its strengths and weaknesses. A strength, weakness, opportunity, threat (SWOT) analysis is a useful tool to identify how capable hospital is of capitalizing on opportunities.

A SWOT analysis is relatively simple to create and usually presents a list of information.

- Create four categories: strengths, weaknesses, opportunities, and threats.
    - The strengths category should include internal systems and processes that are successful, competitive advantages, and assets such as technology, patents, expertise, and cash.
    - Weaknesses include internal factors that keep your business from being more competitive, such as gaps in hiring or lack of funding.
    - Opportunities are external factors that can aid your company such as regulation changes and special events.
    - Threats are external factors your company has no control over.
- List the appropriate information in each category box. Brainstorming is excellent for getting ideas and information onto paper. Save the ideas from the brainstorming sessions

in each applicable box, and create an overall insight for each category. Once complete, pull together all the insights and summarize them.

- When performing SWOT analysis, strengths and weaknesses are derived from an internal evaluation while opportunities and threats involve an external review.

Current business environment: A situational analysis should examine the external and internal environment that impacts hospitals performance. External factors include the economy, competitors, government policies, and regulations. Company culture, employees, business resources, and cash management are internal factors that affect a business.

A PESTLE analysis examines the external situation of a company by looking at political, economic, social, technological, legal, and environmental factors. Examining each category can provide insights into the overall business market. Look at each category of a PESTLE analysis more closely:

- Political factors: the impact of government policies or elections.
- Economic factors: how fiscal trends, current import and export trade ratios, and taxes affect a business.
- Social factors: the effect of customer lifestyles and demographics.
- Technological factors: how technology and innovation impact a business.
- Legal factors: the impact of safety regulations and employment laws.
- Environmental factors: how environmental regulations or climate change affect a company .

5C situation analysis example

A situational analysis should include the internal and external factors that affect a business, and a 5C approach may be the simplest. The 5Cs are company, customers, competitors, collaborators, and climate.

In a 5C analysis, the company segment includes the hospitals vision and goals, its market position, distribution, opportunities, and products. The customers provide key information on current customers, the target market, and the opportunities a company should pursue through a marketing plan.

The competitors' section reveals hospitals strengths and how it can improve, based on competitors' strengths and weaknesses. Collaborators are the partnerships that make products and distribution possible. Climate includes factors like government policy and the economy.

References

1. Kasapoglu OA. Selection of the Forecasting Model in Health Care. J Hosp Med Manage. 2016, 2:2.
2. Ghofran Ayed Almohamadi, Marwan M. Lingga . Forecasting technique to Predict Patient Volumes In Home Healthcare Service. PalArch's Journal of Archaeology of Egypt. 2011;18:15.
3. Steven Harper, Fariss Terry Mousa. Time and Motion Studies. Oxford Bibliographies. www.oxfordbibliographies.com. Assessed on 25th Sept 2021.
4. Mayank Agarwal. Work Study: Meaning, objectives and Types. yourlibrarayarticle.com . assessed on 26thSept 2021.
5. Groover, M. P. *Work Systems and Methods, measurement, and Management of Work*. Pearson Education International, 2007.
6. N D Vohra. Quantitative Techniques in Management. Tata Mc Graw – Hill Publishing Company Limited. New Delhi. Seventh Reprint 1996.
7. Sulaf Almagooshi. Simulation modelling in healthcare: Challenges and trends. ScienceDirect. Procedia Manufacturing 3 (2015) 301 – 307.
8. Tonya Barrier. Systems Analysis. Encyclopedia of information Systems. 2003, 345-349.
9. Tim Stobierski . Harvard Business School online. Online.hbs.edu/blog/post/cost-benefit Analysis. Accessed on 8th May 2022.
10. Cost Effectiveness analysis. Chapter 3 in Priorities in Health. National Library of Medicine. www.ncbi.nlm.nih.gov/NBK10253/
11. Budgeting. Finance Management. efinance management.com/budgeting. Accessed on 9th May 2022.
12. How to perform situational analysis for strategic planning. brex.com/blog/situation-analysis/. Accessed on 22nd May 2022

10

Marketing and Quality

Marketing is a core business strategy fundamental to success of any organization. Good marketing means creating, pricing, providing access to and promoting needed products/services to a target group such that goals of all parties are met. There are no specific strategies for marketing of hospitals. Systematic approach has evolved over years and sound client-provider relationship forms the basis for this. Events both indoor and outdoor play a significant role in marketing of health care institutions. Marketing has since long been considered a taboo for doctors and the only acceptable marketing allowed was "word of mouth" but doctors now use additional avenues to promote themselves. The purpose is to let people know who you are and what you do and where you do it. The dynamic evolution of life has inevitably affected the healthcare marketing as an indispensable element of health brands. In India, health care has become one of the largest sectors in terms of both employment and revenue. People in India have become health conscious off late and healthcare market size is ever increasing. There is a huge potential of Foreign Direct Investment in Indian healthcare market and government has been introducing many policies to get healthcare service to next level. India is emerging as a new destination for availing health care facilities considering its low cost and advance technologies used by foreign medical tourists. Through its specificity, health care marketing is an interdisciplinary field because it uses certain concepts, methods and techniques specific both to classical and social marketing . An effective marketing approach involves in-depth investigation of the patients needs, identifying latent needs and offering new health services that patients have not explicitly requested. The marketing of healthcare services differs primarily through the nature of demand for health services. Secondly, the beneficiary may not be the target of marketing campaign, the physician being the one who decides what, where, when, and how much will be provided for a particular service. The decision maker may be the doctor, the health plan representative, a family member. Health care services also differ where the product can be complex and may not be easily conceptualized. The marketer faces the challenge of attracting customers to healthcare organizations, however without attracting too many from the category of those who are likely to represent economic depts.

Over the past decade, healthcare has experienced many marketing trends that have fundamentally altered marketing. These trends are as follows:

- From mass marketing approach to a more specific approach.
- From image marketing to service marketing.
- From "one measure for all" to personalization.
- From emphasis on a health episode to a long lasting relationship.
- From ignoring the market to market intelligence.
- From low tech to high tech.

Marketers have used many traditional methods that include marketing research, product design, distribution, pricing, advertising, promotional sales and sales management. These methods need to be joined by new ones, related to new technology and new concepts, to attract customers through messages and offers. Although the consumer typically receives most of the information about a product through the commercial media, the most important information comes from recommendations or publicly available independent authorities. Two categories of sources provide complementary functions; commercial media- informs, while personal or expert sources legitimize or potentiate the evaluation process. In an attempt to meet a need, the patient expects certain benefits from chosen health service and provider. The patients attitudes, judgements and preferences about certain brands through a procedure of evaluating the attributes of these brands develop a set of beliefs about the attributes that correspond to each brand. Patient satisfaction must be the main objective of any healthcare organization and this requires a thorough knowledge of their needs and expectations. By acting in a dynamic and unpredictable environment, the health service provider must be able to detect the opportunities and threats of the market on which it operates. In this context, the formulation of a realistic, coherent and explicit strategy by the medical unit is of crucial importance in anticipating its future and reducing uncertainty in the activity. The marketing strategy is the way an organization acts under the influence of environmental factors.

A valuable proposal must have the following characteristics:

- It is true
- The value offered is superior to the one of the competition.
- It is important to the target public.
- It is memorable and easy to remember.
- It is difficult to copy by the competition.

The benefits of implementing marketing strategies are :

- To improve the competitive advantage.
- To increase the visibility.
- To create solid reputation among patients.
- To understand the needs and expectations of consumers.
- To understand the patients perceptions of quality and results of their experience within the medical organization, offering memorable experiences to patients and of course, building a strong, effective, dominant brand on the health services market.

Branding

The branding strategies have since long been used by large industries and now are being increasingly used by hospitals. Branding of hospitals is all about creating a recall in the minds of service consumers and influences through credible reinforcements of key brand elements specific to that particular service provider. Branding of any hospital includes information about the services of the hospital and the word of mouth. Good client- provider relationship is to be observed by all the staff members be it doctors, nurses, technicians or front office staff. To brand you need to position yourself differently from others. Branding is an emotional response to an organization or its services and to achieve this you need strength in five dimensions i.e. name, personality, profile/recognition, positioning and reputation/ track record.

For positioning a hospital or a doctor one may use traditional communication tools such as public relations, media, website/internet, brochures/posters, magazines etc. At present digital content helps build positive brand impressions. The use of new digital marketing strategies is essential to maximize the efficiency of marketing expenses and generate higher return rates. By applying innovative health marketing principles to reinvigorate the medical organization's marketing initiatives, organizations will be able to better position their service offers to consumers. For health care providers, the use of informative blogs or articles published on social media can be effective ways to stay relevant to patients. Moreover infusing targeted keywords into the content can add a marketing boost. It is important to understand today's medical consumer who prefers to look for medical information online, where he also has a wealth of healthcare services, healthcare providers, reviews from patients who contacted the provider, etc. With digital marketing, almost everything can be tracked and measured. The way consumers use the internet to find hospital units and healthcare providers evolves in favor of smart devices. With more than 80% of the patients who frequently use smartphones, to either identify or interact with physicians it is essential to reconfigure marketing initiatives to better fit the era we live in.

Quality Matters

Quality and accreditation standards are becoming mandatory for health care institutions; these will enhance the brand image of institutions. It is therefore important that all health care institutions start identifying their quality needs and implement processes which create transparency in consumer experience. Quality is the way to build an enduring brand name and image. The service the hospital provides must not only satisfy the patient but delight him and this is achieved when the service he receives far exceeds his expectations. It is very important to recruit and train personnel so that they can give quality services at that particular hospital. Packaging of health services is made such that, people enroll themselves thinking that they are getting more tests /services compared to other hospitals at an affordable price. Hospitals are trying to position themselves in a respectable manner in front of their patients and people who take their services.

Successful brand is achieved by:-

I. **Compassionate care:** when a service is being delivered to patient by a hospital not only has that care to be as per the standards set for the ailments but how the service is delivered is also important. The hospital staff have to be caring and courteous towards patients.

II. **Positioning:** if a hospital wants to have a brand name it has to position itself differently from others and this difference has to be maintained. It needs to be proved while treating every new patient.

III. **Quality facilities:** To provide quality service the hospital needs to have the latest state-of-art facilities in the from of hi-tech equipment and best qualified and competent specialists. There will be no takers of obsolete technology.

IV. **Marketing:** Marketing is all about creating a good image to outsiders and insiders. You need to have a strong human resource department to build image among staff and various programs like CMEs for referral doctors, awareness sessions for general public, health camps in community, organizing events on health days and interviews with specialists on media, etc.

V. **Internet:** Hospital needs to have a website of its own where it displays its presence and facilities it provides. Internet is the first place where patient would like to know about institutions providing care to specific diseases.

Marketing Mix

Marketing mix strategy is necessary in medical organizations including its performance measured by patient satisfaction, the coordination of planned marketing efforts to address organizational performance being essential. The marketing strategy is the way an organization acts under the influence of environmental factors. In practical terms, marketing strategies outline a path following the analysis of environmental factors. The marketing policy defines its general framework of action in order to carry out its entire activity, including several strategies. Marketing mix is adopted and is being used as a tool by corporate hospitals . 7P's of marketing mix are used for marketing mix strategy for sustainability .

Product: Product offered by healthcare organization are intangible in nature, hence product mix becomes very important for marketers. In order to provide effective and reliable services the hospital is fully equipped with various facilities rendering services in the form of intangibility ie Emergency Services, Ambulance Services, Diagnostic services, pharmacy services.

Price: Pricing is the most important factor and element in marketing mix in deciding for a particular treatment in a hospital. In case of general diseases it may not be required element since treatment is easily available but when it comes to treatment of complex diseases people opt for quality services at an affordable price eg what has made India hub of medical tourism because quality services are available at low cost as compared to west.

Place: Distribution of medicate services and location of hospital plays a crucial role in attracting patients. It is an element which is associated with channels of distribution of services which can be delivered ie adequate transport, communication facilities, prime location and pollution free environment.

People: Quality of health care personnel in the form of qualification, training and experience plays an important role in attracting clientele and also in maintaining the image of hospital in community.

Physical Evidence: Physical evidence plays an important role in healthcare services, as a core benefit patient seeks proper diagnosis and cure of problem. It is the evidence of environment in which the service is delivered with physical or tangible commodities, where hospital and patients interact. Physical evidence can be in the form of reviews by customers.

Process: Process generally forms the different tasks that are performed by the hospital, the process factor is mainly dependent on the size of the hospital and kind of service it is offering. Ie out patient and inpatient.

References

1. David stones. Marketing and branding your organization. Candle lighters Canada. Presentation given at ICCIPO Workshops, Vancouver, September. 2005.
2. Paras Kapoor. Hospital banding Bharathidasan institute of Management, Trichy.
3. The impact of marketing strategies in healthcare systems. Journal of Medicine and life. 2019: Vol 12(2); 93-96.
4. Nithin R V, Narendranath V, DevaKumar G. An empirical study on marketing mix strategies on health care services in a tertiary care hospital. IJMAS 2016 : 2(10); 19-24.

11

Evaluation

Evaluation in health programme is an integral part of a professional role. The idea is to compare the performance with the standard. The standards are benchmarks which are laid down by experts in the field. Ultimate aim is to provide a basis for development. It is important to add that health professionals, even policy makers and advisers in government service are usually not trained or otherwisc cquipped to perform formal evaluations. The demands of public are increasing, resources shrinking and under constant pressure of containment. The systems have to be responsive to the needs of the population.

Most programmes when properly evaluated turn to be ineffective or at best marginally accomplishing their set aims. There are several possible explanations for this. First, the objectives of the organizations evaluated may have been multiple and difficult to summarize in simple performance criteria. Second, the nature of the service technology preludes accurate measurement. Third, isolating effects of services from extraneous factors is exceedingly difficult. Fourth, effects of services on clients are not readily quantifiable·

In recent years there has been a movement in evaluation practice away from the employment of just a single technique to the utilization of a wide range of methods. Choice of method will depend on the purpose of the evaluation in question.

Table 11.1: Changes in evaluation perspectives

Evaluation Before	Evaluation now
Imposed from above	Regarded as an aid
Is a duty or task	Functions as a tool
Takes time away from "real work"	Perceived as important, worth time
Not integrated in the organization	The organization learns
Highlights only negative results	Shows how we get better
Is complex and requires experts	Is everyone's concern.
Is expensive	Should be part of regular work
Quantity over quality	Quantity and quality both important

Source: Adapted from Menckel, 1993

Evaluation Design

There is no single best design. The design which is the best and most suited to the purposes of evaluation is to be used.

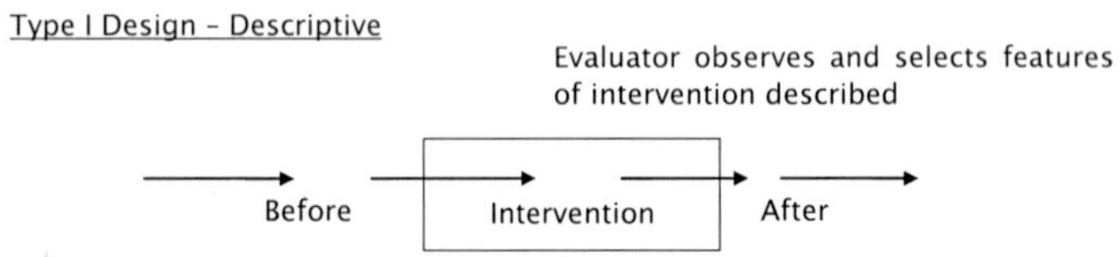

Fig. 11.1: Type I design-descriptive

It is used where managers do not have time and money for an outcome evaluation and only want a description of what is really happening. It may also help other people to set up a similar programme.

Strengths:

(a) Much resources not needed

(b) Can be done in collaboration with service providers and people receiving treatment.

Weaknesses:

(a) Can be ignored as unscientific, biased or trivial and does not give data on effects

(b) Usefulness of such evaluations depends on the skill, knowledge and credibility of the evaluator.

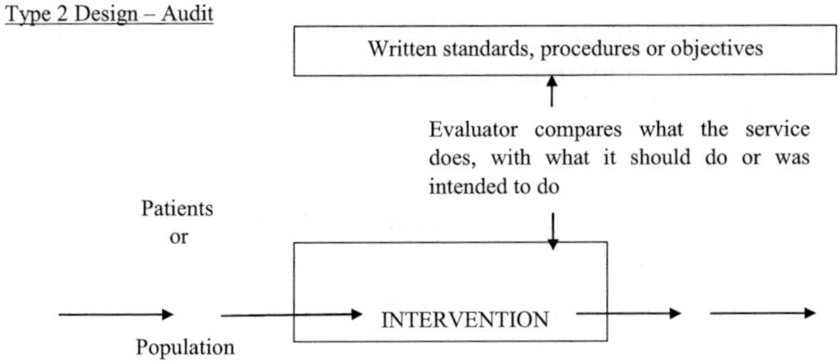

Fig. 11.2: Type 2 design-audit.

The purpose of the design is to compare what people are doing with what they are supposed to do. The audit may be carried out by external evaluators or by the organization itself using established standards.

Strengths:

(a) Few resources needed .

(b) Can be done quickly. Goal for self evaluation.

(c) It can promote understanding of why an intervention fails or succeeds.

(d) Can sometimes give generalized knowledge.

Weaknesses:

(a) Depends on having clearly specified set of standards, procedures or objectives.

(b) The design does not help to judge the value of the intervention, but just whether people follow orders.

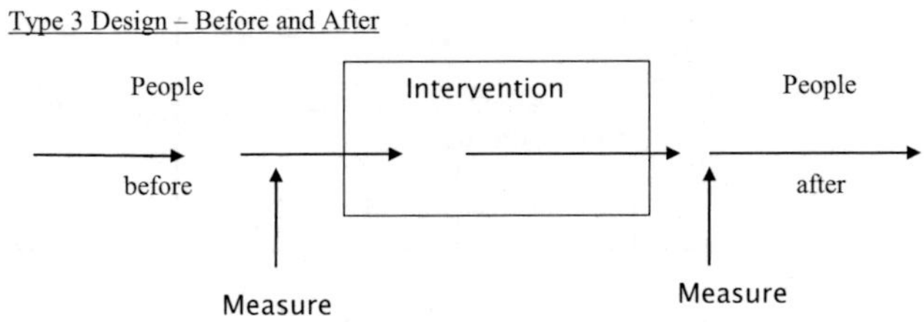

Fig. 11.3: Type 3 design-before and after.

The purpose of the design is to help to judge the value of an intervention by comparing the state of people "before" with their state "after" intervention.

Strengths:

(a) Evaluations can be small scale and relatively quick.

(b) The design can be arranged to use few resources if the evaluator selects a small number of subjects.

Weaknesses:

(a) Cannot give conclusive objective evidence of effects (confounding variables are not controlled for)

(b) The subjects selected may have shown these effects over time in any case.

Type 4 design – Comparative:

The design is like type 3 design but compares the outcomes of two groups undergoing evaluation.

Strengths:

(a) Can suggest which of the two interventions is more effective.

(b) The design is suitable where it is unethical or impractical to trial or intervene in only one group.

Weaknesses:

(a) Is expensive

(b) It is difficult to prove that effects are due to interventions alone rather than other factors.

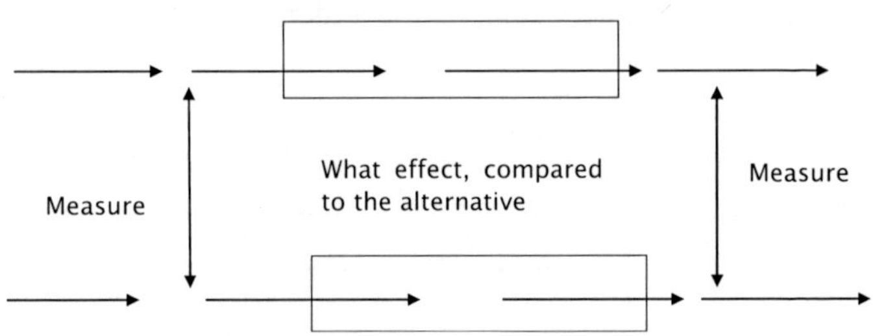

Fig. 11.4: Type 4 design-comparative.

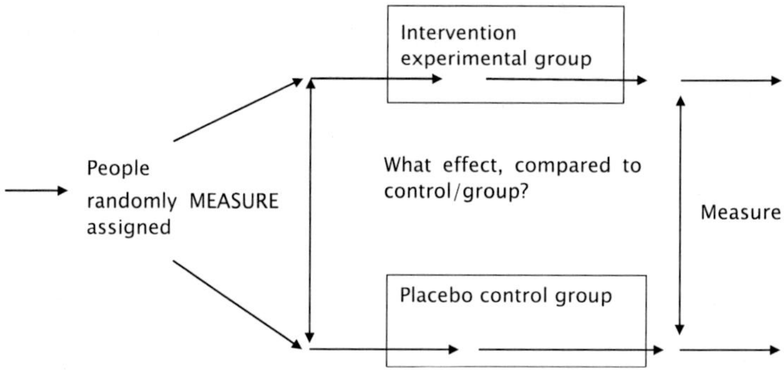

Fig. 11.5: Type 5 design – Randomized Control.

This is the classic evaluation design for evaluation of a treatment or service. In this we create two groups which are similar except that only one group (experimental group) receives the intervention and the other group (control group) receives placebo. The people are randomly assigned to a control and an intervention group. The design gives conclusive evidence of the effect of treatment.

Strengths:

(a) Gives more reliable and valid information about the effect of an intervention than other designs

(b) Results of a well- conducted evaluation of this design usually have high credibility among clinicians.

Weaknesses:

(a) Is expensive, takes time and needs evaluators with experience, skill and statistical expertise to produce credible results.

(b) Evaluations of this design do not take account of patient's subjective experiences and the group average may mask extreme effects on some individuals.

Reference

1. Rossi P.H. (1978). Some issues in the evaluation of human services delivery. In : The management of Human Services (R.C Sarri and Y. Hasen feld, eds). New York: Columbia University Press, pp. 235-61.

2. Weiss, C.H (1972) Evaluation research. Methods for Assessing Program effectiveness. (Methods of Social science series). Engle wood Cliffs, NJ: Prentice-Hall.

3. Menckel, E. (1993) Evaluating and promoting change in Occupational health Service – Models and applications Stockholm: The Swedish Work Environment fund.

4. Jhon Overetveit: Evaluating occupational health interventions In: Evaluation in occupational Health Practice. Butter worth – Heinemann, pp. 38-52.

12

Developing Practices for Safety

Hospitals confront a multitude of risk events in their daily working ranging from untoward incidents occurring to patients, employees and visitors to use of inadequate equipment or procedure to perform a task. It includes (1) property risks such as structural damage, vehicular accidents, technological obsolescence etc; (2) liability risks such as professional negligence, workers compensation etc and (3) employee benefit risks such as disability claims.

Risk management is a program designed to reduce the incidence of preventable accidents and injuries to minimize the financial loss to the institution should an injury or accident occur.

In short risk management is the protection of assets. Risk management personnel usually accomplish this goal by following four steps i.e. risk identification, risk analysis, risk control and risk financing.

Clinical risk management is an approach to improving the quality and safety of health care by identifying circumstances that put the patient at risk and acting to prevent or control those risks. In November 1999, the Institute of Medicine (I0M) released a report "To Err is Human: Building a safer Health System" The report estimated that 98,000 Americans die each year as a result of preventable errors. Deaths due to medical errors is higher than motor vehicle accidents (43,458), breast cancer (42,297) or AIDS (16,516). Approximately 7000 patients are estimated to die from medication errors alone which is 16% higher than deaths attributed to work related injuries. It was stated that medical errors are one of the leading cause of death.

Medical error is defined as "the failure of a planned action to be completed as intended or the use of a wrong plan to achieve an aim, including problems in practice, products, procedures and systems." Medical errors can be active or latent. Active error occurs at the level of the frontline operator and whose effects are felt almost immediately. Latent errors are errors that lie in the organization and its system. These errors lie dormant in the system for lengthy periods of time. They can be improper training of staff, organizational problem etc.

Risk Management

Mission of risk management is to select, coordinate, and efficiently apply interdisciplinary skills to harmful uncertainties which may diminish the future value of public, private or personal resources.

American Society of Health care Risk Management (ASHRM) identified eight minimal components of a risk management program:

1. There must be a designated, trained and experienced risk manger who must obtain at least eight hours of continuing risk management education annually.
2. Risk managers must have access to all necessary credentialing, management and medical data
3. Institutions must commit the necessary resources to risk management through a written policy statement that is adopted by the governing body, medical staff and administration.
4. Facilities must have a system in place for the identification, review and analysis of unanticipated adverse outcomes.
5. Organizations must have the means to centralize risk management data and to share and integrate data collection and analysis with other clinical and administrative departments.
6. Periodically, at least annually, risk managers must provide the organization's governing body a report that reviews and evaluates risk management program activity.
7. Risk managers must ensure that medical staff and new employee educational programs minimize patient's risks and address high risk clinical areas .

8. Risk managers must forward information on individual practitioners such as malpractice claim history, knowledge of adverse outcomes and incident reporting data to the committees that evaluate the competency of medical staff.

Effective risk management strategy should be judged not just in terms of whether it saves the provider money, although that certainity is a legitimate and important goal, but also should be judged against the fundamental objective of contributing to the quality of services. While as risk management is concerned with acceptable levels of care from legal stand point and is focused on legal, insurance and risk financing activities quality assurance is focused on improving care.

Medical Errors and patient safety

The components of the clinical risk management are

(a) Patient Complaints:- Number of areas which need improvement can be identified through patient complaints. These may be about poor or disrespectful communication or about administration of a wrong drug. A copy of the patients rights should be given to the patient at the time of admission and the same need to be displayed at prominent places throughout the hospital. Medicolegal action taken against the hospital should be analyzed to identify preventable factors and find ways to improve systems and processes.

(b) Incident reporting:- Reports are collected from staff across the hospital that identify incidents; these include incidents involving harm or potential harm to patients. Patient safety incidents are common in hospitals, and many of them lead to patient harm or extra cost. All national health services (NHS) hospitals in UK now have routine incident reporting systems as part of their risk management programme. However hospital reporting system may significantly under report-patient safety incidents. To test the performance of these systems researchers compared data from the routine reporting systems with a review of case notes for the same clients in a large NHS hospital in England. From a random sample of 1006 admissions, 324 patient safety incidents were identified. Case note review identified 303 (93%) incidents while the reporting system identified 54(17%) of these 324 incidents out of which 136(42%) resulted in patient harm. All of these were detected by the case note review but only 6 (5%) were detected by reporting systems. The 21 incidents missed by case note review were minor whereas the 130 incidents missed by the reporting system led to patient harm. The routine reporting system in this hospital missed most patient safety incidents that were identified by case note review and detected only 5% of those incidents that resulted in patient harm. This suggests that the routine reporting systems considerably under reports the scale and severity of patient safety incidents.

(c) Root cause Analysis: Root cause analysis (RCA) is a method of identification of organizational deficiencies that may not be immediately apparent and which may have contributed to the cause of the event. The idea is not to find the bad apple but to understand what is lacking in the system that allows such events to occur.

- General characters of RCA include
- Focus on system and process and not on individuals
- Review of relevant literature
- Examine extensively for underlying contributing cause.
- Identify procedure and system modifications.

(d) Sentinel events: These are incidents that were preventable and had a very harmful patient outcome. A root cause analysis technique is to analyse the event to identify processes and systems that can be improved to make sure it does not happen again and something is learned from the event. Sentinel events to be reported are:

- Procedures involving the wrong patient or body part.
- Suicide in an inpatient unit.
- Retained instruments or other material after surgery requiring re-operation or further surgical procedure.
- Intravascular gas embolism.
- Hemolytic blood transfusion reaction resulting from ABO incompatibility
- Medication error leading to the death of patient reasonably believed to be due to incorrect administration of drugs.

- Maternal death or serious morbidity associated with labour or delivery.
- Infant discharged to wrong family
- Other catastrophic events.

(e) Mortality review: - Weekly reviews of deaths would also ensure that safest and best care is provided to patients.

Limited adverse occurrence screening

Medical record is systematically screened using predetermined criteria to identify adverse patient occurrences such as nosocomial infection, transfer to a high dependency unit from a general care ward etc. Ways to improve care are identified.

Patient safety can flourish only when hospital leaders actively listen and when health care practitioners and staff discuss patient safety issues. To build such a safety culture following steps need to be adhered to:

- Create a vigorous method of detecting flaws, analyzing problems and achieving meaningful results.
- Encourage everyone in the hospital to report safety information in a thorough timely fashion.
- Make sure there is no possibility of reprisals against those who make reports.
- When a safety report is submitted make meaningful changes in procedures. Let staff members know the hospitals response to the report. Feedback will encourage others to contribute to the process.
- Provide learning aids for hospital workers, keeping them informed of safety issues and institution's progress.
- Conduct regular walks through your institution including all patient care areas, pharmacies, and laboratories. Speak to your front line staff about safety issues. Learn their concerns and their suggestions first hand. Make them part of safety team.
- Ask about adverse events or near-misses and the issues that may have led to these events and ways to mitigate them.
- Explore if a rapid response team can prevent avoidable deaths.

Patient safety plan.

The patient safety plan is designed to continuously improve patient, visitor and employee safety. The plan has to be implemented through the integration and coordination of patient safety activities of medical staff, clinical departments and support service departments. Each employee plays a crucial role in ensuring patient, visitor and employee safety.

Patient safety committee

Every hospital should have a patient safety committee to primarily look into those aspects of risk which have an impact upon patient care issues. The committee provides a multidisciplinary forum for analysis of risk to patient and the dissemination of information on identified risk for the purposes of improving patient care and reducing morbidity and mortality within hospital. It shall review reports on occurrences typically ranging from "no harm" frequently occurring "near misses" to "sentinel events" with serious adverse outcomes, claims and identified risks which are gathered in accordance with this plan. It shall provide recommendations concerning identified risks and where appropriate shall request and approve plans for corrective action and evaluate the implementation that of. The patient safety committee should have Medical Superintendent as chairman and can be designated as Patient Safety Officer. He shall be responsible for managing all aspects of safety plan. On behalf of the committee he shall provide reports at least annually to the Hospital Council or Hospital Executive Board on the occurrences of medical errors and action taken to improve patient safety both in response to actual occurrences and pro-actively. The patient safety officer shall advice the hospital council regarding clinical issues that may necessitate changes to policies and procedures, orientation, ongoing education or resource allocation. He shall have the responsibility for gathering information on risks to patients. The committee will be comprised of Medical Superintendent as chairman and following would be the members: Heads of Surgical, Medical, Anesthesiology division, Chairperson of Quality Control committee, Infection Control Officer, Deputy Medical Superintendent, Assistant Medical Superintendent, Chief of Nursing, Chief of Pharmacy, Chairperson of Risk Management Committee, Public Relations Officer and Chief of Hospital Security.

Each member of the medical staff should participate in the incident reporting system and in the implementation of corrective action activities in the event of identified risk. There has to be coordination between patient safety committee and quality improvement committee and should share the data regarding potential sources of patient inquiry. The quality improvement committee also needs to monitor incidents of identified risk on behalf of the committee. Patient, family and staff opinions need to be considered by the committee to ensure performance improvement.

Patient safety scenario

Patient safety in American hospitals in a study released by Health Grades in 2004 had not improved significantly since 1999 when it was given top priority in US hospitals. Agency for health care Research and Quality (AHRQ) has developed a set of patient safety indicators (PSI) specifically designed for screening hospital data for incidents of concern related to quality. A study in US showed that the 18 patient safety indicators evaluated contributed to $9.3 billion excess charges and 32,591 deaths in the United States annually. In 2002, AHRQ in collaboration with the University of California- Stanford Evidence-based practice center identified 20 indicators that could be readily identified in hospital discharge data and were deemed potentially preventable patient safety indicators. This tool set of 20 evidence - based PSI's was created and released to the Public in 2003 to be used by various health care stake holders to asses and improve patient safety in US hospital.

List of Patient safety Indicators used in the health grades study

- Accidental puncture or laceration.
- Complications of anesthesia.
- Deaths in low mortality Diagnostic Related Groupings (DRG_S)
- Decubitus ulcer.
- Failure to rescue.
- Foreign body left during procedure.
- Iatrogenic pneumothorax.
- Selected infections due to medical care.
- Post operative hemorrhage or hematoma

- Post operative hip fracture.
- Post operative physiologic and metabolic derangement.
- Post operative pulmonary embolism or deep vein thrombosis.
- Post operative respiratory failure.
- Post operative wound dehiscence.
- Transfusion reaction.

List of AHRQ patient Safety Indicators not used in the Health Grades study

- Birth trauma – injury to neonate.
- Obstetric trauma – caesarian? delivery.
- Obstetric trauma – vaginal delivery with instrument.
- Obstetric trauma – vaginal delivery without instrument.

In order to evaluate overall hospital performance and to identify the best performing hospitals across the U.S. AHRQ'S Patient safety Indicator version 2.1, Revision 3a February 2005 software application was used to evaluate hospitals on 16 PSI'S. It was observed that patient safety incidents were increasing; 82% of the mortalities were potentially preventable. The most commonly occurring Patient safety incidents were failure to rescue, decubitus ulcer and post- operative sepsis.

Lancaster General Hospital uses Bar codes and Motion Tablet PCs to improve patient safety. Doctors, nurses, patients and drugs are assigned unique bar codes. During medication administration a nurse scans his bar coded identification badge to log onto the system and then scans the patient's bar code and medication package to verify through the Motion Tablet PCs that the right patient is receiving the right dose of the right medication at the right time. The medpoint software is interfaced with the hospital's pharmacy information system. Each doctor's written prescription stays with the patient chart and a copy is scanned via a pyxis connect scanner to the pharmacy and entered into information system. The Motion Tablet PCs running the MedPoint software prompts nurses electronically at the point of care to compare and verify the pharmacy transcription with the written physician order. The Joint Commission on Accreditation of Health care organizations has (JCAHO) identified the following seven national patient safety goals as being mandatory requirement for participation in the joint Commission's accreditation program.

1. Improve the accuracy of patient identification.
2. Improve the effectiveness of communication among caregivers.
3. Improve the safety of using high - alert medications.
4. Eliminate wrong site, wrong patient, wrong procedure.
5. Improve the safety of using infusion pumps.
6. Improve the effectiveness of clinical alarm system.
7. Reduce the risk of healthcare- acquired infections.

During the Clinton presidency in US, the Secretary of the Department of Health and Human Services was directed to establish a "Quality inter-agency coordination task force" with responsibility where ever feasible to collaborate on goals, models and time tables consistent with the commission's six " National Aims for Improvement" These are:

- reduce the underlying causes of illness, injury and disability.
- reducing health care errors.
- ensuring the appropriate use of health care services.
- expanding research on the effectiveness of treatments.
- addressing over/under supply of health care resources.
- increasing patient participation in their own care.

National quality forum (NQF) has identified 26 safe practices that are utilized universally in applicable health care settings to reduce the risk of harm to patients. NQF is a private, non-profit public-benefit corporation created in 1999 in response to a need to develop and implement a national strategy for health care quality measurement and reporting. NQF is a voluntary consensus standard setting organization. Established as a unique public-private partnership, the NQF has participation from nearly 170 organizations. NQF report identifies 26 safe practices in five specific categories.

- Promoting a culture of safety.
- Matching health care needs with service delivery capabilities.
- Facilitating information transfer and clear communication.

- Adopting safe practices in specific clinical settings or for specific processes of care and
- Increasing safe medication use.

WHO Patient Safety Solutions

1. Look-Alike, Sound-Alike Medication Names .
2. Patient Identification.
3. Communication During Patient Hand-Overs.
4. Performance of Correct Procedure at correct body site .
5. Control of Concentrated Electrolyte Solutions.
6. Assuring Medication Accuracy at Transitions in Care.
7. Avoiding Catheter and Tubing Mis-Connections.
8. Single Use of Injection Devices.
9. Improved Hand Hygiene to Prevent Health Care Associated Infection.

Measures which can improve patient safety:

1. Improve accuracy of patient identification. At least two patient identifications such as name and medical record number should be used when providing care, treatment or service to a patient. The idea is first to identify the right patient and then to give right service to that patient.
2. Improve the effectiveness of communication among care givers.
3. Ensure that message is conveyed and understood in its original form whenever communicating any patient related information. In-effective communication is the most frequently cited reason of sentinel events. Effective communication which is timely, accurate, complete, unambiguous and understood by the recipient reduces errors and results in improved patient safety. The receiver of information must be made to read back or test back.
4. Take action to improve the timeliness of reporting critical test results and values. The organization should define the acceptable length of time between the ordering of critical tests and reporting the test results and values.

5. Trailing zero e.g. (X.o mg) should not be used in medication orders or mediation related documentation.
6. In hospitals there are number of instances of patient hand offs such as nursing and physician shift changes, anesthesiologist report to recovery room nurse, patient shift from emergency to in patient units. There should be up to date information exchange regarding the patient care, treatment and services, condition and any recent or anticipated changes. There has to be interactive communication between the giver and receiver of patient information
7. Prevent interchange of look-alike and sound-alike drugs. Properly label medications and medication containers.
8. Take all measures to reduce the incidence of nosocomial infections.
9. Treat all unexpected deaths as sentinel events.
10. A complete list of medications should be provided to patients at the time of discharge and also transferred to another facility in case of referral.
11. Organization should ensure to reduce the risk of patient harm resulting from falls. Staff should receive education and training to reduce patient falls.
12. Encourage patient's active involvement in their own care as a patient safety strategy. Communication with patients and their attendants (family) about all aspects of care, treatment and services is an important characteristic of a culture of safety. When patients know what to expect they are more aware of possible errors and can be an important source of information about potential adverse events and hazardous conditions.
13. In psychiatric patients and those with behavioral abnormalities the risk of patient going for suicide needs to be addressed.
14. Wrong site, wrong procedure and wrong person surgery must be prevented. It can be achieved by active involvement and effective communication between members of the patient care team. All relevant documents should be available at the time of the procedure and should be consistent with the patient details as well as procedure to be done. Missing information should be deliberated upon thoroughly before starting the procedure.

Verification of correct patient, correct procedure and correct site should be done at the time of admission into hospital, anytime responsibility of care is transferred to another unit, in the anesthesia room and at the time of surgery. The intended site must be marked such that the mark is visible at the time of assessment.

15. Verification, site marking and thorough assessment must be done even in procedures which are done outside the operating room i.e. bed side procedures.

Swiss cheese model of Health care

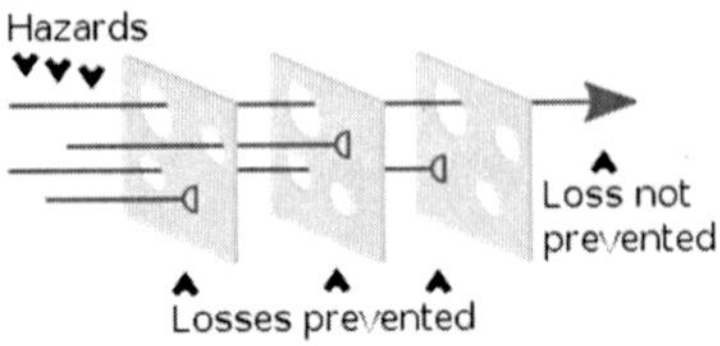

The Swiss cheese model of accident causation illustrates that, although many layers of defense lie between hazards and accidents, there are flaws in each layer that, if aligned, can allow the accident to occur. The **Swiss cheese model** of accident causation is a model used in risk analysis and risk management, including aviation safety, engineering, healthcare, emergency service organizations. It likens human systems to multiple slices of Swiss cheese, stacked side by side, in which the risk of a threat becoming a reality is mitigated by the differing layers and types of defenses which are "layered" behind each other. Therefore, in theory, lapses and weaknesses in one defense do not allow a risk to materialize, since other defenses also exist, to prevent a single point of failure. The model was originally formally propounded by James T. Reason of the University of Manchester, and has since gained widespread acceptance. It is sometimes called the "cumulative act effect". In the Swiss cheese model, an organisation's defenses against failure are modeled as a series of imperfect barriers, represented as slices of cheese, specifically Swiss cheese with holes known as "eyes", such as Emmental cheese. The holes in the slices represent weaknesses in individual parts of the system and are continually varying in size and position across the slices. The system produces failures when a hole in each slice momentarily aligns, permitting (in Reason's words) "a trajectory of accident opportunity", so that a hazard passes through holes in all of the slices, leading to a failure. The model includes active and Passive failures. Active failures encompass the unsafe acts that can be directly linked to an accident. Example of active failure is giving injectible through wrong route. Latent failures include contributory factors that may lie dormant for days, weeks, or months until they contribute to the accident eg lack of proper equipment, shortage of staff, underqualified staff, standard operative procedures not in place . Latent failure could be the similar packaging of two drugs that are then stored close to each other in a pharmacy. This failure would be a contributory factor in the administration of the wrong drug to a patient. Such research led to the realization that medical error can be the result of "system flaws, not character flaws", and that greed, ignorance, malice or laziness are not the only causes of error.

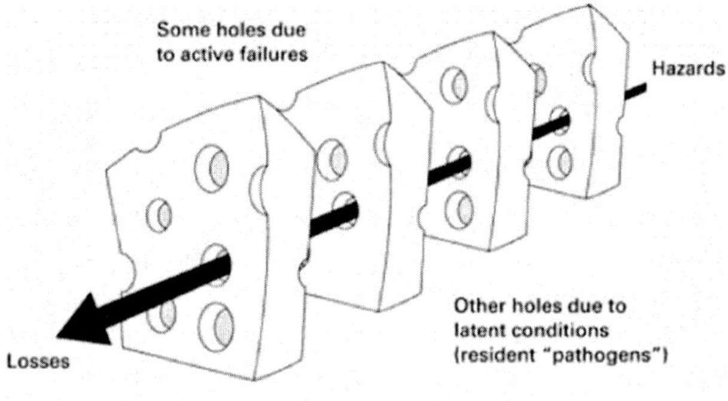

Successive layers of defences, barriers and safeguards

Patient Handoffs

A hand-off is a transfer and acceptance of patient care responsibility achieved through effective communication. It is a real time process of passing patient specific information from one caregiver to another or from one team of caregivers to another for the purpose of ensuring the continuity and safety of the patient's care. There are a number of terms used to describe the handoff process, such as handover, sign-out, signover, cross-coverage, and shift report.

Health care professionals typically take great pride and exert painstaking effort to meet patient needs and provide the best possible care. Unfortunately, too often, this diligence and attentiveness falters when the patient is handed off, or transitioned, to another health care provider for continuing care, treatment or services. A common problem regarding hand-offs, or hand-overs, centers on communication: expectations can be out of balance between the sender of the information and the receiver. This misalignment is where the problem often occurs in hand-off communication. Potential for patient harm ; from the minor to the severe is introduced when the receiver gets information that is inaccurate, incomplete, not timely, misinterpreted, or otherwise not what is needed. The Institute of Medicine (IOM) reported that "it is in inadequate handoffs that safety often fails first". When hand-off communication fails, many factors are involved, such as health care provider training and expectations, language barriers, cultural or ethnic considerations, and inadequate, incomplete or nonexistent documentation, to name just a few. A handoff is largely dependent on the interpersonal communication skills of the caregiver as well as the knowledge and experience level of the caregiver. There is reported variability in quality, lack of structure in how handoffs usually occur, and variances in shift handoffs. Concern has been raised that the transition of care between providers during handoffs will continue to be problematic as research indicates that "only 8 percent of medical schools teach how to hand off patients". The hazard that "fumbled handoffs" pose to patient safety and the delivery of quality health care cannot be ignored. Ineffective handoffs can lead to a host of patient safety problems; research and development of strategies to reduce these problems are required. Physicians and nurses communicate differently. Nurses are focused on the "big picture" with "broad and narrative" descriptions of the situation, whereas physicians are focused on bullets of critical information. A technique that seeks to bridge the gap between the different communication styles of nurses and physician is the situation, background, assessment, recommendation (SBAR) briefing model that is being used successfully to enhance handoff communication.

Handoffs occur across the entire health care continuum in all types of settings. There are different types of handoffs from one health care provider to another, such as in the transfer of a patient from one location to another within the hospital or the transition of information and responsibility during the handoff between shifts on the same unit. Interdisciplinary handoffs occur between nurses and physicians, and nurses and diagnostic personnel, while intradisciplinary handoffs occur between physicians or between nurses. Interfacility handoffs occur between hospitals and among multiple organizations, including home health agencies, hospices, and extended-care facilities.

Handoffs may involve use of specialized technology (e.g., audio recorders, pagers, hand-held devices, and computerized records), fax, written documents, and oral communication. Each type and location of handoff presents similar as well as unique challenges.

Various types of Hand-offs therefore are

- Shift-to-shift handoff
- Nursing unit-to-nursing unit handoff
- Nursing unit to diagnostic area.
- Special settings (operating room, emergency department).
- Discharge and interfacility transfer handoff
- Physician-to-physician handoffs

Handoffs are an extremely complex phenomenon to study as they occur in a variety of settings; stages along the continuum of care; and among various personnel with different skill sets, priorities, and educational levels. Contributors to handoff problems included failed communication, omissions, distractions, lack of or illegible documentation, lack of utilization of transfer forms, incomplete medical records, lack of medication reconciliation, and lack of easy accessibility to information. A variety of environmental issues emerged including designs that served to increase, rather than decrease, the number of handoffs. Interfacility handoffs posed a number of challenges, including cultural differences and lack of integrated systems, thereby increasing the likelihood of transmission difficulties between organizations. Organizational and system failures or lack of systems to support the handoff process emerged as contributors to adverse events. A lack of knowledge was found regarding effective handoff processes, and education on effective handoff strategies was also lacking. Handoff processes need to include consideration of the person involved in the handoff and their level of education, expertise, and comprehension (e.g., the novice nurse's informational needs may be different from the expert nurse). Novices also differ from expert nurses in their use of information.

There must be an organizational commitment to the development and implementation of systems that support effective handoffs as well as a just culture. This includes cultures of safety and learning. A safety culture supports identifications of problems and errors to be addressed to prevent the recurrence. A culture of learning promotes learning from the experiences of the past to prevent a recurrence of tragic fumbled handoffs. Environments and processes need to be designed to promote desired outcomes and enhance patient safety.

Actions suggested by The Joint Commission

Each health care setting has its own issues and challenges related to hand-offs. The Joint Commission emphasizes the importance of health care organizations using a process that identifies causes for hand-off communication failures and barriers to improvement in each setting, and then identifies, implements, and validates solutions that improve performance. The Joint Commission's Targeted Solutions Tool® (TST®) for Hand-off Communications to which Joint Commission-accredited organizations already have access can assist in managing this quality improvement process.

1. *Demonstrate leadership's commitment to successful hand-offs and other aspects of a safety culture.*

   Focus on improving the organization's systemic approach to hand-offs, rather than singling out individual errors. Provide support, time and budget to hand-off quality improvement initiatives. Developing an institutional respect for hand-offs requires action from all disciplines, and all disciplines need to incorporate changes into practice and culture. Make successful hand-offs an organizational priority and expectation.

2. *Standardize critical content to be communicated by the sender during a hand off* – both verbally (preferably face to face) and in written form. Make sure to cover everything needed to safely care for the patient in a timely fashion. Standardize tools and methods (forms, templates, checklists, protocols,

mnemonics, etc.) to communicate to receivers. Avoid making hand-offs using solely electronic or paper communications. If face-to-face communication is not possible, communicate in real time via telephone or video conference. Provide ample time and opportunities to ask questions. Communicate and receive hand-off content in a timely way to ensure delivery of appropriate care and services.

Ensure that, at a minimum, the critical content to communicate to the receiver includes:

- Sender contact information
- Illness assessment including severity
- Patient summary, including events leading up to illness or admission, hospital course, ongoing assessment, and plan of care.
- To-do action list
- Contingency plans
- Allergy list
- Code status
- Medication list
- Dated laboratory tests
- Dated vital signs

3. *Conduct face-to-face hand-off communication and sign-outs* between senders and receivers in locations free from interruptions, and include multidisciplinary team members and the patient and family, as appropriate.
4. *Standardize training on how to conduct a successful hand-off – from both the standpoint of the sender and receiver.*
5. Use electronic health record (EHR) capabilities and other technologies such as apps, patient portals and telehealth to enhance hand-offs between senders and receivers.
6. Monitor the success of interventions to improve hand-off communication, and use the lessons to drive improvement.
7. Sustain and spread best practices in handoffs, and make high-quality hand-offs a cultural priority.

Safe Surgery

Worldwide, 45% of medical errors occur in the operating theatre and nearly half of these are preventable. Faced with evidence of avoidable harm, attitudes and practices need to change to promote safer healthcare. Five Steps to Safer Surgery is a surgical safety checklist. It involves briefing, sign-in, timeout, sign-out and debriefing. Specific checklists have since been issued by the NPSA for maternity, ophthalmology, neurosurgery and interventional radiology procedures.

Table 12.1: Five Steps to Safer Surgery

Step	Timing of intervention	What to discuss	Comments/Challenges
1. Briefing	Before list or each patient (if different staff for each patient, eg emergency list)	Introduction of team/ individual roles List order Concerns relating to staff/equipment/surgery/ anaesthesia	Local arrangements will determine when the first patient on list is sent for. May also include aspects from steps 2 and 3. Could be an opportunity to discuss anticipated breaks during the list (eg lunch) May be difficult to get the team together.
2. Sign-in	Before induction of anaesthesia	Confirm patient/procedure/ consent form, Allergies, Airway issues, Anticipated blood loss, Machine/ medication check	Aspects of step 3 may be done here. Surgical site marking should be checked bŷ the surgeon at this point
3.Timeout (stop moment)	Before the start of surgery	Team member introduction. Verbal confirmation of patient information. Surgical/ anaesthetic/nursing issues, Surgical site infection bundle, Thromboprophylaxis, Imaging available.	In practice most of this information is discussed before, so this is used as a final check. Surgeons may use this opportunity to check that antibiotic prophylaxis has been administered
4. Sign out	Before staff leave theatre	Confirmation of recording of procedure: Instruments, swabs and sharps correct, Specimens correctly labelled, Equipment issues addressed, Post operative management discussed and handed over.	Should include all team members (including surgeons and anaesthetists)
5. Debriefing	At the end of the list	Evaluate list, Learn from incidents,Remedy problems, eg equipment failure can be used to discuss five-step process	Can be difficult to gather people together to do this. Evaluation of the list includes a discussion of what went well.

Adapted from : Ann R Coll Surg Engl 2011; 93: 501–503.

References

1. Smith, D.G and Wheeler, J.R.C (1992) Strategies and structures for hospital risk management programs. Health Care Management review 17(3): 9-17.
2. Youngberg B.J (1994) The Risk Manager's Desk Reference. Gaithersburg, Md: Aspen, PP. 13-26; Harpster, L.M and Veach, M.S eds (1990) Risk Management Handbook for Health Care Facilities. Chicago. American Hospital Publishing, pp. 28-30.
3. Medical errors and Patient safety. Position paper. ASCLS August 2001.
4. Quality Interagency coordination Task Force, Doing what counts for patient safety; Federal Actions to Reduce Medical errors and their Impact (Washington Qulc Task Force 2000)
5. Jonathan A. Handler, 'Defining, Identifying and Measuring error in Emergency Medicine" Academic Emergency Medicine 2000; volume 7, Number 11, 1183-1188.
6. Hagg, S.R (1990) Elements of a risk management Program. In Risk Management Handbook for health care Facilities, edited by L.M Harpster and M.S Veach. Chicago; American Hospital publishing, pp. 23-33.
7. Kapp M.B (1990) Health care risk Management. The challenge of measuring costs and benefits. Quality Review Bulletin. 16(5): 166-169.
8. Ovlikoff J.E and Landou G.B (1981). Why risk management and quality assurance would be integrated. Hospitals 55(11): 54-55.
9. Patient Safety indicators, version 2.1, Revision 1. March 2004. Agency for Health care Research and Quality, Rockville, MD.
10. Zhan C, Miller MR. Excess length of stay, charges and Mortality Attributable to Medical Injuries during Hospitalization. JAMA. 2003: 290(14): 1868-74.
11. w.w.w.Jcaho.com/accredited+organizations/patient+safety/npsg/04_ npsg.htm.
12. The white House, office of the press Secretary, Establishment of the Quality interagency coordination Task Force, March 13, 1998.
13. Emma Dickinson. Hospital Miss Most patient safety Incidents. Medical News today Dec 2006.
14. Florence Kavaler, Allen D. Spiegel. Progressive steps in the Risk Management process in Risk management in Health care Institutions Second edition, Jones and Bartlett publishers (1) 3-26-2000.
15. Patient safety in American Hospitals Health Grades Quality study July 2004.
16. National Patient safety Goals. Hospital version 2007.
17. Patient Safety Solutions Preamble-May 2007. WHO Collaborating Centre for Patient Safety Solutions. World Health Organization 2007.
18. Sentinel Event Alert, © The Joint Commission Published by the Department of Corporate Communications. Issue 58 Page 2. www.jointcommission.org.

19. Reason 1990.
20. Douglas A. Wiegmann & Scott A. Shappell (2003). A human error approach to aviation accident analysis: the human factors analysis and classification system. Ashgate Publishing. pp. 48–49. ISBN 0754618730.
21. Patricia Hinton-Walker; Gaya Carlton; Lela Holden & Patricia W. Stone (2006-06-30). "The intersection of patient safety and nursing research". In Joyce J. Fitzpatrick & Patricia Hinton-Walker (eds.). Annual Review of Nursing Research Volume 24: Focus on Patient Safety. Springer Publishing. pp. 8–9. ISBN 0826141366.
22. Tim Amos & Peter Snowden (2005). "Risk management". In Adrian J. B. James; Tim Kendall & Adrian Worrall (eds.). Clinical Governance in Mental Health and Learning Disability Services: A Practical Guide. Gaskell. p. 176. ISBN 1904671128.
23. Thomas V Perneger. BMC Health Serv Res 2005; 5:71; 2005 Nov 9. doi: 10.1186/1472-6963-5-71.
24. Stranks, J. (2007). Human Factors and Behavioural Safety. Butterworth-Heinemann. pp. 130–31. ISBN 9780750681551.
25. Mary Ann Friesen; Susan V. White; Jacqueline F. Byers. Handoffs: Implications for Nurses. In Patient Safety and Quality: An Evidence-Based Handbook for Nurses. Chapter 34.
26. Rachel Vickers. Five steps to safer surgery . Jyoti Shah, Jo Fitz-Henry Series Editors. peri-operative care series : Ann R Coll Surg Engl 2011; 93: 501–503.
27. Safe Surgery Saves Lives. Implementation Manual WHO Surgical Safety Checklist 2009. Patient Safety . WHO.

13

Health Care Financing

Health care expenditures have risen from 3% of world GDP in 1948 to 7.9% in 1997. Providing access to all citizens has long been a cornerstone of modern health financing systems in many countries. To ensure that individuals have access to health services, three interrelated functions of health system financing are crucial: revenue collection, pooling of resources and purchasing of interventions.

Revenue collection: is the process by which the health system receives money from house holds and organizations or companies, as well as from donors. Health systems have various ways of collecting revenue such as general taxation, mandated social health insurance contributions (usually salary related and almost never risk related), voluntary private health insurance contributions (usually risk related), out of pocket payments and donations. Most high income countries rely on either general taxation or mandated social health insurance. In contrast low income countries depend far more on out of pocket financing.

Pooling: is the accumulation and management of revenues in such a way as to ensure that the risk of having to pay for health care is borne by all members of the pool and not by each contributor individually. Pooling is traditionally known as insurance function. Its main purpose is to share the financial risk associated with health interventions for which the need is uncertain. In this way it differs from collecting, which may allow individuals to continue bearing their own risks from their own pockets or savings. When people pay entirely out-of-pocket, no pooling occurs. Pooling reduces uncertainty both for citizens and providers. By increasing and stabilizing demand and the flow of funds, pooling can increase the likelihood that patient will be able to afford services and that a higher volume of services will justify new provider investments.

Purchasing : Is the process by which pooled funds are paid to providers in order to deliver a specified or unspecified set of health interventions. Purchasing can be performed passively or strategically. Passive purchasing implies following a predetermined budget or simply paying bills when presented. Strategic purchasing involves a continuous search for the best ways to maximize health system performance by deciding which intervention should be purchased, now and from whom. This means actively choosing interventions in order to achieve the best performance both for individuals and the population as a whole by means of selective contracting and incentive schemes.

Private financing particularly in developing countries is largely synonymous with out–of-pocket spending or with contributions to small, voluntary and often highly fragmented pools. In contrast public or mandatory private financing (from general taxation or from contribution to social security) is always associated with prepayment and large pools. The level of prepayment is mainly determined by the predominant revenue collection mechanism in the systems. General taxation allows for maximum separation between contributions and utilization, while out-of-pocket payment represents no separation. The reason why later is used so generally in developing countries is that separation of contributions from utilization requires the agencies responsible for collection to have very strong institutional and organizational capacity, the attributes which are lacking in many developing countries. Thus although the highest possible level of prepayment is desirable, it is usually very difficult to attain in low income settings where institutions are weak. General taxation as the main source of health financing demands an excellent tax or contribution collecting capacity. This is usually associated with a largely formal economy where as in developing countries the informal sector is often predominant. While it is true that benefits may come as a result of the use of funds, under taxation these benefits are not directly linked to the taxes. Only full scale economic analysis using heroic assumptions can link the benefits resulting from the spending of taxes to the costs of taxes themselves. Taxation can be direct or indirect. Direct taxes are those that are directly levied on income. They cannot therefore, be shifted i.e. the burden cannot be made to fall on some one other than the taxpayer. Indirect taxes on goods and services can be shifted to some degree. Two types of taxes are commonly used to finance health care: payroll tax and sales tax. A pay roll tax is a tax that is levied on wages. Sales tax is a tax on a product or service. Most states use sales tax as a major source of revenue.

All other prepayment mechanisms including social security contributions and voluntary insurance premiums are easier to collect, as the benefit of participating is linked to actual contributions. In most cases, participation in social insurance schemes is restricted to formal sector workers who contribute through salary deductions at the work place. This makes it easier for social security organizations to identify them, collect contributions and possibly exclude them from benefits if no contribution is made. Similarly identification and collection is easier for voluntary health insurance and community pooling arrangements. Nevertheless such prepayment still requires large organizational and institutional capacity compared to out-of-pocket financing. Health insurance can be incrementally adopted in the social and economic environment of low and middle income countries. First small voluntary health insurance schemes can serve as learning models. Then principle of compulsion is followed to incrementally expand coverage to other groups and regions till universal coverage is achieved. Mandated benefit package should be adopted incrementally in accordance with changing needs, values and economic circumstances in order to ensure sustainability of social health insurance. Insurance can be obtained through the workplace either by being paid directly by the employees (through pay roll deductions) or by the employers. There is no controversy over incidence of premiums paid by employees or by individuals, the purchasers bear the cost of their insurance purchases. The cost of insurance benefit packages are viewed by employers as an expense much like the wages. If benefits are increased then the employer will reduce wages. Thus the economic burden of all health insurance benefits will fall on the employee either directly (out-of-pocket) or indirectly (through lower wage). Because of desirability of separating contribution from utilization out-of-pocket payment should not be used unless no other alternative is available. Although prepayment and pooling are a significant improvement over purely out-of- pocket financing they do not take questions of income into account. As a result of large pools society takes advantage of economics of scale, the law of large numbers and cross-subsidies from low-risk to high-risk individuals. Pooling by itself allows for equalization of contributions among members of the pool regardless of their financial risk associated with service utilization. Societies interested in equity are not indifferent to who is subsidized by whom. In addition to ensuring cross subsidies from low to high-risk, health financing should also ensure subsidy for greater equity. Existence of multiple pools allows members of pools to have different risk and income profiles. Without some compensatory mechanisms such arrangements would offer incentives for pooling organizations to select low risks and to exclude the poor and the sick. Brazil has introduced compensatory mechanisms in the allocation of revenues from the central to state governments to reduce such differences.

Reimbursement

There are various types of reimbursements: fee-for-service, per case, per capita, and salary reimbursement.

Fee-for-Service Reimbursement: In this a physician is paid a specific sum for each individual service he provides to the patient. The services are broken down into units such as a complete physical exam; a follow up visit, a tonsillectomy and so on. Each category of service is assigned a relative value in accordance with some criterion. Another method of fee setting is referred to as the UCR (usual, customary and reasonable). Usual refers to the usual or typical fee charged by the billing physician, customary refers to fees charged by all physicians in the community and reasonable refers to allowances for particular circumstances. The customary fee is derived from the frequency distribution of the fees charged by all physicians in the community for the procedure. The insurer then decides which percentile to use to set an allowable maximum fee. Indeed fee-for-service reimbursement is believed to encourage physicians to provide medical care. The degree of encouragement will depend on the relation between the fee and the service's marginal cost. Some analysts believe that fee-for-service reimbursement encourages many unnecessary practices. The fee schedule is a potentially powerful tool that third parties can use to influence both the type of practices performed and where they are performed. If a third party wanted to discourage certain procedure which is thought to be unnecessary e.g. tonsillectomy it could lower the amount of reimbursement. If a third party wanted of encourage certain procedures to be performed on an outpatient rather than on inpatient basis, it could reimburse physicians differently for the same procedure.

In recent years there has been a swing toward prospective reimbursement i.e. predetermined rates and away from retrospective payment. Until the early 1980s hospitals were reimbursed on a retrospective basis, that is a third party insurer would reimburse a hospital for the expenses it had already incurred or the charges it had already billed. Whatever the arrangement retrospective reimbursement has one over-riding effect on supply and on costs: it encourages an organization to expand. Increase in both the scope and quality of services tend to occur. It can lead to higher costs, more services and higher quality services. Prospective reimbursement involves setting the basis of reimbursement before the reimbursement period. As a result this payment scheme puts the provider at risk for any excess of cost over revenue. In retrospective payment provider has an incentive to increase the quality and volume of service as it will be reimbursed for these, it bears no financial risk. In order to protect itself financially, the payer must incur expenses to set standards and monitor and enforce them. These contracting costs can be quite high because of the technical nature of medical care. In prospective fee-for-service system almost all of the financial risk is imposed on the payer. This is because all services provided by the hospital will be paid for. As long as the per service rate exceeds the hospital's marginal cost, the provider will have an incentive to add additional services. The payer would have to set standards and monitor and enforce them, thus incurring costs.

Per case reimbursement:- In this a physician is paid a fixed amount for each type of case treated. The physician bears the cost of any services he or she provides and is paid a sum for the entire case.

If the physician reduces the number of services, more money will be left over as profit. Per case reimbursement for physicians is not being considered at this time because studies have shown wide variations in services for a single case type which would result in difficulties in establishing rates. While reimbursing a hospital all per case payment systems make use of case mix groups. Each group contains cases that use roughly the same amount of resources and payers reimburse the hospitals the same sum for all cases within the group. Under such a system, the risk to the payer is considerably reduced. However there is still a wide range of costs within each diagnostic group, sometimes the within group variation in resource use is due to severity. Hospitals that attract higher severity cases either because they are referral centers or inner city hospitals may lose money due to higher costs. They may therefore refuse to accept such cases without some kind of severity adjustment. In order to reduce costs imposed on providers who accept more severe cases payers have developed a two part system. Cases within each diagnostic group are divided into two groups i.e. typical cases and outliers. Using the distribution of stays within each diagnostic group, a trim point is established that separates long stay outliers from typical cases. The actual setting of the trim point is arbitrary and depends on how much pressure the payer wants to impose on the provider to reduce its stays. Outliers are reimbursed in two parts: a per case portion to cover those days inside the trim and an additional per diem payment to cover the additional days. Thus the risk of very high cost cases due to very long stays will be borne in a large part by the payer.

Per capita and Salary reimbursement: the incentives for physicians who are paid on a per capita or a salary basis do exist if they provide no more than the basic minimum level of series. However a physician who intends to remain in practice for a long time could not afford to allow the quality of services to fall to a low level.

Per diem fees: under this arrangement there will be a sharing of financial risks between the payer and the hospital. The longer the hospital keeps the patient, the more it will be reimbursed since the later part of most hospital stays are less costly than the earlier portion, the per diem rates are likely to exceed the marginal costs of the later part of a stay.

Per admission method: Hospital gets payment for adding more patients. Payers usually adjust the payment by a case mix or severity index because cases differ considerably by diagnosis and severity.

Slowing Growth of Health Care costs

Health care costs continue to be an important concern throughout the world. They remained a central issue of 2008 presidential campaign in U.S. There are three basic assumptions. First, health care spending has high intrinsic social value and the primary driver of cost increases is technical progress. The aging of the population and increasing number of patients with chronic illnesses contribute to the problem. Second the unconstrained growth in medical spending is threatening the income of individual patients, the cost structures of employer and the fiscal balance of government. Third the high social value of health care limits policy options for containing health care spending. In short, we want cost control but we also want broad access to health care and continued innovation in medical sciences. Trade offs among these goals are inevitable, and they can be minimized only through thoughtful policies. Nevertheless, the pressures to address increasing costs are so intense that policy decisions cannot be delayed until long-term studies are completed. Several types of payment reforms have been suggested and are being tried throughout the country. All of them are potentially disruptive to providers whose business are based on fee-for-service payments. Payment reform is likely to be most effective when providers are organized into delivery systems that can accept responsibility for cost mitigation goals. Health information system that include electronic records have significant potential for cost savings and enjoy strong political support. Policy makers often focus on the personal health record but the greatest cost reducing effect of electronic record will result from improved coordination among health care providers and from decision support that improves clinician's use of tests and treatments. Such decision support has the potential to decrease variation among physicians in the use of health care services, thereby reducing both baseline costs and cost trends. The potential is largely unrealized to date, however. Critical barriers include the requirements for capital investment and standardization of administrative and clinical data. Even more daunting is the need for cultural change among physicians, who must be willing to use decision-support system if electronic records are to improve their care. The improved care of patients with chronic conditions such as diabetes mellitus and coronary artery disease is a promising focus for cost reduction because about 70% of health care costs are generated by 10% of patients, most of whom have one or more chronic disease. Improved reliability and coordination of care of these patients could reduce their need for hospitalization. The observation that health care costs are concentrated in the period just before the patient's death raises concern that our health system uses excessive resources to extend the life of dying patients. Medicare data from oregen indicate that the use of hospitalization and intensive care units in the last months of life can be decreased without compromising the care of dying patients and their families. However any serious attempt to change end–of-life care requires deep cultural change that extends well beyond the provider community.

Two familiar targets for cost-reduction are malpractice and drug pricing reform, but the potential savings from these approaches are probably small. Although the current malpractice system is an inefficient way to protect patients from negligent care, the direct cost of malpractice and estimated costs of defensive medicine are not major factors in overall health care spending. In any case political support for malpractice reform is weak because of resistance to major changes. Costs can be reduced through more restrictive drug formularies and tougher price negotiations, but the savings are modest because pharmaceuticals account for just 10-15% of health care spending. Enhanced primary prevention efforts have strong support and could lead to important general health benefits. James J. Mongan etal recommend modification in reimbursement with explicit goal of rewarding the practice of evidence based medicine, reductions in variance among physicians in the use of services, and improvement in the care of patients with chronic conditions. They recommend consideration of blended arrangements including pay-for-performance programs, case rates and even adequately funded and appropriately risk-adjusted capitation. They recommend enhancing standardization of health care transactions to drive down administrative costs.

Ayushman Bharat – Pradhan Mantri Jan Arogya Yojana

Ayushman Bharat - Pradhan Mantri Jan Arogya Yojana (AB-PMJAY) is a Centrally Sponsored Scheme having central sector component under Ayushman Bharat Mission anchored in the Ministry of Health and Family Welfare (MoHFW). It is an umbrella of two major health initiatives, namely Health and wellness Centres and National Health Protection Scheme. AB PM- JAY was launched on 23rd September 2018 at Ranchi, Jharkhand.

In-patient hospitalization expenditure in India has increased nearly 300% during last ten years. (NSSO 2015). More than 80% of the expenditure are met by out of pocket (OOP) expenditure. Rural households primarily depended on their 'household income / savings' (68%) and on 'borrowings' (25%), the urban households relied much more on their 'income / saving' (75%) for financing expenditure on hospitalizations, and on '(18%) borrowings. (NSSO 2015). Out of pocket (OOP) expenditure in India is over 60% which leads to nearly 6 million families getting into poverty due to catastrophic health expenditures. AB-PMJAY will have major impact on reduction of Out Of Pocket (OOP) expenditure.

Health and Wellness Centres

Under this 1.5 lakh existing sub centres bring health care system closer to the homes of people in the form of Health and wellness centres. These centres provide comprehensive health care, including for non-communicable diseases and maternal and child health services. This comprehensive Primary Health Care is Universal and free to users, with a focus on wellness and the delivery of an expanded range of services closer to the community. The emphasis of health promotion and prevention is designed to bring focus on keeping people healthy by engaging and empowering individuals and communities to choose healthy behaviors and make changes that reduce the risk of developing chronic diseases and morbidities.

List of Services to be provided at Health & Wellness Centre

- Pregnancy care and maternal health services
- Neonatal and infant health services
- Child health

- Chronic communicable diseases
- Non-communicable diseases
- Management of mental illness
- Dental care
- Eye care
- Geriatric care Emergency medicine

National Health Protection Mission (AB-PMJAY)

Benefits

- AB-PMJAY provides a defined benefit cover of Rs. 5 lakh per family per year. This cover takes care of almost all secondary care and most of tertiary care procedures.
- To ensure that nobody is left out (especially women, children and elderly) there is no cap on family size and age in the scheme.
- The benefit cover also includes pre and post-hospitalisation expenses. All pre-existing conditions are covered from day one of the policy. A defined transport allowance per hospitalization is also permitted to be paid to the beneficiary.
- Benefits of the scheme are portable across the country and a beneficiary covered under the scheme is allowed to take cashless benefits from any public/private empanelled hospitals across the country.
- The beneficiaries can avail benefits in both *public and empanelled private facilities*. All public hospitals in the States implementing AB-PMJAY, are deemed empanelled for the Scheme. Hospitals belonging to Employee State Insurance Corporation (ESIC) may also be empanelled based on the bed occupancy ratio parameter.
- To control costs, the payments for treatment is done on package rate (defined by the Government) basis. The package rates include all the costs associated with treatment. For beneficiaries, it is cashless, paper less transaction. Keeping in view the State specific requirements, States/ UTs have the flexibility to modify these rates within a limited bandwidth.

Eligibility criteria

- AB-PMJAY is an entitlement based scheme with entitlement decided on the basis of deprivation criteria in the SECC database.
- The different categories in rural and urban areas include
  - families having only one room with kucha walls and kucha roof;
  - families having no adult member between age 16 to 59;
  - female headed households with no adult male member between age 16 to 59;
  - disabled member and no able bodied adult member in the family;
  - SC/ST households;
  - landless households deriving major part of their income from manual casual labour,
  - Families in rural areas having any one of the following: households without shelter, destitute, living on alms, manual scavenger families, primitive tribal groups, legally released bonded labour.
  - For urban areas, 11 defined occupational categories are entitled under the scheme - Occupational Categories of Workers, Rag picker, Beggar, Domestic worker, Street vendor/ Cobbler/hawker / Other service provider working on streets, Construction worker/ Plumber/ Mason/ Labour/ Painter/ Welder/ Security guard/, Coolie and another head-load worker, Sweeper/ Sanitation worker / Mali, Home-based worker/ Artisan/ Handicrafts worker / Tailor, Transport worker/ Driver/ Conductor/ Helper to drivers and conductors/ Cart puller/ Rickshaw puller, Shop worker/ Assistant/ Peon in small establishment/ Helper/Delivery assistant / Attendant/ Waiter, Electrician/ Mechanic/ Assembler/ Repair worker, Washerman/ Chowkidar.

As per the SECC 2011, the following beneficiaries are automatically excluded:

- Households having motorized 2/3/4 wheeler/fishing boat

- Households having mechanized 3/4 wheeler agricultural equipment
- Households having Kisan Credit Card with credit limit above Rs. 50,000/ -
- Household member is a government employee
- Households with non - agricultural enterprises registered with government
- Any member of household earning more than Rs. 10,000/ - per month
- Households paying income tax
- Households paying professional tax
- House with three or more rooms with pucca walls and roof
- Owns a refrigerator
- Owns a landline phone
- Owns more than 2.5 acres of irrigated land with 1 irrigation equipment
- Owns 5 acres or more of irrigated land for two or more crop season
- Owning at least 7.5 acres of land or more with at least one irrigation equipment

Implementation Strategy

At the national level to manage, a National Health Agency has been set up. States/ UTs are advised to implement the scheme by a dedicated entity called State Health Agency (SHA). AB-PMJAY will have major impact on reduction of Out Of Pocket (OOP) expenditure on ground of:

- Increased benefit cover to nearly 40% of the population, (the poorest & the vulnerable)
- Covering almost all secondary and many tertiary hospitalizations. (except a negative list)
- Coverage of 5 lakh for each family, (no restriction of family size)

This leads to increased access to quality health and medication. In addition, the unmet needs of the population which remained hidden due to lack of financial resources are catered to. This leads to timely treatments, improvements in health outcomes, patient satisfaction, improvement in productivity and efficiency, job creation thus leading to improvement in quality of life.

The expenditure incurred in premium payment is shared between Central and State Governments in specified ratio as per Ministry of Finance guidelines in vogue. The total expenditure depends on actual market determined premium paid in States/ UTs where AB-PMJAY is implemented through insurance companies.

Number of Beneficiaries

AB-PMJAY targets about 10.74 crore poor, deprived rural families and identified occupational category of urban workers' families as per the latest Socio-Economic Caste Census (SECC) data covering both rural and urban. AB-PMJAY will be rolled out across all States/UTs in all districts with an objective to cover all the targeted beneficiaries.

Guidelines for implementation of Ayushman Bharat-Pradhan Mantri Jan Arogya Yojana in Public Hospitals

All public hospitals empanelled under Ayushman Bharat Pradhan Mantri Jan Arogya Yojana are required to provide inpatient services to the entitled beneficiaries free of cost. Following is the list of benefits to be provided to the entitled beneficiaries:

1. Registration Charges.
2. Bed Charges (General Ward)
3. Nursing and boarding Charges.
4. Surgeons, Anesthetists, Medical Practitioner, Consultants fees etc.
5. Anesthesia, Blood Transfusion, Oxygen, O.T Charges, Cost of Surgical Appliances etc.
6. Medicines and Drugs.
7. Cost of Prosthetic devices, implants etc.
8. Pathology and Radiology tests: radiology to include but not limited to X-Ray, MRI, CT scan etc.
9. Diagnosis and Tests.
10. Food to Patient.

11. Pre and Post Hospitalization expenses : Expenses incurred for consultation, diagnostic tests and medicines before the admission of the patient in the same hospital and cost of diagnostic tests and medicines and up to 15 days of the discharge from the hospital for the same ailment/surgery.
12. Any other expenses related to the treatment of the patient in the hospital.

Strengthening of Hospital Drug stores and Laboratories

Drugs

To the extent possible only generic medicines need to be prescribed in public hospitals. To the extent possible medicines shall be provided from the Essential Drug List (EDL) in the hospital store to the AB-PMJAY beneficiaries. If there is shortage in the EDL, medicines shall be procured from Jan Aushadhi stores or any other government store strictly as per procurement guidelines.

A technical committee under the chairmanship of M.S/BMO and Nodal Officer AB-PMJAY, Administrative officer/Accounts & Store Superintendent/Store Keeper as members shall select Non – Emergency Drug list drugs and other consumables including surgical items, implants etc to be stored in the Hospital Pharmacy. Select list of non-EDL drugs shall be sent to State Health Agency (SHA) for approval. Where a drug that is not in the EDL/ Non -EDL list approved by SHA, is to be purchased, the treating /hospital doctor must prepare a request stating the reason why the specific drug is needed and get it approved by the technical committee which shall record the decisions and get the approvals from SHA subsequently on case to case basis.

Investigations

AB-PMJAY requires Standard Treatment Guidelines to be followed and necessary documents leading to the diagnosis are required to be uploaded to the claim server on compulsory and daily basis. All Hospitals have to strengthen the labs inside the Hospital Premises for services not available in the hospital lab. AB-PMJAY funds have not to be used for unnecessary investigations from outside laboratories but to augment diagnosis and therapeutic facilities inside hospitals.

The hospital level Chikitsa Prabandhan Samiti (CPS) / Hospital Management Committee (HMC) /Rogi Kalyan Samiti (RKS) can use the AB-PMJAY funds for purchase of new equipments, improve capacity or features of existing equipment, extend Annual Maintenance Contract (AMC), carry out maintenance not covered by AMC or any other contract, purchase consumables/reagents or spare parts, carry out infrastructural modifications for proper use of these equipment and hire technical personnel only after getting express permission from SHA. All hiring should be done as per the NHM rules. In exceptional circumstances, RKS can contract out certain lab services which are not available in the hospital ; through open tender process to select single firm or empanel certified labs who are ready to work on CGHS rates, with prior approval of SHA. Expenditure on purchase of drugs / diagnostics in no case shall exceed 50% of claim amount.

Accounting for Claims

Ayushman Bharat cell at each hospital have to upload claims for all procedures done in respect of entitled in patient beneficiaries and shall follow it up till the claim is finally settled. The cell has to invariably report on monthly basis to State Health Agency about the claim through respective M.S/CMO and in case of rejected claims shall furnish details including the reasons for rejection/ non-settlement. All the procedures followed in getting the claims settled are subjected to audit. M.S /BMO/medical officer incharge shall facilitate the State Health Agency and Insurance Agency in conducting hospital audits, treatment audits and other verifications at hospital as prescribed in AB-PMJAY guidelines.

Account Maintenance

Respective empanelled public hospitals have to maintain a dedicated bank account and books for the amount accrued as claim under the scheme. The bank account opening and maintenance has to be as per the general applicable rules in this matter and shall not require any special approval. Receipts from insurance reimbursements are subject to audit and must be properly accounted for and deposited in a separate bank account operated jointly by the Medical Superintendent/ Block Medical Officer (MS/BMO) and any other administrative officer. These are not to be deposited directly into the

RKS account. The funds have to be utilized in accordance with laid down framework for administrative/technical/financial rules besides the guidelines/norms and ceilings of AB-PMJAY. All the withdrawals and reimbursements from the account for all PM-Jay related matters have to be done by approved banking instrument (Cheque/draft/bank order etc) only. Cash payments should not be done.

Executive Committee for Insurance funds

Executive committee with the following composition is to be constituted in all public hospitals.

Medical Superintendent/BMO/MOIC	Chairperson
Deputy Superintendent /RMO Vice	Chairman
Nodal Officer AB-PMJAY	Member Secretary
(to be Nominated by the chairperson)	
Administrative Officer/Accounts officer	Member
HODs of all Departments & Consultants	Member
Matron/Nursing Superintendent	Member
Stores Officer	Member

Chairperson may co-opt any other officer as may be deemed necessary.

The empanelled public hospitals may make minor changes if necessary, in the composition of the committee as per local content.

Utilization of insurance funds in the Hospitals

Insurance Fund shall be credited into the dedicated AB-PMJAY bank account. Insurance Fund (settled amount) has to be divided into three heads namely RKS share(75), Incentive share (20%) and SHA share (5%). The RKS Head share shall further be divided into Tied and Untied RKS Heads. Tied RKS Head bears expenses vis-à-vis routines, like patient Registration, Bed Charges, Diet and Stationary, Cost of Drugs and diagnostics and Untied RKS Head has to be used for all purposes except mentioned above. Incentive share part is calculated based on the settled claims by Insurance company on case to case basis. SHA share of 5% shall be on Settled claims, calculated on monthly basis. The empanelled Public hospitals have to deposit the share on monthly basis in the SHA account. This remains as a corpus fund with State Health agency in a dedicated account maintained by SHA for the purpose. The fund has to be utilized by SHA in accordance with the laid down framework for administrative, technical, financial rules besides the guidelines/norms and ceilings of AB-PMJAY.

Incentive Share

Incentive has to be paid only if expenses of the concerned claim are not above 75% of the package rates. Twenty percent of the insurance fund (on case to case basis) earmarked as the staff incentive share shall be distributed as per the following general guidelines.

1. Surgeon/Main physician/doctor treating the case: 25%
2. Surgeon assisting the surgery/other physician/doctors involved intreating the case; 10%
3. Anesthetist/doctor of other departments actively involved in the case management of medical cases : 20%
4. MS/BMO/MOIC : 5%
5. Consultation/call duty etc : 5%
6. Staff nurses: 15%
7. Nursing Assistants/ Hospital Attendant : 10%
8. Lab Technician : 3%
9. X-Ray/USD/CT Scan Technician : 3%
10. Others if any : 4%

Lab technicians are eligible for incentives if lab investigations are done in hospital lab for these cases. Doctors involved in the USG, CT Scan are covered as consultation component of incentive. Unspent amount in the incentive share shall become part of Untied Head of RKS Share. Executive Committee on Insurance funds constituted in the hospital acts as Grievance Redressal Cell with regard to grievances related to incentives of doctors and other staff and implementation of AB-PMJAY. The books of account have to be maintained by the public hospitals for all the three components.

Administrative and service delivery guidelines

Empanelled public hospitals have to set up a dedicated helpdesk for AB-PMJAY preferably in the reception area of hospital. In-patient tickets issued to patients have to depict clearly as to whether the patients are entitled to benefits under AB-PMJAY or not. State hospitals have to designate an existing MBBS doctor as dedicated Medical Co-ordinator for submitting the claims .

The Pradhan Mantri Arogya Mitras (PMAMs) will be selected based on the following criteria:

(a) Completed 10+2 from a recognized institution (Preferably Graduate) (b) Basic proficiency in computer operations (c) Completed the Pradhan Mantri Arogya Mitra Training Course and passed the respective course exam/certification. (d) Possessing fluent communication skills in Hindi/ English and Local language of the State/ region (e) Having adequate functional computer literacy which shall include understanding of Microsoft Office Suite and navigating through Internet Portals.

Preference to be given to Female Candidates for the position of Pradhan Mantri Arogya Mitra. Qualified ASHA workers may be given preference for the position of PMAM (if interested).

Existing staff of Government hospitals can also be nominated to act as Pradhan Mantri Arogya Mitra by the State Government.

Recruitment of Pradhan Mantri Arogya Mitra

(a) The State Health Agency (SHA)/Hospitals will have the flexibility to recruit PMAM through third party agency/agencies or through any other mechanism for public facilities. Based on the number of PMAMs required, the SHA shall pay them through a third-party agency / agencies/hospital or any other mechanism. In case of requirement of extra PMAMs, the SHA/Selected Agency/Hospital should have the capability to promptly scale up its capacity and provide the required number of PMAMs. (b) SHA can directly hire PMAMs at State/ District or hospital level. (c) If the State Government requires, they can even nominate existing staff of public hospitals as PMAMs. (d) For Private EHCP, the recruitment and placement of PMAM should be done by the health care provider itself. The cost of the PMAM in that facility should be borne by the Private EHCP. (e) The monthly remuneration of PMAMs including fixed component and incentives (if any) should not be less than the minimum wages in the State as prescribed by the Minimum Wages Act.

Placement of Pradhan Mantri Arogya Mitra

PMAMs will be placed at every public and private EHCP. The exact numbers of PMAMs to be placed shall be dependent on the average case-load per day. A suggestive placement of PMAMs based on cases registered per day is given below.

(a) 0-10 Cases – 1 PMAM (b) 10-20 Cases – 2 PMAMs (c) 20-30 Cases – 3 PMAMs (d) 30-40 Cases – 4 PMAMs

The State or EHCP can revise the number of PMAMs based on local conditions, however, they will ensure that services are available to the beneficiaries 24x7 in the hospital.

Roles and Responsibilities

PMAM plays three main roles under AB PM-JAY. First as a Trusted Partner of Beneficiaries, then as a Representative of Authorities and finally as a System Operator. The PMAM is the primary contact for the beneficiaries at every EHCP.

The PMAM shall be responsible for the following broad areas:

(a) Guiding the Beneficiary about the overall benefits under AB PM-JAY and providing information about receiving prompt treatment at EHCP

(b) Operating the Beneficiary Identification System to identify and verify the beneficiaries entitled under AB PM-JAY

(c) Operating the Transaction Management System such as submitting requests for PreAuthorization, Updating Surgery/ Treatment Details and Filing for Claims d) Ensure the privacy and confidentiality of personal and sensitive beneficiary information is maintained while operating IT systems under AB PM-JAY

For ensuring timely access to medical care, PMAM is responsible for operating the Beneficiary Identification System (BIS) to identify, authenticate and verify the beneficiaries entitled under the AB PM-JAY.

Reference

1. Health systems: Improving performance. The WORLD HEALTH REPORT WHO 2000.
2. Financing Health care in THE ECONOMICS OF HEALTH AND MEDICAL CARE 5TH Edition Jones and Bartlett publishers (13) 291-305. 2004.
3. Provider payment in THE ECONOMICS OF HEALTH AND MEDICAL CARE 5TH Edition Jones and Bartlett Publishers (7) 147-172. 2004.
4. F.A Jan, N.A Pandit, Q.A. Qayoom. Health Insurance The Indian Perspective. JIMSA 16(4) 213-214, 2003.
5. James J. Mongan, Timothy G. Ferris, Thomas H. Lee. Options for solving the Growth of health care costs. N. ENG J MED 358; 14:1509-1514 April 2008.
6. Institute of Medicines. Rewarding provider performance aligning incentives in Medicare. Washington DC :National Academics Press 2006.
7. Davis K. Paying for care episodes and Care coordination. New Eng J. Med; 356: 1166-8: 2007.
8. The Dartmouth Atlas Project. The care of patients with severe chronic illness: an online report on the Medicare program 2006. (Http://www.dartmouthatlas.org)
9. Studdert DM, Mello MM, Gawande AA, et al claims errors and compensation payments in medical malpractice litigation. N.eng J. Med; 354:2004-33 2006.
10. Rubin RJ, Mendelson DN How much does defensive medicine cost? J AM Health policy 4:7-15; 1994.
11. Huskamp A/A, Epstein AM, Blumenthal The impact of a national prescription drug formulary on prices, market share and spending: lesson for medicine? Health A/s (3) 22: 149-58 2003.
12. National Health Agency.
13. Guidelines for Pradhan Mantri Arogya Mitra. National Health Authority.
14. Guidelines for implementation of Ayushman Bharat Pradhan Mantri Jan Arogya Yojana in Public Hospitals of J& K. Notification no; 01- HME of 2019.

14

Private-Public Partnerships in Health Care

With shrinking budgetary allocations and fiscal problems most of the governmental organizations are finding it difficult to cater to the growing health care needs of the populations. Many governments are exploring options to improve equity, efficiency, accountability, quality and accessibility of the entire health system and one of the options available is promoting private-public partnerships. Private sector in India is most unregulated, but is easily accessible.

A good working definition of partnerships would include three points: First, these partnerships involve at least one private-for-profit organization and at least one not-for-profit or public organization. Second, the partners have some shared objectives for the creation of social values often for disadvantaged populations. Finally, the core partners agree to share both efforts and benefits. However the governmental organization can interface with the non-profit private sector for technical expertise or outreach. A chief factor encouraging these partnerships is that neither side alone can achieve its specific goals. Partnerships need to be differentiated from privatization which involves permanent transfer of control through transfer of ownership right or an arrangement in which the private sector share holder has waived its right to subscribe. Public-private partnership also needs to be differentiated from outsourcing. PPP usually entails a combination of services, for example, design, construction and maintenance whereas outsourcing is usually for one or relatively simple services.

Partnerships between public/governmental entities, private/ commercial entities and civil society have a contribution to make in improving the health of the poor by combining the different skills and resources of various organizations in innovative ways. Public agencies clearly benefit from working in collaboration with the private sector in areas where the public sector lacks expertise and experience.

Partnerships are more justified in areas of disease control product development, disease control product distribution, strengthening health services, commercializing traditional medicine, health program co-ordination, health service delivery etc. Partnership with for-profit sector is not appropriate in areas of policy making and development of regulations. Private-public partnerships should not be expected to substitute for action on responsibilities that properly rest elsewhere. In particular public sector agencies should continue to fund fundamental research, set standards for product safety, efficacy and quality, establish systems whereby citizens have adequate access to health products and services, use public resources in an efficient manner and create environments in which commercial enterprise is appropriately motivated to meet the needs of whole populations.

There are different models of public-private partnership in hospital provision:

(a) Franchising: Public authority contacts a private company to manage existing hospital. Private company takes over management of an existing public hospital.

(b) DBFO (Design, build, finance, operate): Private partner designs facilities based on public authority's specific requirements, builds the facility, finances the capital cost and operates their facilities. In DBFO model private sector finances any funding short falls for the project; designs, constructs and operates specified services within the facility for a specified time. The government establishes service performance objectives and private sector partner is paid based on its performance as measured against the objectives. The capital and operational costs in DBFO are blended together in a service payment to the private sector over a period of up to 30 years. Adding responsibility for capital maintenance to the private sector is central theme in most DBFO projects causing private owner/operator to make the operating versus capital lifecycle cost trade offs while consistently delivering a project that meets user needs. The majority of the payments the government makes to the private sector are set in advance for the whole contract period with adjustments based on inflation, performance by the private sector and hospital consumption. If the private sector does not perform to the standards agreed to in the contract, deductions are taken off. The deductions are related to the seriousness of the breach and are based upon a pre-established performance regime. Often publicity owned facilities age too fast due to lack of proper capital for maintenance but DBFO prevents this as the maintenance of asset is included in the contract. At the end of the contract the facilities are returned to the public sector in a good state as specified in the contract.

(c) BOO (Build, Own. Operate): Public authority purchases services for fixed period (say 30 years) after which ownership remains with private provider.

(d) BOOT (Build, Own, Operate, Transfer): Public authority purchases services for fixed period after which ownership reverts to public authority.

(e) BOLB (Buy, Own, Lease back): Private contractor builds hospital; facility is leased back and managed by public authority.

(f) Alzira model: Private contractor builds and operates hospital with contract to provide care for a defined population in return for an annual per capita payment.

Private partner selection and obligations of the partners.

Competitive process of selecting a private sector partner is less effective than an invited or negotiated partnership. While competing to win a contract, the private partner proposes low cost in order to clinch the bid. The public sector managers on the other hand are more concerned about satisfying procedural requirements than meeting the needs. The tendering process in government invariably chooses the lowest bid who later on fail to provide same level of quality as mentioned in the contract. Some of the successful partnership projects documented point to the importance of prior negotiations with the potential partners.

Both the partners in private-public partnership have to be committed to mutual responsibilities. Another corner stone of partnership is the relative autonomy enjoyed by both the partners on day-to-day operations as well as in the over all management of the partnership. Autonomy is seen as non-intrusiveness by the public sector and the freedom of the private agency to take operational decisions without having to resort to cumbersome bureaucratic approvals or being constantly told about do's and don'ts.

Quality of Services

One of the major grey areas in any public-private partnership has been specific conditions related to quality. Although quality of service is talked about at the time of drafting an agreement, specific terms as to how quality of care is to be achieved and monitored need to be properly included in the contract document.

For the under-developed and developing countries public-private partnership is being considered a feasible solution to the current ills of the health care delivery system. Utilizing private capital to relieve some of the burden on the public health care system would make a significant contribution in resolving some of the current challenges being faced by health and medical care system. Currently lack of stable, long-term funding is jeopardizing long-term planning in the traditional system of health care delivery. Thus the need of the hour is that policy makers, planners and administrators of the health and medical care systems explore the possibilities of suitable public-private partnerships to make medical care systems efficient, effective and suited to the needs of its rightful beneficiaries.

Outsourcing

Currently outsourcing of health services is a hot topic in most countries. Outsourcing is a cost effective procedure in health care that leads to increased service quality services. Many operations in health care have been outsourced during the years. These include housekeeping, laundry, dietary services, payroll, billing, human resource, marketing and so on. Recently many of par clinic services as radiology practices have been outsourced. While public private partnership is partnership between government and private sectors where public sector still retains the upper hand, outsourcing includes introducing private sector management to a state-owned enterprise through management services agreement or contracting of services to the private sector. Outsourcing in industrialized countries began outside the healthcare sector, but is now well developed model for health service providers. Off-shoring which is another type of outsourcing simply means having the outsourced business functions done in another country. Off-shoring is one situation in which developing countries that are able to adopt standards, processes and language of developed countries can benefit from liberalization of the movement of goods and services.

Critical reasons of outsourcing are as follows:

- Gaining competitive advantage.
- Access to key technologies.
- Reducing operational costs.
- Reducing risk and sharing risk.
- Access to capital resources.
- Focus on goals.

According to Modern Healthcare's 27th Annual Outsourcing Survey in USA, the number of outsourcing contracts for respondents continues to rise. Laundry jumped ahead of housekeeping as the top hospital department management contract. European healthcare IT outsourcing market revenues continue to rise. In Taiwanese hospitals among non-medical items services outsourced are Medical waste, Common waste, Gift Store, Linen, Restaurant, security guard, IT, Medical equipment Maintenance. Among Medical services items frequently outsourced are Ambulance, Hemodialysis, Laser, Shake wave, Laboratory and Radiology. However other medical services such as nursing, pharmacy show much lower rate of outsourcing ie around 3%. Even though outsourcing has many benefits, it will fail if not managed successfully . Hospital executives must choose outsourcing providers who hold the necessary leadership capabilities. Managing outsourcing requires an understanding of outsourcing strategy, the benefits and risks of outsourcing, the evaluation process and the methods to managing outsourcing providers. Before negotiating any outsourcing transaction, hospital executives should carefully analyze the legal and regulatory implications, which will vary according to the type of services and the vendor involved .

However not all of the outsourcing is beneficial to hospitals. Negative perceptions about the contract management groups of emergency department outsourcing persist among some physicians. The March 2003 severe acute respiratory syndrome (SARS) outbreak from China to Taiwan has had an obvious impact on local hospitals out sourcing ability. Director of Centre of Disease Control in Taiwan ordered the shutdown of the outsourcing system due to rapid transmission of virus through hospitals by the carelessness of the housekeeping and laundry services during SARS outbreak.

Refernces

1. Nishtar Sania. Public-private "partnership" in health a global call to action. Health research policy and systems 2004,2:5.
2. Reich.R.Michael. Public private partnerships for public health in public private partnerships for public health. Harvard University press. April 2002: 1; 1-18.
3. Raman. A.Venkat, B Jorkman. J. Warner. Public/Private partnership in Health care services in India. Research study funded by the Indo-Dutch programme on alternatives in Development. (project 5.3.96)
4. Farooq. A. Jan, G.J. Qadri. Public-Private Partnership in Health Care. DAK voice 2007 Vol 4 Issue 4: 34-37.
5. Margzin Mckee, Nigel Edwards, Rifat Atun. Bulletin of World Health Organization 2006.84(11): 890-896.
6. Roy Widdus. Public-Private partnerships for health: their main targets, their diversity and their future directions. Bulletin of the World Health Organization, 2001, 79: 713-720
7. Standing Senate Committee on social Affairs, Science and Technology. The Health of Canadians. The federal role volume. Five: Principles and recommendations for reform part 1 April 2002. P14.
8. Saeed Karimi, Zahra Agharahimi, Maryam Yaghoubi. Impacts of outsourcing in educational hospitals in Iran: A study on Isfahan University of Medical Sciences-2010. J Edu Health Promot 2012;1:25.
9. Chih-Tung Hsiao, Jar-Yuan Pai, Hero Chiu. The study on the outsourcing of Taiwan's hospitals: a questionnaire survey research. BMC Health services Research 2009,9:78.
10. Vahit Yigit, Dilaver Tengilimoglu, Adnan Kisa, Mustafa Zeedan Younis. Outsourcing and its implications for Hospital Organizations in Turkey. J Health Care Finance 2007; 33(4): 86-92.

15

Indian Public Health Standards for District and Sub-District Hospitals

To meet national and international commitments, it is essential for public health facilities to deliver quality services. To meet these objectives, the IPHS were launched to deliver quality services to all citizens with dignity and respect. Thus, the IPHS for Sub Health Centres, Primary Health Centres (PHCs), Community Health Centres (CHCs), Sub District Hospitals (SDH) and District Hospitals (DH) were published in 2007 and revised in 2012. They are the reference point for public health care infrastructure planning and upgradation in the States and UTs. They are designed to provide guidance on the health system components such as infrastructure, human resource, drugs, diagnostics, equipment, quality, and governance requirements for delivering health services at these facilities. The provision of uniform health care forms the cornerstone for a successful public health delivery system. The High-Level Expert Group on UHC (constituted by the Government of India) defined it as "ensuring equitable access for all Indian citizens in any part of the country, regardless of income level, social status, gender, caste or religion, to affordable, accountable and appropriate, assured quality health services (promotive, preventive, curative and rehabilitative) as well as services addressing wider determinants of health delivered to individuals and populations, with the Government being the guarantor and enabler, although not necessarily the only provider of health and related services." To ensure quality provision of close-to-client health services, an organised provider network is essential. Approach of IPHS 2022 is a target-based and outcome-oriented approach rather than an input-based and normative approach to reach under serviced areas. Since the last revision of the IPHS in 2012, several new initiatives, interventions, programmes and projects have been introduced in the public health system. The introduction of comprehensive primary care through strengthened Sub Health Centres and PHCs (now known as Health and Wellness Centres or HWC), similarly, in urban areas, Urban Health and Wellness Centres or UHWC, speciality UPHCs (polyclinics), quality improvement initiatives (Kayakalp, LAQSHYA, Grievance Redressal Systems) and the progression from the Millennium Development Goals (MDGs) to the Sustainable Development Goals (SDGs) have also been key developments in recent few years. The revised and updated 2022 IPHS norms retain the earlier approach of supporting government health facilities to attain a minimum acceptable functional standard (indicated as 'Essential') while striving and aspiring for improvement (indicated as 'Desirable') so as to accelerate India's progress towards achievement of uniform health care and sustainable development goals. The revised 2022 IPHS include the various components related to service delivery, i.e., infrastructure requirements, HR norms and capacity building, drugs, diagnostics and equipment, administrative and support services, quality assurance and improvement, monitoring and related governance issues. Indian Public Health Standards-Volume I contains norms for DH and SDH combined together as they both provide secondary care services.

The National Health Policy, 2017 recommends two beds per 1000 population. It is therefore proposed that the provision of one bed per 1000 population is an 'Essential' norm for every district while two beds per 1000 is a target they should aspire towards 'Desirable'. However, while calculating the patient-bed ratio in a district, it should primarily rely on the facilities from PHC to DH since tertiary care facilities (Medical Colleges) do not cater only to the district where it is located, but to other districts too. . As a thumb rule, all such beds that are available and functional for a patient for more than 24 hours, have been calculated as in-patient hospital beds (including critical care beds). The remaining beds such as Emergency, LDR, dialysis, day-care and pre & post-operative beds have not been counted as in- patient hospital beds. However, all such beds will be counted for budgetary allocation, provision of HR, and also clinical and other support services.

Table 15.1: Beds per Population

Population	Essential beds	Desirable beds
Less than 2 lakh	50 beds + 15 additional (Emergency and day care beds)	100
Between 2–5 lakh	100 beds + 25 additional (Emergency and day care beds)	200
Between 5–10 lakh	200 beds + 38 additional (Emergency and day care beds)	300
Between 10–20 lakh	300 beds + 49 additional (Emergency and day care beds)	400
Between 20–30 lakh	400 beds + 60 additional (Emergency and day care beds)	500
More than 30 lakhs	500 beds + 65 additional (Emergency and day care beds)	700

This grading is useful as it provides a systematic basis for identifying resources required at the DH according to the size of the facility. Districts with less than 5 lakh population with a functional DH do not need a Sub District hospital. Districts with populations between 5-10 lakh can have one SDH. Thereafter, one SDH for every 10 lakh population can be considered for the provision of comprehensive secondary care health services. Every district should have at least one district hospital which should be comprehensively functional for providing secondary care services as defined in the guidelines. While all secondary care services are important, certain critical services like emergency, High Dependency Unit (HDU)/Intensive Care Unit (ICU), Operation Theatre (OT), Labour Delivery & Recovery complex, Special Newborn Care Unit (SNCU), lab and imaging services, etc. need to be prioritised. Although the present IPHS has considered requirement of the total number of beds in a district, it also provisions for additional beds during the time of emergency/disaster. States can still propose for additional beds, depending on disease burden, programme requirements, etc. However, any such addition can only be considered if the Bed Occupancy Rate (BOR) is more than 70%. This will ensure optimal utilisation of bed. Accordingly, provision of commensurate human resource and logistic support system should also be ensured. IPHS prescribes norms for allopathic services. However, AYUSH services have been retained in IPHS 2022 as desirable. The HRH, medicines, and other inputs required for AYUSH services shall be given by Ministry of AYUSH. The present IPHS has considered the requirement of MCH beds in the total number of beds itself so that stand-alone MCH beds are not created randomly. States, however, can still propose MCH wings if they are unable to accommodate a holistic district plan which includes the requirement of maternal and child health needs. A Citizens' Charter should be prominently displayed near the entrance of the facility. District hospital services have three pillars; clinical care, a knowledge hub for capacity development of HR in health, and public health programme to ensure the continuum of care and reduce the disease burden. Clinical care includes curative, palliative, and rehabilitative services along with services for implementation of national programmes (as appropriate), provision of drugs, diagnostic services, administrative/maintenance services and other support services. Apart from curative services, there should be a strong focus on health promotion, prevention, palliation and rehabilitation at all district and Sub District hospitals. District hospitals should aim to become the knowledge hub of their corresponding districts by providing services like medical courses including Diplomate of National Board (DNB), nursing schools, ANM training centres, district training centres for miscellaneous training, and a resource centre equipped with computers, information resources and telemedicine capability. This may be managed through a partnership with universities.

The suggestive flow of services as underneath should be followed for IPHS compliance in any SDH & DH.

Enquiry Registration → Waiting → Nursing station → Clinic → Dressing room/Injection room → Diagnostics (lab/imaging) → Drug dispensation → Message to the patient for Mera Aspatal feedback → Exit.

Infrastructure

The infrastructure for all facilities should follow the rules and regulations as laid down in National Building Code and in the state by-laws.

Factors to be considered while building a new facility either at the same site or selecting a new site for a facility include:

- Accessibility to the public (with good road connectivity) .
- Ensuring the facility is not in a low-lying flood-prone area.
- Ensuring it is adequately serviced by public utilities such as water, electricity and telephone connectivity, sewage and

storm-water disposal. In areas where these are not available, appropriate substitutes should be identified such as a deep well for water, generators for electricity and radio communication for telephony.

- Ensuring elderly and disabled-friendly access .
- Minimizing exposure to air, noise, water and land pollution and having facilities with vector-breeding proof buildings.
- Reviewing land utilization in adjoining areas, the general topography, proximity to the local bus stands, railway station and other modes of transport and obtaining the necessary environmental (including seismic safety), fire safety and administrative clearance.
- The local agency by-laws and rules should be strictly adhered to. While adhering to these, 60% of the total area of the facility should be reserved for landscaping, play area, circulation area etc. and the remaining 35-40% should be the plinth area (including residential areas). The built-up portion will include areas for core clinical services, support services such as the Central Sterile Services Department (CSSD), kitchen and mechanised laundry, residential areas and the knowledge hub (teaching and training sites). An estimated 80% of the built-up areas should be dedicated to core patient services and clinical areas. Use of this space for administrative and related services (e.g., offices and general stores) should be avoided.
- Wherever possible, new buildings should be constructed vertically than horizontally (within state norms and compliant with the National Building Code) so that there is more space available for creating green spaces.

Where lack of space is a particular concern (as in urban areas or pre-existing spaces), the possibility of expansion vertically based on floor area ratio (FAR) rather than horizontally should be seriously considered, while bearing in mind that at least 10 metre of space all around the boundary wall should be left open. Adequate width to allow easy access to the fire engine should be provisioned for and in no case should it measure less than 6 metre.

As a general principle and wherever possible, clinical areas especially Emergency services, LDR complex, OPD should be on the ground floor. Administrative offices, teaching and training areas and general store rooms should be located on higher floors. Emphasis should be given to creating a positive, client-friendly ambiance around the facility. This includes due consideration to the provision of facilities for patient registration, waiting areas, clear way-finding, and sign-posting, parking, gardens, washrooms, drinking water, and disabled-friendly facilities. The facility should be environment friendly with scope for adequate natural light, water harvesting and solar energy, if appropriate. The foundation of the health facility infrastructure should be strong enough to meet the requirement of the seismic zones of that area and any future vertical expansion. It should strictly adhere to the statutory fire safety norms.

General appearance and upkeep

The facility should have a high boundary wall with at least two gates for entry/exit. There should be no unwanted/outdated posters or hoardings on the walls of the building and the boundary of the facility. There should be no encroachment in and around the facility. As per The Noise Pollution (Regulation & Control) Rules, 2000; an area of 100 metres around the hospital should be defined as a "Silence Zone". Clear access to vehicles should be maintained. No vehicle should be parked outside the gate and no waiting areas should be allowed for autos, buses etc. The Public Address System must be installed for efficient traffic management in and around the facility. Adequate lighting should be ensured so that the facility is clearly visible from the approach road. The facility should be plastered and painted in a uniform colour scheme and free from seepage, cracks and broken window panes. The floors should be anti-skid and non-slippery.

Way- finding and Signage

Adequate and clear signage should be displayed on the main and connecting roads to the facility. The layout of the hospital should be displayed near the entrance. Safety, hazard and caution signs should be prominently displayed at relevant places. A fluorescent fire exit plan should be considered where appropriate. Tactile pathways should be made for visually incapacitated visitors.

Parking

Clear access for vehicles and ambulances should be maintained, especially near the emergency department. Wherever possible, separate parking spaces should be allotted for staff parking and visitor parking. Fringe parking can be created, if such space is available.

Landscaping

Gardens, landscaping and open spaces give a positive, healing environment that reduces stress, anxiety and mental fatigue. So, wherever possible, identify and promote greenery and open spaces. Herbal gardens should be promoted on the campus. A dedicated play area for children should also be identified.

Facility Entrance

This should take into consideration the flow of facility traffic at different speeds from the walking wounded and patients on wheelchairs to fast-moving ambulances. There should be a clear, separate entrance for the emergency area, OPD area and the main entrance for other clinical services, including in-patient areas. Entrance for service areas such as supplies and logistics, equipment should be separate.

Environmental friendly features

The facility should be environment-friendly and energy-efficient. Where possible, the use of rainwater harvesting, solar energy and energy-efficient bulbs/equipment should be encouraged. Use of low-energy LED lighting or alternate low-energy option to save indoor lighting energy costs is recommended. The facility should have a plan for the usage of renewable energy with battery backup during times of storms, floods, or power blackouts. Refrigerants used in the Heating, Ventilation & Air-conditioning (HVAC) equipment should be CFC (Chloro Fluoro Carbon) free, with a low Greenhouse Warming Potential (GWP) when available. When choosing the technology, guidelines and standards issued by the Ministry of New and Renewable Energy must be adhered to.

Disabled and elderly friendly

For easy access of non-ambulant (wheelchair, stretcher), semi-ambulant, visually disabled, and elderly people, infrastructural norms in line with the 'Guidelines and Space Standards for the barrier-free built environment for Disabled and Elderly Persons' of the Government of India should be followed. Also, provisions of the 'Rights of Person with Disability Act 2016' should be implemented. A dedicated section in OPD for geriatric patients with provision for sample collection and report area should also be provisioned to ensure convenient elder-friendly access.

Circulation areas, corridors and ramps

The flooring of circulation areas such as corridors, lifts, ramps, staircases and other common spaces should be anti-skid and non-slippery. Corridors should be at least 3 metres wide. All two-way swing doors or doors in general circulation areas should be provided with vision panels giving visibility from a height of 800 mm to 1500 mm. Ramps shall have a slope of 1:15 to 1:18 and should be checked for maneuverability of beds and trolleys at turning points.

Disaster and emergency preparedness

They should also be capable of handling sudden healthcare needs during disasters and unforeseen emergencies/epidemics/ pandemics etc. While creating infrastructure seismicity of zones needs to be considered. Wherever the health facilities are already existing possible retrofitting should be planned.

Electric power supply

Public health facilities should have access to adequate, affordable, and reliable electricity supply.

Fire Safety

Compliance as per state and central government guidelines for fire regulations should be ensured while planning for a SDH/DH. Availability of open spaces, clearly visible fire exits with proper illumination and lighting (even during an interruption in electric supply) are some of the important considerations for creating fire-safe infrastructure.

Illumination

The illumination and lighting in the SDH/DH should be according to the prescribed standards (BIS) given below. Shadowless lights in the operation theatre and delivery rooms should be provided. Emergency portable light units should be provided in the wards and departments. Illumination in different areas should be as follows

1 Reception and waiting room : 150 lux

2 Wards:

  2a General 100 lux

  2b Beds 150 lux

3 Operation Theatre:

  3a General 300 lux

  3b Tables Shadow less light

4 Laboratories : 300 lux

5 Radiology : 100 lux

6 Casualty and Outpatient Departments : 150 lux

7 Stairs and Corridor : 100 lux

8 Dispensaries : 300 lux

Water Supply

The arrangement should be made for round the clock piped water supply along with an overhead water storage tank with a provision to store at least three days of water requirement. Water supply preferably through two independent sources must be ensured. A separate water tank for critical care areas should be made available. It should have pumped and boosting arrangements. Approximately 450 to 500 litres of water per bed (including day care, emergency, dialysis and LDR beds) per day is required for a district hospital. Separate provision for firefighting and water softening plants is to be made available. Cleaning of all water tanks should be ensured on a regular basis (at an interval of a maximum of three months) and records should be maintained accordingly. In view of the critical shortage of water, conservation of water by rain water harvesting and by use of recycled water to the maximum extent possible is required. Hospitals must encourage the use of a safe clean rainwater harvesting system to help reduce the municipal water demand and enhance the ground water table.

Drainage and Sanitation

A separate drainage system for effluents being generated from various service areas to Effluent Treatment Plant (ETP) needs to be in place, so that all effluents are treated before discharge. Provision for an Effluent Treatment Plant (ETP) based on the estimated effluent load (and separate from the treatment of sewage) should also be provided at the district hospital and larger public health facilities. As per Bio Medical Waste Management Rules (BMW) rules, it is mandatory to establish a Sewage Treatment Plant at a health facility with more than 10 beds.

Waste management

Should be done as per Biomedical Waste Management and Handling Rules.

Infrastructure for Clinical Services

1. Out Patient Services : The facility should be planned keeping in mind the maximum peak hour patient load and should have scope for future expansion, if possible. The OPD wing should have an approach from the main road with signage visible from a distance.

- Registration area : It should be well ventilated, lit, and spacious with each counter ensuring a minimum space of 15-20m2.

Type of Hospital Number of Counters

SDH 100 beds : 3 Counters.

DH 50 beds : 3 Counters

DH 100 beds : 3 Counters

DH 200 beds : 4 Counters

DH 300 beds : 4 Counters

DH 400 beds : 6 Counters

DH 500 beds : 6 Counters

- Waiting area : The waiting area should be organized in designated areas such as near the registration counter, OPD, and outside critical areas. This should be built to a scale of 1 sq. ft. per one-third of peak hour load for the registration area and about one-half of peak hour load for OPD areas. A minimum of 400 sq. ft. of area should be provided. Adequate seating arrangements preferably such, which are less space occupying and easy to maintain should be placed. The waiting area for paediatric OPD can have colourful wall paintings with cartoon characters. The play area can be equipped with toys, games, puzzles, etc. to create an environment where children enjoy themselves and learn while waiting to be treated.

Patient amenities in waiting areas should include

- Essential amenities

  Fans

  Clean drinking water

  Clean and gender-sensitive toilets

- Desirable amenities

  Air-conditioning

Television/LCD in waiting area displaying facility-related information, health-related IEC.

2. Nursing Station : A common nursing station in the OPD complex is required where nurses will record vitals of patients such as Blood Pressure, temperature, etc., and guide patients before they enter the consultation/examination room. They should also keep with them emergency resuscitation kits and tray for management of anaphylactic shock. Separate stations for high case load OPDs (such as OBGY, immunization, family planning, and NCD services) to be provisioned. A common nursing station for the remaining OPD clinics should also be made available. The stations should have space to seat nurses, keep equipment/consumables to measure vitals, and maintain records. Digital record-keeping is preferred.

3. Consultation room : This should have enough space with a minimum area of 12 sq. m.to accommodate the required furniture and examination equipment so that interaction with patients can be conducted with privacy and dignity. It should be well lit and ventilated with minimum furniture in the room which is compact so that there is adequate space for the patient and/or attendants. An examination table,

X-ray view box, single curtain screens and hand washing facilities should be provided, as needed.

4. Examination room : It should be co-located with the consultation room or both can be part of the same room with arrangements for privacy for examination of the patient (a curtained off area). It should have adequate space for an examination table, curtains (wheeled, wall-mounted, single-piece), free movement around the examination table, and a wall-mounted cupboard where essential equipment and registers can be kept. Three colours should not be used in clinical service areas of a health facility namely– red/pink, blue and yellow to avoid Service Provision | 25 interference with examining pallor, cyanosis, and icterus respectively. Larger examination rooms/OPDs will be needed for certain specialities, e.g., Dentistry (for dental chair) and Eye care (for vision testing). Ultrasound services, nursing station and separate toilet should be attached/at one place for obstetrics and gynaecology services. The Ultrasound room attached to the obstetric services should contain a patient couch, a chair and adequate space for the equipment. The lighting must be adequate for proper examination. The hand washing facility and toilet should be attached to the ultrasound room. Immunization clinic with waiting room having an area of 3 m × 4 m and cold chain facility in Maternity Wing/Paediatric Clinic should be provided.

5. Counselling room.

6. Sound treated room for audiometry: The inside of the cubicle should not be less than 8ft x 8 ft and have acoustic treatment on wall and ceiling.

7. PFT/ECG room.

8. Health and Wellness room: The health and wellness room is ideally a platform for community interaction for all health education and promotional activities. The room should be provisioned with adequate space to accommodate 18-20 persons and facilities to conduct yoga, group counselling sessions on health, nutrition, adolescent and other health promotional activities. The room should be equipped with training, audio-visual and IEC material.

9. Integrated Clinical and Public Health Laboratory : The layout of the lab should ensure logical flow of specimens from receipt to

disposal. Zoning should clearly identify areas i.e. testing for routine, emergency and critical care cases. There must also be demarcated areas for collection and delivery of reports, sample collection, sample processing, haematology, biochemistry, pathology, and microbiology. A minimum area of 150 m2 is suggested for a lab load with 100 collections.

10. Medical Imaging : Imaging services should be located in a place that is accessible to both OPD and wards and also to the emergency and operation theatre complex. It is essential to install digital imaging facility at all health care facilities which are installing new system. Appropriate structural shielding should be provided for walls, doors, ceilings and floors of the room housing the imaging equipment so that radiation exposures received are kept to the minimum and do not exceed the respective limits for annual effective doses as per directives issued by the Competent Authority. Appropriate overlap of shielding materials should be provided at the joints or discontinuities. Appropriate radiation protection devices such as barriers, aprons, goggles, and thyroid shields should be used during the operation of imaging equipment. TLD badges should be provided to all the operators and workers involved during the imaging procedure. During non-working hours, TLD cards must be stored along with Control TLD card outside the X-ray room (in a radiation-free area). Mobile X-ray equipment, when used as fixed X-ray equipment, shall comply with all the requirements of those of fixed X-ray installation. The movement of mobile X-ray equipment shall be restricted within the institution for which it is registered.

11. Drug Dispensing Counter: The drug dispensing counter should be located in an area conveniently accessible from all clinics. It should be well ventilated, lit, and spacious with each counter ensuring a minimum space of 15-20 square meter.

12. Emergency Care : The emergency wing of a district hospital should be comprehensively created to meet the emergency needs and management of medical, surgical, accidental, burn, and trauma cases. Every DH should have a separate burn unit and all burn cases should directly go there. Similarly, obstetric emergencies should go directly to Labour Delivery Recovery Complex while neonatal emergencies should go directly to SNCU. Polytrauma cases will be directed to

the Polytrauma unit (demarcated in larger facilities – 400-500 bed DH). If such units are not available, all these cases will also report to Emergency. Sub District Hospital and District Hospital should conform to the layout plan as per "Operational and Technical Guidelines on Emergency Services at District Hospitals".

(a) The emergency wing should be planned to keep in mind easy accessibility and quick response.

(b) Emergency service provision through adequately trained human resources for health should be available round-the-clock.

(c) It should preferably have a distinct entry independent of OPD main entry so that minimum time is lost in attending to cases that need resuscitation and also to others requiring emergency management. There should be easy approach and access for ambulances with adequate space for the free passage of vehicles and a covered area for alighting patients.

(d) Stretchers, wheelchairs, and trolleys should be available at the entrance of the emergency at a designated area.

(e) Lay out should be such that it follows the functional flow for clinical management of the patient.

(f) Signage of emergency should be displayed at the entry of the hospital with additional signage at key points.

(g) The Emergency should have a dedicated triage and four clinical management zones (red, yellow, green, black). The triage area should have dedicated space with wall-mounted multipara monitors and medical gas outlets.

(h) Emergency beds earmarked is as follows

Type of Hospital	*No of emergency beds*
SDH 100 beds	11
DH 50 beds	7
DH 100 beds	11
DH 200 beds	21
DH 300 beds	26
DH 400 beds	37
DH 500 beds	44

(i) Separate provision for examination of gender-based violence victims should be made available in the emergency as per GoI guidelines. Provisions for privacy and confidentiality must be maintained.

(j) A separate area for medico-legal cases should be identified.

(k) Duty rooms for doctors/nurses/allied health professionals should be available.

(l) Sufficient separate waiting areas and public amenities for patients and relatives should be available and located in such a way that it does not disturb the effective functioning of the emergency department.

(m) The emergency area should have close linkages with the emergency OT, procedure room, dressing room, plaster room, lab and radiology services, and critical care areas (HDU/ICU). There should be ready access to vital diagnostic and supportive equipment such as ECG, Pulse Oximeter, Cardiac Monitor with Defibrillator, and Multipara Monitor.

(n) An open space equipped with multiple electrical plug points for placing equipment should be earmarked for disaster preparedness. Multiple points should also be available for oxygen and suction apparatus to be used during disasters.

(o) Two isolation beds should be identified for potentially infectious patients.

13. Burn Unit: Burn Unit in a district hospital should preferably be located in a quiet environment, free from noise and other disturbances, contamination, and possible cross-infection. A 3 bedded unit would have 2 beds in ward and one bed earmarked for acute care, six-bedded unit consists of 4 beds in a ward and 2 beds earmarked for acute care and 10 bedded unit 4 should be marked for acute care.

14. Dialysis Unit : The dialysis station should be designed to provide an adequate space area and safe treatment as well as to ensure the privacy of patients. An area of 120 sq. ft. per machine should be provided. The nursing station should be located in an area that allows adequate surveillance of patients on haemodialysis machines. The facilities such as observation rooms, recovery rooms, isolation rooms, RO room should be provisioned.

Type of Hospital	*Number of Dialysis Beds*
SDH 100 beds :	4
DH 50 beds:	4
DH 100 beds:	4
DH 200 beds:	4
DH 300 beds:	8
DH 400 beds:	8
DH 500 beds :	8

15. Critical Care : Critically ill patients requiring highly skilled lifesaving medical aid and nursing care will be admitted here. This will include the continuing management of major surgical, medical cases, severe injuries, head injuries, severe haemorrhage, acute coronary occlusion, kidney, and respiratory catastrophe, poisoning, etc. Generally, HDU beds are for patients which do not require invasive ventilation where any specialist can monitor and manage their condition. ICU beds are for patients whose lives are in danger, requiring ventilator support with backup for super and multispecialty care. every DH should have a hybrid critical care area (HDU +ICU) with both ventilatory and non-ventilatory beds. Ideally creation of a hybrid model having both HDU and ICU beds helps in optimal utilisation of HR and other resources.

Type of Hospital	*Total number of dialysis beds*
SDH 100 beds	16
DH 50 beds	5
DH 100 beds	16
DH 200 beds	22
DH 300 beds	30
DH 400 beds	40
DH 500 beds	45

The room for Hybrid HDU/ICU should be sound treated and air-conditioned with facilities of environmental control for each room. Air-conditioning should ensure 45 -65% humidity, and 23±2°C temperature. Ceilings, flooring and walls should be constructed of materials with high sound adsorption capabilities. The recommended noise level should be in the range of 35-50 decibels. There should be 10-12 air changes per hour and positive air pressure maintained. ICU bed needs a floor space of 25-30 sq mt, paediatric ICU bed needs 12 sq mt and HDU requires 20-24 sq mt per bed. There should be space of 0.9 mt between head end and wall and 3.5 mt between centre of adjacent beds.

16. Operation Theatre Complex: The location of Operation Theatre Complex should be in a quiet environment, free from noise and other disturbances, contamination, and possible cross-infection. Close linkages with the surgical ward, high dependency/ICU, imaging, laboratory, blood bank/storage unit, CSSD/TSSU, and mechanised laundry should be ensured. This unit also needs constant specialised services such as piped suction and medical gas supply, electric supply, heating, air-conditioning (air handling unit), ventilation, and efficient lift service, if the theatres are located on upper floors. Ductless air handling units should be preferred. Zoning should be maintained to keep the theatres free from microorganisms. There should be four well-defined zones of varying degrees of cleanliness/asepsis namely, Protective Zone, Clean Zone, Aseptic or Sterile Zone, and Disposal or Dirty Zone. Normally there are three types of traffic flow, namely, patients, staff, and supplies. All these should be properly channelized. An Operation Theatre Complex should also have a Reception, Pre-operative Room, and Post-Operative Resting Room. The operating room should be made dust-proof. The temperature should be maintained at 21 + 3 degrees Celsius inside the theatre at all times. Corresponding relative humidity should be between 50-60%. Ideally, 20 air exchanges, and out of these, four should be fresh air exchanges per hour. Appropriate devices should be installed inside the OT to monitor and display these conditions. Following parameters needs to be assessed and monitored regularly to ensure effective management of OT complex: y Temperature, humidity inside the OT y Differential pressure inside and outside OT y Maintenance record of Air Handling Unit, frequency of air exchange per hour and cleaning its filter y Last HEPA filtration report and HEPA validation report There should also be a scrub-up room where the operating team washes and scrubs their hands and arms. A pair of surgeon's sinks and elbow or knee operated taps are Essential in the scrub area. There should be a trolley change area for shifting the patient from protective to clean and from clean to

the sterile zone. Laminar flow should be maintained in the operation theatre. It should have a single leaf door with a self-closing device and a viewing window for communication. The Operation Theatre Complex should also have a Sub-Sterilizing Unit (TSSU) attached to the operation theatre limiting its role to cleaning of surgical instruments on an emergency basis only. There should be a storage room to keep functional equipment. This will ensure adequate space inside the theatre. A separate documentation room and pantry for staff are also desirable. Theatre refuses, such as dirty linen, used instruments and other disposable/non-disposable items should be removed in separate zipped bags to a designated room (dirty utility room) after each surgery via hatch box and dirty utility corridor. Non-disposable instruments after an initial wash are given back for instrument sterilization and the rest of the disposable items are disposed of and destroyed. Dirty linen is sent to the laundry through a separate exit/dumb waiter. This room should be provided with a sink, slop sink, workbench, and draining boards. A separate room for trolley wash is also to be provisioned.

Type of Hospital	*Total number of OT's*
SDH 100 beds	3
DH 50 beds	2
DH 100 beds	3
DH 200 beds	4
DH 300 beds	5
DH 400 beds	5
DH 500 beds	5

17. Labour room complex

Since the country has achieved more than 90% institutional deliveries, the focus is now to achieve quality in the delivery of MCH services. Privacy of women must be ensured by having walls between labour beds. Area requirement for one LDR unit (consisting of one labour bed and space for alternate birthing positions) is 225-350 sq. ft. Natural light and views by means of a window are Essential as windows are an important aspect of sensory orientation and psychological well being of mothers. Lighting in the suite should be dimmable. The suite should be located in the labour room complex near the obstetric operation theatres and preferably on the ground floor.

Taking an average length of stay in the LDR as 12 hours and CBR as 20 for a district, the following number of LDR bed requirements have been estimated:

Type of Hospital	*Number of LDR beds*
SDH 100 beds	3
DH 50 beds	3
DH 100 beds	4
DH 200 beds	6
DH 300 beds	10
DH 400 beds	15
DH 500 beds	15

Some of the other important points for consideration of a Labour room complex are:

- It should not be a thoroughfare and have provisions to change footwear at the entry.
- A dedicated triage space should be ensured.
- The unit should be airconditioned with an attached toilet with each labour bed. Drinking water and hot water facilities should be available.
- Separate areas for dirty linen and decontamination should be clearly demarcated.
- Other facilities such as Doctors Duty Room, Nursing Station, Staff changing room, Store with the capacity to keep consumption worth not more than one week should be provisioned.
- Cleanliness shall always be maintained by regular washing and mopping with disinfectants and should be done after every delivery. Close linkages with CSSD and mechanised laundry to be adhered to ensure autoclaved delivery kits and other instruments.
- The area should be away from the draught of air and should have a power connection for plugging in the radiant warmer. A clear floor area should be provided in the room for the newborn corner. It is a space within the labour room, (20-30 sq. ft in size), where a functional radiant warmer is present.

18. Special New-born Care Unit & Mother and New-born Care Unit

Special New-born Care Unit (SNCU) is a neonatal unit that will provide special care (all care except major surgery) for sick newborns. Along with SNCU, certain beds will be designated as neonatal intensive care beds (NICU) for assisted ventilation. In addition to this unit, a ward for mothers and babies to stay together – Mother and New-born Care Unit (MNCU) should also be provided which should not be less than SNCU beds. Adjustable beds to facilitate kangaroo mother care should be made available in the MNCU. The location of the unit should be in a quiet environment, free from noise and other disturbances, contamination, and possible cross-infection. Close linkages with the labour room complex, nutritional rehabilitation centre, and district early intervention centre should be ensured. The unit should comprise of Triage and Reception area for receiving cases and assessing in the triage area. A Waiting Area in front of MNCU with simple amenities like comfortable sitting space, safe drinking water, AV system, Tea/ Coffee vending machine, and a washroom for the parents or attendants should be provided. Follow up area to be provisioned for with AV facilities and adequate space for daily counselling, during discharge and imparting Family Participatory Care (FPC) training.

Type of Hospital	*Number of SNCU beds*	*Number of beds with assisted Ventilation (NICU)*
SDH 100 beds	12	-
DH 50 beds	6	-
DH 100 beds	12	4
DH 200 beds	16	4
DH 300 beds	20	6
DH 400 beds	24	6
DH 500 beds	24	8

19. DEIC: District Early Intervention Centre

Developmental impairment is a common problem in children's health that occurs in approximately 10% of the childhood population and even more among "at-risk" children discharged from the sick newborn care unit. Research has proved that the period from birth to 6 years are the most critical years for all children. After screening and identification of any of the 4Ds i.e. Defects at Birth, Deficiencies, Diseases and Developmental delays including disabilities, the cases get referred to the DEIC. DEIC should comprise of the following space/ rooms (ideal size of DEIC would be approx. 4900-5000 sq. feet):

- Waiting space
- Play/therapy area
- Reception space for Registration including anthropometry
- Paediatrician and Medical officer room
- Dental examination room (Dental Doctor/Dental technician)
- Vision testing room
- Hearing testing room: soundproof room having two partitions -One smaller and separated by one way looking glass with carpeted and double doors
- Speech room with looking mirror extending from the floor to one and a half feet above the level of the table
- Early intervention room cum occupational therapy room
- Psychological testing room
- Laboratory
- Nursing/nutrition room cum Feeding room
- Sensory integration room
- ECG cum Echo room
- Computer room (Manager/DEO) including Store
- Pantry and space for drinking water and washing
- Toilets (gender based, staff - all equipped with facilities for handicapped)
- Open space
- Outer sensory garden (Desirable)

20. Nutritional Rehabilitation Centre (NRC)

Nutrition Rehabilitation Centre (NRC) is a unit in a health facility where sick children with Severe Acute Malnutrition (SAM) are admitted and managed. It should comprise of following areas:

- Reception

- Play Area
- Counselling Area
- Nursing Station
- Kitchen with cooking demonstration aids
- Store
- Toilets

21. Inpatient wards

For larger facilities, a typical ward would accommodate about 30 patients. The beds should be placed either on one side or both sides of a nursing station ensuring good visibility and ventilation. Wherever possible, segregation of beds based on gender to maintain dignity and ensure privacy (with access to separate toilets and bathing spaces) should be ensured. Toilets should be conveniently located. Every ward should have a procedure room, a small store that can accommodate supplies of drugs and linen for five to seven days, a pantry and a janitors/housekeeping room. A changing room will help ensure the privacy and dignity of patients. All beds in the ward should have a wall fitted cupboard for the patient's belongings. Call bells with switches for all beds should be provided in all types of wards with indicator lights and with the location indicator situated in the nurse's duty room. In every ward, one-third of the beds should be demarcated with a separate port for oxygen, suction and air so that patients can be provided emergency or short-term support. Apart from general wards, certain beds for patients should be demarcated for isolation. The number will depend on the total number of beds in the district hospital. The table depicting the number of isolation beds is given above. The isolation rooms should be separated from general wards, have negative air pressure and at least 6 air changes per hour.

22. Record keeping room

In light of the Right to Information Act 2005 in the health facilities a proper system of collection, sorting, filing, indexing and storage of documents along with quick retrieval should be designed for effective and efficient record keeping management. Digitization of records wherever possible should be done while adhering to the data security guidelines of GOI.

23. Store-room

Health facilities should have adequate and spacious stores located away from patient traffic with facilities for storing drugs, consumables, linen, furniture, equipment, and sundry articles. Based on the nature and number of items, the main store may be divided into sub-stores such as medical and drug stores, surgical stores, furniture, and equipment, general, linen, and stationery stores. Depending on the volume of items requiring temperature control during storage, an adequate number of refrigerators/walk-in coolers should be available. A separate inspection and stock holding section/area should be provisioned for so that there is no chance of mixing old and new stocks.

24. Knowledge hub

District hospitals should aim to be developed as knowledge hubs in order to enhance the quality of health workers' education and training. Infrastructure for conducting medical, nursing, and allied health teaching and training as based on their respective curriculum requirements should be developed. The infrastructure for the knowledge hub at a district hospital includes the below-mentioned areas

- Medical courses (DNB) including Teaching/Seminar rooms, Faculty room/Staff Room, Library (with internet facility), Hostel, Canteen/Pantry etc.
- Skill Lab
- Training for Allied Health Professionals
- B.Sc. Nursing Schools & Post Nursing specialities.

25. Administrative unit.

Administrative block with the provision of the Medical Superintendents Office and the following areas should be provided:

- Office including administrative rooms for MS, Nursing I/c, Hospital Manager.
- Meeting Hall
- Record Room
- Staff Room/cubicles including Establishment and Accounts (number to be based on number of administrative staff)
- Pantry

The administrative unit/block should be located on the top floor of the main hospital building and away from clinical areas, wherever feasible.

26. Nurses

Nurse bed ratio is as given below: (Beds: Nurse)

General ward- 1:6

ICU - 1:1

HDU- 1:2

SNCU- 1:3

NICU/PICU/Ped HDU- 1:2 (Considering an 8-hour shift, three shifts to cover a 24-hour period).

27. Medical Lab Technologist/Lab Technicians

All Medical lab technologist/Lab technicians will perform integrated functions even if their source of salary is from different programmes. All district labs will be functional 24x7. For the Blood bank, number of lab staff also provisioned for as per Schedule F, Part XII B, Drugs and Cosmetics Act, 1940.

28. Pharmacist

It has been estimated that a pharmacist will dispense about 120 prescriptions/day. Additionally, a senior pharmacist also needs to maintain drug and equipment inventory.

Other support areas required are as follows:

- Blood Bank& Blood Storage Units
- Central Sterile services unit
- Laundry
- Dietary Services
- Manifold and Medical Gas pipeline.
- Residential quarters
- Guest House
- Mortuary

Minimum performance standards for Specialist & Health care staff

Medical Officer OPD = 75 patient/day

IPD assistance with specialists

OT assistance, emergency and other duties

General Medicine OPD = 60 pts/day

IPD = 20 pts/day

10 procedures/week

General Surgery OPD= 60 pts/day

IPD= 20 pts/day

OT= 7 major surgeries/week

Obstetrics & Gynecologist

OPD= 60 pts/day

IPD= 20 pts/day

OT= 7 major surgeries/week

Pediatrician

OPD= 60 pts/day

IPD= 20 pts/day

10 Procedures/week

Orthopedic OPD= 60 pts/day

IPD= 20 pts/day

OT= 7 major surgeries/week

Anesthesiologist As per the surgical requirement in OT's, in-charge and emergency services, pain clinics

Ophthalmologist OPD= 60 pts/day

IPD= 20 pts/day

OT= 10 major surgeries/week

Dentist OPD = 20 pts/day

Dental Procedures= 8-10

ENT OPD= 60 pts/day

IPD= 20 pts/day

OT= 7 major surgeries/week

Psychiatry OPD= 20-30 pts/day

IPD= Admitted Psychiatric cases

Consultation for referred patient

Radiologist Reporting on imaging (X-ray, CT scan, Ultrasound etc.) – 20-30pts/day

Conducting diagnostic tests, supervising and mentoring technicians

Technical advice to doctors/nurses

Teaching and training

Service Provision

Staff (Desirable) Break up of activities

Dermatologist OPD= 60 patient/day

IPD= Technical advice for in-patients

Minor surgeries (Skin biopsies, cauterization etc.)

Cardiologist OPD= 40 pts/day

Conducting and supervising Echocardiography, Doppler test, Treadmill test and other cardiac tests.

Nephrologist y OPD = 40 pts/day

Monitoring dialysis patient (Morning and evening)

IPD = 20 pts/day

Urologist OPD= 40 pts/day

IPD= 15 pts/day

OT= 7 major surgeries/week

Cystoscopy and other procedures

Gastroenterologist (surgical and medical)

OPD= 40 pts/day

IPD= 15 pts/day

Endoscopy, Coloscopy and other procedures

Assuming an 8-hour shift and 75% of productivity and efficiency, it is estimated that there will be 6 hour working time for 6 days a week.

Both surgical and medical specialist are expected to conduct IPD rounds every day.

If a doctor is nominated as the nodal officer for a National Health Programme, one day per week may be dedicated to provide support to that programme (Administrative duties, monitoring, training, supervision etc. This could also be spread out on a day to day basis (e.g. 2 hours/day for national programme work).

It is assumed that each surgical specialist would be having 3 OPD days and 3 OT days each week. Each surgical specialist is expected to perform at least 7 major surgeries in a week. For medical specialist with no OT duties, the OPD will be all days in a week. Both medical and surgical specialist are expected to make IPD rounds every day.

One GDMO for each specialist has been proposed to strengthen the service delivery and also to support the specialist in teaching and training. These GDMOs will work only in that speciality for which they are hired for.

Reference

1. INDIAN PUBLIC HEALTH STANDARDS; SUB DISTRICT HOSPITAL and DISTRICT HOSPITAL : 2022; Volume I, National Health Mission : Ministry of Health & Family Welfare.

16

Important Legislations

The Right to Information Act (15th June 2005)

This act is called the Right to Information Act, 2005. An act is to provide for setting out the practical regime of right to Information for citizens to secure access to information under the control of public authorities in order to promote transparency and accountability in the working of every public authority. Subject to the provisions of this act, all citizens have the right to information.

Every public authority shall—

(a) maintain all its records duly catalogued and indexed in a manner and the form which facilitates the right to information under this Act and ensure that all records that are appropriate to be computerised are, within a reasonable time and subject to availability of resources, computerised and connected through a network all over the country on different systems so that access to such records is facilitated; b) publish within one hundred and twenty days from the enactment of this Act,—

(i) the particulars of its organisation, functions and duties; (ii) the powers and duties of its officers and employees; (iii) the procedure followed in the decision making process, including channels of supervision and accountability; (iv) the norms set by it for the discharge of its functions; (v) the rules, regulations, instructions, manuals and records, held by it or under its control or used by its employees for discharging its functions; (vi) a statement of the categories of documents that are held by it or under its control; (vii) the particulars of any arrangement that exists for consultation with, or representation by, the members of the public in relation to the formulation of its policy or implementation thereof; (viii) a statement of the boards, councils, committees and other bodies consisting of two or more persons constituted as its part or for the purpose of its advice, and as to whether meetings of those boards, councils, committees and other bodies are open to the public, or the minutes of such meetings are accessible for public; (ix) a directory of its officers and employees; (x) the monthly remuneration received by each of its officers and employees, including the system of compensation as provided in its regulations; (xi) the budget allocated to each of its agency, indicating the particulars of all plans, proposed expenditures and reports on disbursements made; (xii) the manner of execution of subsidy programmes, including the amounts allocated and the details of beneficiaries of such programmes; (xiii) particulars of recipients of concessions, permits or authorisations granted by it; (xiv) details in respect of the information, available to or held by it, reduced in an electronic form; (xv) the particulars of facilities available to citizens for obtaining information, including the working hours of a library or reading room, if maintained for public use; (xvi) the names, designations and other particulars of the Public Information Officers; (xvii) such other information as may be prescribed; and thereafter update these publications every year;

(c) publish all relevant facts while formulating important policies or announcing the decisions which affect public; d) provide reasons for its administrative or quasi-judicial decisions to affected persons.

(2) It shall be a constant endeavour of every public authority to take steps in accordance with the requirements of clause (b) of sub-section (1) to provide as much information suo motu to the public at regular intervals through various means of communications, including

internet, so that the public have minimum resort to the use of this Act to obtain information.

(3) For the purposes of sub-section (1), every information shall be disseminated widely and in such form and manner which is easily accessible to the public.

(4) All materials shall be disseminated taking into consideration the cost effectiveness, local language and the most effective method of communication in that local area and the information should be easily accessible, to the extent possible in electronic format with the Central Public Information Officer or State Public Information Officer, as the case may be, available free or at such cost of the medium or the print cost price as may be prescribed.

Every public authority has to designate as many officers as the Central Public Information Officers or State Public Information Officers, as the case may be, in all administrative units or officers under it as may be necessary to provide information to persons requesting for the information under this Act. A person, who desires to obtain any information in national or in the official language of the area in which the application is being made, accompanying such fee as may be prescribed, to public authority requesting for an information, which is held by another public authority but is closely related, the public authority to which such application is made, has to transfer the application or such part of it as may be appropriate to that other public authority and inform the applicant immediately about such transfer. Public Information Officer, as the case may be, on receipt of a request must, as expeditiously as possible, and in any case within thirty days of the receipt of the request, either provide the information on payment of such fee as may be prescribed or reject the request for any of the reasons specified in sections 8 and 9. Provided that where the information sought for concerns the life or liberty of a person, the same should be provided within forty-eight hours of the receipt of the request. Where a request has been rejected public Information Officer should communicate to the person making the request, the reasons for such rejection and the period within which an appeal against such rejection may be preferred. There shall be no obligation to give any citizen information, disclosure of which would prejudicially affect the sovereignty and integrity of India, the security, strategic, scientific or economic interests of the state, relation with foreign state or lead to incitement of an offence, information including commercial confidence, trade secrets or intellectual property, the disclosure of which would harm the competitive position of a third party or any other reason as specified in law. The Central Information Commission consists of Chief Information Commissioner and such number of Central Information Commissioners, not exceeding ten, as may be deemed necessary. The Chief Information Commissioner and Information Commissioners are appointed by the president on the recommendation of a committee consisting of Prime Minister who is the chairperson of the committee, the Leader of Opposition in the Lok Sabha and a Union cabinet Minister to be nominated by the Prime Minister. The chief Information commissioner and information Commissioners are persons of eminence in public life with wide knowledge and experience in law, science and technology, social service, management, journalism, mass media or administration and governance. They must not hold any other office of profit or be connected with any political party or carry on any business or pursue any profession. The State Information commission consists of the State chief information commissioner, and such number of State Information commissioners, not exceeding ten, as may be deemed necessary. The State Chief Information commissioner and the State Information Commissioners are appointed by the Governor on the recommendation of a committee consisting of Chief Minister who is the Chairperson of the committee, the Leader of Opposition in the Legislative Assembly and a Cabinet Minister to be nominated by the Chief Minister. The State Chief Information Commissioner and State Information Commissioners are persons of eminence in public life with wide knowledge and experience in law, science and technology, social service, management, journalism, mass media or administration and governance. They do not hold any other office of profit or connected with any political party or carry on any business or pursue any profession.

If the Central Public Information Officer or State Public Information Officer, as the case may be, fails to give decision on the request for information within the period specified under sub-section (1), the Central Public Information Officer or State Public Information Officer, as the case may be, shall be deemed to have refused the request.

Where a decision is taken to provide the information on payment of any further fee representing the cost of providing the information, the Central Public Information Officer or State Public Information Officer, as the case may be, shall send an intimation to the person making the request, giving—

(a) the details of further fees representing the cost of providing the information as determined by him, together with the calculations made to arrive at the amount in accordance with fee prescribed under subsection (1), requesting him to deposit that fees, and the period intervening between the dispatch of the said intimation and payment of fees shall be excluded for the purpose of calculating the period of thirty days referred to in that sub-section;

(b) information concerning his or her right with respect to review the decision as to the amount of fees charged or the form of access provided, including the particulars of the appellate authority, time limit, process and any other forms.

Where access to the record or a part thereof is required to be provided under this Act and the person to whom access is to be provided is disabled, the Central Public Information Officer or State Public Information Officer, as the case may be, shall provide assistance to enable access to the information, including providing such assistance as may be appropriate for the inspection.

Where access to information is to be provided in the printed or in any electronic format, the applicant shall, subject to the provisions of sub-section (6), pay such fee as may be prescribed:

Provided that the fee prescribed under sub-section (1) of section 6 and sub-sections (1) and (5) of section 7 shall be reasonable and no such fee shall be charged from the persons who are of below poverty line as may be determined by the appropriate Government.

Notwithstanding anything contained in sub-section (5), the person making request for the information shall be provided the information free of charge where a public authority fails to comply with the time limits specified in sub-section (1).

Before taking any decision under sub-section (1), the Central Public Information Officer or State Public Information Officer, as the case may be, shall take into consideration the representation made by a third party under section 11.

Where a request has been rejected under sub-section (1), the Central Public Information Officer or State Public Information Officer, as the case may be, shall communicate to the person making the request,—

(i) the reasons for such rejection; (ii) the period within which an appeal against such rejection may be preferred; and (iii) the particulars of the appellate authority.

An information shall ordinarily be provided in the form in which it is sought unless it would disproportionately divert the resources of the public authority or would be detrimental to the safety or preservation of the record in question.

Notwithstanding anything contained in this Act, there shall be no obligation to give any citizen,—

(a) information, disclosure of which would prejudicially affect the sovereignty and integrity of India, the security, strategic, scientific or economic interests of the State, relation with foreign State or lead to incitement of an offence;
(b) information which has been expressly forbidden to be published by any court of law or tribunal or the disclosure of which may constitute contempt of court.
(c) information, the disclosure of which would cause a breach of privilege of Parliament or the State Legislature;
(d) information including commercial confidence, trade secrets or intellectual property, the disclosure of which would harm the competitive position of a third party, unless the competent authority is satisfied that larger public interest warrants the disclosure of such information;
(e) information available to a person in his fiduciary relationship, unless the competent authority is satisfied that the larger public interest warrants the disclosure of such information;
(f) information received in confidence from foreign Government;
(g) information, the disclosure of which would endanger the life or physical safety of any person the source of information or

assistance given in confidence for law enforcement or security purposes;

(h) information which would impede the process of investigation or apprehension or prosecution of offenders;

(i) cabinet papers including records of deliberations of the Council of Ministers, Secretaries and other officers:

Provided that the decisions of Council of Ministers, the reasons thereof, and the material on the basis of which the decisions were taken shall be made public after the decision has been taken, and the matter is complete, or over:

Provided further that those matters which come under the exemptions specified in this section shall not be disclosed;

(j) information which relates to personal information the disclosure of which has no relationship to any public activity or interest, or which would cause unwarranted invasion of the privacy of the individual unless the Central Public Information Officer or the State Public Information Officer or the appellate authority, as the case may be, is satisfied that the larger public interest justifies the disclosure of such information:

Provided that the information which cannot be denied to the Parliament or a State Legislature shall not be denied to any person.

Notwithstanding anything in the Official Secrets Act, 1923 nor any of the exemptions permissible in accordance with sub-section (1), a public authority may allow access to information, if public interest in disclosure outweighs the harm to the protected interests.

Subject to the provisions of clauses (a), (c) and (i) of sub-section (1), any information relating to any occurrence, event or matter which has taken place, occurred or happened twenty years before the date on which any request is made under secton 6 shall be provided to any person making a request under that section: Provided that where any question arises as to the date from which the said period of twenty years has to be computed, the decision of the Central Government shall be final, subject to the usual appeals provided for in this Act.

Without prejudice to the provisions of section 8, a Central Public Information Officer or a State Public Information Officer, as the case may be, may reject a request for information where such a request for providing access would involve an infringement of copyright subsisting in a person other than the State. Where a request for access to information is rejected on the ground that it is in relation to information which is exempt from disclosure, then, notwithstanding anything contained in this Act, access may be provided to that part of the record which does not contain any information which is exempt from disclosure under this Act and which can reasonably be severed from any part that contains exempt information.

Where access is granted to a part of the record under sub-section (1), the Central Public Information Officer or State Public Information Officer, as the case may be, shall give a notice to the applicant, informing—

> (a) that only part of the record requested, after severance of the record containing information which is exempt from disclosure, is being provided; (b) the reasons for the decision, including any findings on any material question of fact, referring to the material on which those findings were based; (c) the name and designation of the person giving the decision; (d) the details of the fees calculated by him or her and the amount of fee which the applicant is required to deposit; and (e) his or her rights with respect to review of the decision regarding non-disclosure of part of the information, the amount of fee charged or the form of access provided, including the particulars of the senior officer specified under sub-section (1) of section 19 or the Central Information Commission or the State Information Commission, as the case may be, time limit, process and any other form of access. If the record is voluminous, citizen has a right to inspect the records of a public authority. For inspection of records, the public authority shall charge no fee for the first hour but a fee of rupees five for each subsequent hour shall be charged. However only such information is required to be supplied under the act which already exists and is held by the public authority. PIO is not supposed to create information or to interpret information or to solve the problems raised by theapplicants or to furnish replies to hypothetical questions.

Where a Central Public Information Officer or a State Public Information Officer, as the case may be, intends to disclose any information or record, or part thereof on a request made under this Act, which relates to or has been supplied by a third party and has been treated as confidential by that third party, the Central Public Information Officer or State Public Information Officer, as the case may be, shall, within five days from the receipt of the request, give a written notice to such third party of the request and of the fact that the Central Public Information Officer or State Public Information Officer, as the case may be, intends to disclose the information or record, or part thereof, and invite the third party to make a submission in writing or orally, regarding whether the information should be disclosed, and such submission of the third party shall be kept in view while taking a decision about disclosure of information:

(2) Where a notice is served by the Central Public Information Officer or State Public Information Officer, as the case may be, under sub-section (1) to a third party in respect of any information or record or part thereof, the third party shall, within ten days from the date of receipt of such notice, be given the opportunity to make representation against the proposed disclosure.

(3) Notwithstanding anything contained in section 7, the Central Public Information Officer or State Public Information Officer, as the case may be, shall, within forty days after receipt of the request under section 6, if the third party has been given an opportunity to make representation under sub-section (2), make a decision as to whether or not to disclose the information or record or part thereof and give in Grounds for rejection to access in certain cases.

(4) A notice given under sub-section (3) shall include a statement that the third party to whom the notice is given is entitled to prefer an appeal under section 19 against the decision.

Where the Central Information Commission or the State Information Commission, as the case may be, at the time of deciding any complaint or appeal is of the opinion that the Central Public Information Officer or the State Public Information Officer, as the case may be, has, without any reasonable cause, refused to receive an application for information or has not furnished information within the time specified under sub-section (1) of section 7 or malafidely denied the request for information or knowingly given incorrect, incomplete or misleading information or destroyed information which was the subject of the request or obstructed in any manner in furnishing the information, it shall impose a penalty of two hundred and fifty rupees each day till application is received or information is furnished, so however, the total amount of such penalty shall not exceed twenty-five thousand rupees:

Provided that the Central Public Information Officer or the State Public Information Officer, as the case may be, shall be given a reasonable opportunity of being heard before any penalty is imposed on him: Provided further that the burden of proving that he acted reasonably and diligently shall be on the Central Public Information Officer or the State Public Information Officer, as the case may be.

The Central Information Commission or State Information Commission, as the case may be, shall, as soon as practicable after the end of each year, prepare a report on the implementation of the provisions of this Act during that year and forward a copy thereof to the appropriate Government.

Each report shall state in respect of the year to which the report relates,—

the number of requests made to each public authority; (b) the number of decisions where applicants were not entitled to access to the documents pursuant to the requests, the provisions of this Act under which these decisions were made and the number of times such provisions were invoked; (c) the number of appeals referred to the Central Information Commission or State Information Commission, as the case may be, for review, the nature of the appeals and the outcome of the appeals; (d) particulars of any disciplinary action taken against any officer in respect of the administration of this Act; (e) the amount of charges collected by each public authority under this Act; (f) any facts which indicate an effort by the public authorities to administer and implement the spirit and intention of this Act; (g) recommendations for reform, including recommendations in respect of the particular public authorities, for the development, improvement, modernisation, reform or amendment to this Act or other legislation or common law or any other matter relevant for operationalising the right to access information.

The right to information (amendment) act, 2019 no. 24 of 2019 an Act to amend the Right to Information Act, 2005. Be it enacted by Parliament in the Seventieth Year of the Republic of India as follows:— 1. (1) This Act may be called the Right to Information (Amendment) Act, 2019. (2) It shall come into force on such date as the Central Government may, by notification in the Official Gazette, appoint. 2. In the Right to Information Act, 2005 (hereinafter referred to as the principal Act), in section 13,— (a) in sub-section (1), for the words "for a term of five years from the date on which he enters upon his office", the words "for such term as may be prescribed by the Central Government" shall be substituted; (b) in sub-section (2), for the words "for a term of five years from the date on which he enters upon his office", the words "for such term as may be prescribed by the Central Government" shall be substituted.

THE PRE-NATAL DIAGNOSTIC TECHNIQUES (REGULATION AND PREVENTION OF MISUSE) ACT, 1994 Amended 2003

An act to provide for the regulation of the use of pre-natal diagnostic techniques for the purpose of detecting genetic or metabolic disorders or chromosomal abnormalities or certain congenital malformation or sex linked disorders and for the prevention of the misuse of such techniques for the purpose of pre-natal sex determination leading to female foeticide, and for matters connected there with or incidental thereto. "Pre-natal diagnostic test" means ultrasonography or any test or analysis of amniotic fluid, chorionic villi, blood or any tissue of a pregnant woman conducted to detect genetic or metabolic disorders or chromosomal abnormalities or congenital anomalies or haemoglobinopathies or sex-linked diseases. No Genetic Counselling Centre, Genetic Laboratory or Genetic Clinic unless registered under this act, shall conduct or associate with, or help in conducting activities relating to prenatal diagnostic technique or employ any person who does not possess the prescribed qualifications. No medical geneticist, gynaecologist, paediatrician, registered medical practitioner or any other person shall conduct or aid in conducting by himself or through any person, any prenatal diagnostic technique at a place other than a place registered under this act. No prenatal diagnostic technique shall be conducted except for the purposes of detection of any of the following abnormalities, namely chromosomal abnormalities, genetic metabolic diseases, haemoglobinopathies, sex-linked genetic disease. No prenatal diagnostic technique shall be used or conducted unless the person qualified to do so is satisfied that any of the following conditions are fulfilled, namely: 1)age of the pregnant woman is above thirty five years II) the pregnant woman has undergone two or more spontaneous abortions or fetal loss, III) the pregnant woman had been exposed to potentially teratogenic agents such as drugs, radiation, infections or chemicals, (iv) the pregnant woman has a family history of mental retardation or physical deformities such as spasticity or any other genetic disease. No person, being a relative or the husband of the pregnant woman shall seek or encourage the conduct of any pre-natal diagnostic techniques on her except as specified in the act. No person conducting pre-natal diagnostic procedure shall communicate to the pregnant woman concerned or her relatives the sex of the fetus by words, signs or in any other manner.

Main provisions in the act are: The Act provides for the prohibition of sex selection, before or after conception.

It regulates the use of pre-natal diagnostic techniques, like ultrasound and amniocentesis by allowing them their use only to detect:

- genetic abnormalities
- metabolic disorders
- chromosomal abnormalities
- certain congenital malformations
- haemoglobinopathies
- sex linked disorders.

  • No laboratory or centre or clinic will conduct any test including ultrasonography for the purpose of determining the sex of the foetus.
  • No person, including the one who is conducting the procedure as per the law, will communicate the sex of the foetus to the pregnant woman or her relatives by words, signs or any other method.
  • Any person who puts an advertisement for pre-natal and pre-conception sex determination facilities in the form

of a notice, circular, label, wrapper or any document, or advertises through interior or other media in electronic or print form or engages in any visible representation made by means of hoarding, wall painting, signal, light, sound, smoke or gas, can be imprisoned for up to three years and fined Rs. 10,000.

The Central Supervisory Board is constituted by central government to exercise the powers and perform the function conferred on the Board under this act. The board consists of Minister in-charge of the Ministry or Department of Family welfare who is the Chairman, Secretary to the Government of India in-charge of the department of family Welfare, who shall be the Vice-Chairman, two members appointed by the Central Government to represent the Ministries of central Government in-charge of Woman and Child Development, law and Justice, Director of Health Services of the Central Government, ten members to be appointed by the Central Government, two each from amongst eminent medical geneticists, eminent gynaecologists and obstetricians, eminent paediatricians, eminent social scientists and representatives of woman welfare organizations, three women of Parliament of whom two are elected by the House of the People and one by the Council of State, four members appointed by the Central Government by rotation to represent the State and Union territories. The board performs following function: advice the Government on policy matters relating to use of pre-natal diagnostic techniques, review implementation of the act and the rules made there-under and recommend changes in the said act and rules to the Central Government, create public awareness against the practice of prenatal determination of sex and female foeticide, lay down code of conduct to be observed by persons working at Genetic Counselling Center, Genetic Laboratories and Genetic Clinics and any other functions as may be specified under the act. Any deviation from law by any individual would mean fine of an amount from ten thousand to fifty thousand and imprisonment for a period of three to five years.

TRANSPLANTATION OF HUMAN ORGANS ACT 1994 (Amended 2003, 2011,2014)

These rules are called the Transplantation of Human Organs and Tissues Rules, 2014.

Subject to the provisions of Section 3 of the Act, a living person may authorise the removal of any organ or tissue of his or her body during his or her lifetime as per prevalent medical practices, for therapeutic purposes in the manner and on such conditions as specified.

For the purpose of certifying the brain-stem death, the Appropriate Authority shall maintain a panel of experts, in accordance with the provisions of the Act, to ensure efficient functioning of the Board of Medical Experts and it remains fully operational.

Duties of the registered medical practitioner.—

(1) The registered medical practitioner of the hospital having Intensive Care Unit facility, in consultation with transplant coordinator, if available, shall ascertain, after certification of brain stem death of the person in Intensive Care Unit, from his or her adult near relative or, if near relative is not available, then, any other person related by blood or marriage, and in case of unclaimed body, from the person in lawful possession of the body the following, namely:-

(a) whether the person had, in the presence of two or more witnesses (at least one of who is a near relative of such person), unequivocally authorised before his or her death as specified in Form 7 or in documents like driving license, etc. wherein the provision for donation may be incorporated after notification of these rules, the removal of his or her organ(s) or tissue(s) including eye, after his or her death, for therapeutic purposes and there is no reason to believe that the person had subsequently revoked the aforesaid authorization.

(b) where the said authorisation was not made by the person to donate his or her organ(s) or tissue(s) after his or her death, then the registered medical practitioner in consultation with the transplant coordinator, if available, shall make the near relative or person in lawful possession of the body, aware of the option to authorise or decline the donation of such human organs or tissues or both (which can be used for therapeutic purposes) including eye or cornea of the deceased person and a declaration or authorisation to this effect shall be ascertained from the near relative or person in lawful possession of the body as per Form 8 to record the status of consent, and in case of an unclaimed body, authorisation shall be made in Form 9 by the authorised official as per sub-section (1) of section 5 of the Act.

(c) after the near relative or person in lawful possession of the body authorises removal and gives consent for donation of human organ(s) or tissue(s) of the deceased person, the registered medical practitioner through the transplant coordinator shall inform the authorised registered Human Organ Retrieval Centre through authorised coordinating organisation by available documentable mode of communication, for removal, storage or transportation of organ(s) or tissue(s).

(2) The registered medical practitioner shall, before removing any human organ or tissue from a living donor, shall satisfy himself –

(a) that the donor has been explained of all possible side effects, hazards and complications and that the donor has given his or her authorisation in appropriate Form 1 for near relative donor or Form 2 for spousal donor or Form 3 for donor other than near relative.

(b) that the physical and mental evaluation of the donor has been done, he or she is in proper state of health and it has been certified that he or she is not mentally challenged and that he or she is fit to donate the organ or tissue provided that in case of doubt regarding mentally challenged status of the donor the registered medical practitioner may get the donor examined by a psychiatrist and the registered medical practitioner shall sign the certificate as prescribed in Form 4 for this purpose.

(c) that the donor is a near relative of the recipient, as certified in Form 5, and that he or she has submitted an application in Form 11 jointly with the recipient and that the proposed donation has been approved by the competent authority as defined at rule 2(c) and specified in Form 19 and that the necessary documents as prescribed and medical tests, as required, to determine the factum of near relationship, have been examined to the satisfaction of the registered medical practitioner and the competent authority.

(d) that in case the recipient is spouse of the donor, the donor has given a statement to the effect that they are so related by signing a certificate in Form 2 and has submitted an application in Form 11 jointly with the recipient and that the proposed donation has been approved by the competent authority under the provisions of sub-rule (2) of rule 7.

(e) that in case of a donor who is other than a near relative and has signed Form 3 and submitted an application in Form 11 jointly with the recipient, the permission from the Authorisation Committee for the said donation has been obtained.

(f) that if a donor or recipient is a foreign national, the approval of the Authorisation Committee for the said donation has been obtained.

(g) living organ or tissue donation by minors shall not be permitted except on exceptional medical grounds to be recorded in detail with full justification and with prior approval of the Appropriate Authority and the State Government concerned.

(3) A registered medical practitioner, before removing any organ or tissue from the body of a person after his or her death (deceased donor), in consultation with transplant coordinator, shall satisfy himself the following, namely:-

(a) that caution has been taken to make inquiry, from near relative or person in lawful possession of the body of a person admitted in Intensive Care Unit, only after certification of Brain Stem death of the person that the donor had, in the presence of two or more witnesses (at least one of whom is a near relative of such person),unequivocally authorised before his or her death as specified in Form 7 or in documents like driving license etc. (wherein the provision for donation may be incorporated after notification of these rules), the removal of his or her organ(s) or tissue(s) after his or her death, for therapeutic purposes and it has been ascertained that the donor has not subsequently revoked the aforesaid authorisation, and the consent of near relative or person in lawful possession of the body shall also be required notwithstanding the authorization been made by deceased donor provided that if the deceased person who had earlier given authorisation but had revoked it subsequently and if the person had given in writing that his organ should not be removed after his death, then, no organ or tissue will be removed even if consent is given by the near relative or person in lawful possession of the body.

(b) that the near relative of the deceased person or the person lawfully in possession of the body of the deceased donor has signed the declaration as specified in Form 8.

(c) that in the case of brain-stem death of the potential donor, a certificate as specified in Form 10 has been signed by all the members of the Board of Medical Experts referred to in sub-section (6) of section 3 of the Act Provided that where a neurologist or a neurosurgeon is not available, an anesthetist or intensivist who is not part of the transplant team nominated by the head of the hospital duly empanelled by Appropriate Authority may certify the brain stem death as a member of the said Board.

(d) that in the case of brain-stem death of a person of less than eighteen years of age, a certificate specified in Form 10 has been signed by all the members of the Board of Medical Experts referred to in sub-section (6) of section 3 of the Act and an authority as specified in Form 8 has been signed by either of the parents of such person or any near relative authorised by the parent.

(4). Procedure for donation of organ or tissue in medicolegal cases.

It shall be ensured that, by retrieving organs, the determination of the cause of death is not jeopardised. The medical report in respect of the organs or tissues being retrieved shall be prepared at the time of retrieval by retrieving doctor and shall be taken on record in postmortem notes by the registered medical practitioner. Wherever it is possible, attempt should be made to request the designated postmortem registered medical practitioner, even beyond office timing, to be present at the time of organ or tissue retrieval doing postmortem.

(5) Authorisation Committee

The medical practitioner who will be part of the organ transplantation team for carrying out transplantation operation shall not be a member of the Authorisation Committee. When the proposed donor or recipient or both are not Indian nationals or citizens whether near relatives or otherwise, the Authorisation Committee shall consider all such requests and the transplantation shall not be permitted if the recipient is a foreign national and donor is an Indian national unless they are near relatives.

When the proposed donor and the recipient are not near relatives, the Authorisation Committee shall,-

(i) evaluate that there is no commercial transaction between the recipient and the donor and that no payment has been made to the donor or promised to be made to the donor or any other person.

(ii) prepare an explanation of the link between them and the circumstances which led to the offer being made.

(iii) examine the reasons why the donor wishes to donate.

(iv) examine the documentary evidence of the link, e.g. proof that they have lived together, etc..

(v) examine old photographs showing the donor and the recipient together.

(vi) evaluate that there is no middleman or tout involved.

(vii) evaluate that financial status of the donor and the recipient by asking them to give appropriate evidence of their vocation and income for the previous three financial years and any gross disparity between the status of the two must be evaluated in the backdrop of the objective of preventing commercial dealing.

(viii) ensure that the donor is not a drug addict.

(ix) ensure that the near relative or if near relative is not available, any adult person related to donor by blood or marriage of the proposed unrelated donor is interviewed regarding awareness about his or her intention to donate an organ or tissue, the authenticity of the link between the donor and the recipient, and the reasons for donation, and any strong views or disagreement or objection of such kin shall also be recorded and taken note of.

(x) Cases of swap donation referred to under subsection (3A) of section 9 of the Act shall be approved by Authorisation Committee of hospital or district or State in which transplantation is proposed to be done and the donation of organs shall be permissible only from near relatives of the swap recipients.

(xi) When the recipient is in a critical condition in need of life saving organ transplantation within a week, the donor or recipient may approach hospital in-charge to expedite evaluation by the Authorisation Committee.

(6) Removal and preservation of organs or tissues.—The removal of the organ(s) or tissue(s) shall be permissible in any registered retrieval or transplant hospital or centre and preservation of such removed organ(s) or tissue(s) shall be ensured in registered retrieval or transplant centre or tissue bank according to current and accepted scientific methods in order to ensure viability for the purpose of transplantation.

(7) Application for living donor transplantation.— (1) The donor and the recipient shall make jointly an application to grant approval for removal and transplantation of a human organ, to the competent authority or Authorisation Committee as specified in Form 11 and the papers for approval of transplantation would be processed by the registered medical practitioner and administrative division of the Institution for transplantation.

(8) Composition of Authorisation Committees.—(1) There shall be one State level Authorisation Committee. Additional Authorisation Committees in the districts or Institutions or hospitals may be set up as per norms given below, which may be revised from time to time by the concerned State Government or Union territory Administration by notification. No member from transplant team of the institution should be a member of the respective Authorisation Committee. Authorisation Committee should be hospital based if the number of transplants is twenty five or more in a year at the respective transplantation centres, and if the number of organ transplants in an institution or hospital are less than twenty-five in a year, then the State or District level Authorisation Committee would grant approval(s).

The hospital based Authorisation Committee shall, as notified by the State Government in case of State and by the Union territory Administration in case of Union territory, consist of,—

(a) the Medical Director or Medical Superintendent or Head of the institution or hospital or a senior medical person officiating as Head - Chairperson;

(b) two senior medical practitioners from the same hospital who are not part of the transplant team – Member;

(c) two persons (preferably one woman) of high integrity, social standing and credibility, who have served in high ranking Government positions, such as in higher judiciary, senior cadre of police service or who have served as a reader or professor in University Grants Commission approved University or are self-employed professionals of repute such as lawyers, chartered accountants, doctors of Indian Medical Association, reputed non-Government organisation or renowned social worker - Member;

(d) Secretary (Health) or nominee and Director Health Services or nominee from State Government or Union territory Administration - Member.

Composition of State or District Level Authorisation Committees.— The State or District Level Authorisation Committee shall, as notified by the State Government in case of State and by the Union territory Administration in case of Union territory, consist of,—

(a) a Medical Practitioner officiating as Chief Medical Officer or any other equivalent post in the main or major Government hospital of the District – Chairperson;

(b) two senior registered medical practitioners to be chosen from the pool of such medical practitioners who are residing in the concerned District and who are not part of any transplant team– Member;

(c) two persons (preferably one woman) of high integrity, social standing and credibility, who have served in high ranking Government positions, such as in higher judiciary, senior cadre of police service or who have served as a reader or professor in University Grants Commission approved University or are self-employed professionals of repute such as lawyers, chartered accountants, doctors of Indian Medical Association, reputed non-Government organisation or renowned social worker - Member;

(d) Secretary (Health) or nominee and Director Health Services or nominee from State Government or Union territory Administration–Member :

Provided that effort shall be made by the State Government concerned to have most of the members' ex-officio so that the need to change the composition of Committee is less frequent.

The quorum of the Authorisation Committee should be minimum four and the quorum shall not be complete without the participation of the Chairman, the presence of Secretary (Health) or nominee and Director of Health Services or nominee.

(9) Verification of residential status, etc.—When the living donor is unrelated and if donor or recipient belongs to a State or Union territory, other than the State or Union territory where the transplantation is proposed to be undertaken, verification of residential status by Tehsildar or any other authorised officer for the purpose with a copy marked to the Appropriate Authority of the State or Union territory of domicile of donor or recipient for

their information shall be required, as per Form 20 and in case of any doubt of organ trafficking, the Appropriate Authority of the State or Union territory of domicile or the Tehsildar or any other authorized officer shall inform police department for investigation and action as per the provisions of the Act.

(10) Procedure in case of near relatives.—

(a) Where the proposed transplant of organs is between near relatives related genetically, namely, grandmother, grandfather, mother, father, brother, sister, son, daughter, grandson and granddaughter, above the age of eighteen years, the competent authority as defined at rule 2(c) or Authorisation Committee (in case donor or recipient is a foreigner) shall evaluate;

(i) documentary evidence of relationship e.g. relevant birth certificates, marriage certificate, other relationship certificate from Tehsildar or Sub-divisional magistrate or Metropolitan Magistrate or Sarpanch of the Panchayat, or similar other identity certificates like Electors Photo Identity Card or AADHAAR card; and

(ii) documentary evidence of identity and residence of the proposed donor, ration card or voters identity card or passport or driving license or PAN card or bank account and family photograph depicting the proposed donor and the proposed recipient along with another near relative, or similar other identity certificates like AADHAAR Card (issued by **Unique Identification Authority of India**).

(b) If in the opinion of the competent authority, the relationship is not conclusively established after evaluating the above evidence, it may in its discretion direct further medical test, namely, Deoxyribonucleic Acid (DNA) Profiling.

(c) The test referred to in sub-rule (2) shall be got done from a laboratory accredited with National Accreditation Board for Testing and Calibration Laboratories and certificate shall be given in Form 5.

(d) If the documentary evidences and test referred to in sub-rules (1) and (2), respectively do not establish a genetic relationship between the donor and the recipient, the same procedure be adopted on preferably both or at least one parent, and if parents are not available, the same procedure be adopted on such relatives of donor and recipient as are available and are willing to be tested, failing which, genetic relationship between the donor and the recipient will be deemed to have not been established.

(e) Where the proposed transplant is between a married couple the competent authority or Authorisation Committee (in case donor or recipient is a foreigner) must evaluate the factum and duration of marriage and ensure that documents such as marriage certificate, marriage photograph etc. are kept for records along with the information on the number and age of children and a family photograph depicting the entire family, birth certificate of children containing the particulars of parents and issue a certificate in Form 6 (for spousal donor).

(f) Any document with regard to the proof of residence or domicile and particulars of parentage should be relatable to the photo identity of the applicant in order to ensure that the documents pertain to the same person, who is the proposed donor and in the event of any inadequate or doubtful information to this effect, the Competent Authority or Authorisation Committee as the case may be, may in its discretion seek such other information or evidence as may be expedient and desirable in the peculiar facts of the case.

(g) The medical practitioner who will be part of the organ transplantation team for carrying out transplantation operation shall not be a competent authority of the transplant hospital.

(h) The competent authority may seek the assistance of the Authorisation Committee in its decision making, if required.

(11) Procedure in case of foreigners.—

When the proposed donor or the recipient are foreigners;

(a) a senior Embassy official of the country of origin has to certify the relationship between the donor and the recipient as per Form 21 and in case a country does not have an Embassy in India, the certificate of relationship, in the same format, shall be issued by the Government of that country;

(b) the Authorisation Committee shall examine the cases of all Indian donors consenting to donate organs to a foreign national (who is a near relative), including a foreign national of Indian origin, with greater caution and such cases should be considered rarely on case to case basis: Provided that the Indian living donors wanting to donate to a foreigner other than near relative shall not be considered.

(12) Registration of hospital or tissue bank.— (1) An application for registration shall be made to the Appropriate Authority as specified in Form 12 or Form 13 or Form 14 or Form 15, as applicable and the application shall be accompanied by fee as specified below, payable to the Appropriate Authority by means of a bank draft, which may be revised, if necessary by the Central or State Government, as the case may be:-

(i) for Organ or Tissue or Cornea Transplant Centre: Rupees ten thousand;

(ii) for Tissue or Eye Bank: Rupees ten thousand;

(iii) for Non-Transplant Retrieval Centre: Nil.

The Appropriate Authority shall, after holding an inquiry and after satisfying itself that the applicant has complied with all the requirements, grant a certificate of registration as specified in Form 16 and it shall be valid for a period of five years from the date of its issue and shall be renewable.

Before a hospital is registered under the provisions of this rule, it shall be mandatory for the hospital to appoint a transplant coordinator. An application for the renewal of a certificate of registration shall be made to the Appropriate Authority at least three months prior to the date of expiry of the original certificate of registration and shall be accompanied by a fee as specified.

Transplant coordinator: The transplant coordinator shall be an employee of the registered hospital having qualification such as:

(a) graduate of any recognised system of medicine; or

(b) Nurse; or

(c) Bachelor's degree in any subject and preferably Master's degree in Social work or Psychiatry or Sociology or Social Science or Public Health. The concerned organisation or institute shall ensure initial induction training followed by retraining at periodic interval and the transplant coordinator shall counsel and encourage the family members or near relatives of the deceased person to donate the human organ or tissue including eye or cornea and coordinate the process of donation and transplantation. The transplant coordinator or counselor in a hospital registered for eye banking shall also have qualification specified in sub-rule (1).

The Central Government and the State Government, as the case may be, shall constitute by notification an Advisory Committee under Chairpersonship of administrative expert not below the rank of Secretary to the State Government for a period of two years to aid and advise the Appropriate Authority and the two medical experts referred to in clause(b) of sub-section(2) of section 13A of the Act shall possess a postgraduate medical degree and at least five years' experience in the field of organ or tissue transplantation.

National registry will have to be maintained as Organ Transplant Registry, Organ Donation Registry and Tissue Registry.

BIOMEDICAL WASTE MANAGEMENT & HANDLING RULES 1998 (Amended 2003, 2011,2016,2018,2019)

These rules apply to all persons who generate, collect, receive, store, transport, treat, dispose, or handle bio-medical waste in any form.

Biomedical waste means any waste, which is generated during the diagnosis, treatment or immunization of human beings or animals or in research activities pertaining thereto or in the production or testing of biologicals (means any preparation made from organisms or micro-organisms or product of metabolism and biochemical reactions intended for use in the diagnosis, immunization or the treatment of human beings or animals or in research activities pertaining thereto).

This rule applies to all institutions generating biomedical waste which includes hospitals, nursing homes, clinics, dispensaries, veterinary hospitals, animal house, pathological lab, and Blood Bank, etc. The Biomedical Waste (Management and Handling) Rules 1998, explicitly state that waste handling and treatment facilities shall have to be established within stipulated deadlines or earlier, for all waste generating establishments. While BMW management handling rules 2003 noted that the hospitals/clinics/nursing homes/ dispensaries etc., which treat below 1000 patients/month though do not have to apply for authorization, shall take all steps to ensure that such waste is handled without any adverse effect to human health and the environment; latest amendments makes it mandatory for all health care establishments to apply for authorization. BMW management and handling rules 2016 mandated that no occupier shall establish on-site treatment and disposal facility, if a service of common biomedical waste treatment facility is available at a distance of seventy-five kilometer. In cases where service of the common bio-medical waste treatment facility is not available, the occupiers shall set up requisite biomedical waste treatment equipment like incinerator, autoclave or microwave, shredder prior to commencement of its operation, as per the authorization given by the prescribed authority. Every occupier, where required, shall set up requisite bio-medical waste treatment facilities like incinerator, autoclave, microwave system for the treatment of waste, or, ensure requisite treatment of waste at a common bio-medical waste treatment facility or any other waste treatment facility. It shall be the duty of every occupier to take all necessary steps to ensure that bio-medical waste is handled without any adverse effect to human health and the environment and in accordance with these rules, make a provision within the premises for a safe, ventilated and secured location for storage of segregated biomedical waste in colored bags or containers in the manner as specified to ensure that there shall be no secondary handling, pilferage of recyclables or inadvertent scattering or spillage by animals and the bio-medical waste from such place or premises shall be directly transported in the manner as prescribed in these rules to the common bio-medical waste treatment facility or for the appropriate treatment and disposal, as the case may be, in the manner as prescribed. Pre-treat the laboratory waste, microbiological waste, blood samples and blood bags through disinfection or sterilisation on-site in the manner as prescribed by the World Health Organisation (WHO) or National AIDS Control Organisation (NACO) guidelines and then sent to the treatment facility for final disposal. Phase out use of chlorinated plastic bags, gloves and blood bags within two years from the date of notification of these rules. Provide training to all its health care workers and others, involved in handling of bio medical waste at the time of induction and thereafter at least once every year and the details of training programmes conducted, number of personnel trained and number of personnel not undergone any training shall be provided in the Annual Report. Immunise all its health care workers and others, involved in handling of bio-medical waste for protection against diseases including Hepatitis B and Tetanus that are likely to be transmitted by handling of bio-medical waste. Establish a Bar- Code System for bags or containers containing bio-medical waste to be sent out of the premises or place for any purpose within one year from the date of the notification of these rules. Ensure segregation of liquid chemical waste at source and ensure pre-treatment or neutralization prior to mixing with other effluent generated from health care facilities and ensure treatment and disposal of liquid waste in accordance with the Water (Prevention and Control of Pollution) Act, 1974 (6 of 1974). ensure occupational safety of all its health care workers and others involved in handling of biomedical waste by providing appropriate and adequate personal protective equipments. Conduct health check up at the time of induction and at least once in a year for all its health care workers and others involved in handling of bio- medical waste and maintain the records for the same. Maintain and update on day to day basis the bio-medical waste management register and display the monthly record on its website according to the bio-medical waste generated in terms of category and colour coding as specified. Make available the annual report on its web-site and all the health care facilities shall make own website within two years from the date of notification of these rules. Establish a system to review and monitor the activities related to bio-medical waste management, either through an existing committee or by forming a new committee and the Committee shall meet once in every six months and the record of the minutes of the meetings of this committee shall be submitted along with the annual report to the prescribed authority and the healthcare establishments having less than thirty beds shall designate a qualified person to review and monitor the activities relating to bio-medical waste management within that establishment and submit the annual report. Maintain all record for operation of incineration, hydro or autoclaving etc., for a period of five years. Existing incinerators to achieve the standards for treatment and disposal of bio-medical waste as specified for retention time in secondary chamber and Dioxin and Furans within two years from the date of this notification.

Who so ever is running the equipment should maintain a log book for each of its treatment equipment according to weight of batch; categories of waste treated; time, date and duration of treatment cycle and total hours of operation. After ensuring treatment by autoclaving or microwaving followed by mutilation or shredding, whichever is applicable, the recyclables from the treated bio-medical wastes such as plastics and glass, shall be given to recyclers having valid consent or authorisation or registration from the respective State Pollution Control Board or Pollution Control Committee. Microbiology waste and all other clinical laboratory waste shall be pre-treated by sterilisation or disinfection as per the World Health Organisation guidelines before packing and sending to the common bio-medical waste treatment facility.

Segregation, Packing, Transportation and Storage:-Bio-medical waste shall not be mixed with other wastes. Bio-medical waste shall be segregated into containers/bags at the point of generation prior to its storage, transportation, treatment and disposal. The containers shall be labeled biomedical waste. Untreated biomedical waste shall be transported only in such vehicles as may be authorized for the purpose by the competent authority as specified by the government. No untreated bio-medical waste shall be kept/stored beyond a period of 48 hours. Provided that, if for any reason, it becomes necessary to store the waste beyond such period, the authorized person must take permission of the prescribed authority and take measures to ensure that the waste does not adversely affect human health and the environment.

Annual Report

Every occupier or operator of common bio-medical waste treatment facility shall submit an annual report to the prescribed authority on or before the 30th June of every year. The prescribed authority shall compile, review and analyse the information received and send this information to the Central Pollution Control Board on or before the 31st July of every year. The Central Pollution Control Board shall compile, review and analyse the information received and send this information, along with its comments or suggestions or observations to the Ministry of Environment, Forest and Climate Change on or before 31st August every year. The Annual Reports shall also be available online on the websites of Occupiers, State Pollution Control Boards and Central Pollution Control Board. Every authorised person shall maintain records related to the generation, collection, reception, storage, transportation, treatment, disposal or any other form of handling of bio-medical waste, for a period of five years.

Authorization

Every occupier of an institution generating, collecting, receiving, storing, transporting, treating, disposing and/or handling bio-medical waste in any other manner, except such occupier of clinic, dispensaries, pathological laboratories, blood banks providing treatment/service to less than 1,000 (one thousand) patients per month, shall make an application in Form 1 to the prescribed authority for grant of authorization.

Biomedical wastes categories and their segregation, collection, treatment, processing and disposal options

Category	Type of Waste	Type of Bag or Container to be Used	Treatment and Disposal options
Yellow	**(a) Human Anatomical Waste:** Human tissues, organs, body parts and fetus below the viability period (as per the Medical Termination of Pregnancy Act 1971, amended from time to time). **(b) Animal Anatomical Waste:** Experimental animal carcasses, body parts, organs, tissues, including the waste generated from animals used in experiments or testing in veterinary hospitals or colleges or animal houses. **(c) Soiled Waste:** Items ontaminated with blood, body fluids like dressings, plaster casts, cotton swabs and bags containing residual or discarded blood and blood components. **(d) Expired or Discarded Medicines:** Pharmaceutical waste like antibiotics, cytotoxic drugs including all items contaminated with cytotoxic drugs along with glass or plastic ampoules, vials etc. **(e) Chemical Waste:** Chemicals used in production of biological and used or discarded disinfectants. **(e) Chemical Waste:** Chemicals used in production of biological and used or discarded disinfectants. **(f) Chemical Liquid Waste :** Liquid waste generated due to use of chemicals in production of biological and used or discarded disinfectants, Silver X-ray film developing liquid, discarded Formalin, infected secretions, aspirated bodyfluids, liquid from laboratories and floor washings, cleaning, house-keeping and disinfecting activities etc. (g) Discarded linen, mattresses, beddings contaminated with blood or body fluid.	Yellow coloured non-chlorinated plastic bags Yellow coloured non-chlorinated plastic bags or containers Separate collection system leading to effluent treatment system.	Incineration or Plasma Pyrolysis or deep burial. Incineration or Plasma Pyrolysis or deep burial In absence of above facilities, autoclav-ing or micro-wav-ing/ hydroclaving followed by shred-ding or mutilation or combination of sterilization and shredding. Expired `cytotoxic drugs and items contaminated with cytotoxic drugs to be returned back to the manufacturer or supplier for incineration at temperature >1200 0C or to common bio-medical

			waste treatment facility or hazardous waste treatment, storage and disposal facility for incineration at >12000C Or Encapsulation or Plasma Pyrolysis at >12000C. All other discarded medicines shall be either sent back to manufacturer or disposed by incineration
		Non-chlorinated yellow plastic bags or suitable packing material	Disposed of by incineration or Plasma Pyrolysis or Encapsulation in hazardous waste treatment, storage and disposal facility.
		Autoclave safe plastic bags or containers	After resource recovery, the chemical liquid waste shall be pre-treated before mixing with other wastewater. The combined discharge shall conform to the discharge norms given in Schedule.
			Non- chlorinated chemical disinfection followed by incineration or Plazma Pyrolysis or for energy recovery. In absence of above facilities, shredding or mutilation or combination of sterilization and shredding. Treated waste to be sent for

			energy recovery or incineration or Plazma Pyrolysis. Pre-treat to sterilize with nonchlorinated chemicals on-site as per National AIDS Control Organisation or World Health Organisation guidelines thereafter for Incineration.
Red	**Contaminated Waste(Recyclable)** (a) Wastes generatedfrom disposable items-such as tubing, bottles,intravenous tubes andsets, catheters, urinebags, syringes (withoutneedles and fixed needlesyringes) andvaccutainers with theirneedles cut) and gloves.	Red colourednon-chlorinatedplastic bags orcontainers	Autoclaving or micro-waving/hydroclaving followed by shredding ormutilation or combination ofsterilization and shredding. Treatedwaste to be sent to registered orauthorized recyclers or for energyrecovery or plastics to diesel or fuel oilor for road making, whichever ispossible.Plastic waste should not be sent tolandfill sites.
White (Translucent)	**Waste sharpsincluding Metals:** Needles, syringes withfixed needles, needlesfrom needle tip cutter orburner, scalpels, blades,or any othercontaminated sharpobject that may causepuncture and cuts. Thisincludes both used,discarded andcontaminated metalsharps	Puncture proof,Leak proof,tamper proof-containers	Autoclaving or Dry Heat Sterilizationfollowed by shredding or mutilation orencapsulation in metal container orcement concrete; combination ofshredding cum autoclaving; and sent forfinal disposal to iron foundries (havingconsent to operate from the StatePollution Control Boards or PollutionControl Committees) or sanitarylandfill or designated concrete wastesharp pit.

Blue	(a) Glassware:Broken or discarded andcon-taminated glassinclud-ing medicine vialsand ampoules exceptthose contaminated withcy-totoxic wastes.	Cardboard boxeswith bluecolored marking	Disinfection (by soak-ing the washedglass waste after cleaning withdetergent and Sodium Hypochlorite-treatment) or through autoclaving ormicro-waving or hydroclav-ing and thensent for recycling.

Disposal by deep burial is permitted only in rural or remote areas where there is no access to common bio-medical waste treatment facility. This will be carried out with prior approval from the prescribed authority and as per the Standards specified . The deep burial facility shall be located as per the provisions and guidelines issued by Central Pollution Control Board from time to time.

As per BMW management and handling rules 2018 above limits are applicable to the occupiers of Health Care Facilities (bedded) which are either connected with sewerage network without terminal sewage treatment plant or not connected to public sewers. For discharge into public sewers with terminal facilities, the general standards as notified under the Environment (Protection) Act, 1986 (29 of 1986) shall be applicable. Health Care Facilities having less than ten beds shall have to install Sewage Treatment Plant by 31st December, 2019. Non-bedded occupiers shall dispose infectious liquid wastes only after treatment by disinfection".

STANDARDS FOR TREATMENT AND DISPOSAL OF BIO-MEDICALWASTES

1. STANDARDS FOR INCINERATION.-

All incinerators shall meet the following operating and emission standards-

A. Operating Standards

1). Combustion efficiency (CE) shall be at least 99.00%.

2). The Combustion efficiency is computed as follows:

%C02

C.E. = ------------ X 100

%C02 + % CO

(3) The temperature of the primary chamber shall be a minimum of 800 0C and the secondary chamber shall be minimum of 10500C + or - 500C.

(4) The secondary chamber gas residence time shall be at least two seconds.

B. Stack Height: Minimum stack height shall be 30 meters above the ground and shall be attached with the necessary monitoring facilities as per requirement of monitoring of 'general parameters' as notified under the Environment (Protection) Act, 1986.

- The existing incinerators shall comply with the standards for Dioxins and Furans of 0.1ngTEQ/Nm3, within two years from the date of commencement of these rules.
- Ash from incineration of biomedical waste shall be disposed of at common hazardous waste treatment and disposal facility. However, it may be disposed of in municipal landfill, if the toxic metals in incineration ash are within the regulatory quantities as defined under the Hazardous Waste (Management and Handling and Transboundary Movement) Rules, 2008 as amended from time to time.
- Incinerators (combustion chambers) shall be operated with such temperature, retention time and turbulence, as to achieve Total Organic Carbon content in the slag and bottom ashes less than 3% or their loss on ignition shall be less than 5% of the dry weight.

STANDARDS FOR AUTOCLAVING OF BIO-MEDICAL WASTE.-

The autoclave should be dedicated for the purposes of disinfecting and treating bio-medical waste.

(1) When operating a gravity flow autoclave, medical waste shall be subjected to:

(i) a temperature of not less than 121° C and pressure of 15 pounds per square inch (psi) for an autoclave residence time of not less than 60 minutes; or

(ii) a temperature of not less than 135° C and a pressure of 31 psi for an autoclave residence time of not less than 45 minutes; or

(iii) a temperature of not less than 149° C and a pressure of 52 psi for an autoclave residence time of not less than 30 minutes.

(2) When operating a vacuum autoclave, medical waste shall be subjected to a minimum of three pre-vacuum pulse to purge the autoclave of all air. The air removed during the pre-vacuum, cycle should be decontaminated by means of HEPA and activated carbon filtration, steam treatment, or any other method to prevent release of pathogen. The waste shall be subjected to the following:

(i) a temperature of not less than 121°C and pressure of 15 psi per an autoclave residence time of not less than 45 minutes; or

(ii) a temperature of not less than 135°C and a pressure of 31 psi for an autoclave residence time of not less than 30 minutes.

STANDARDS FOR DEEP BURIAL.- (1) A pit or trench should be dug about two meters deep. It should be half filled with waste, then covered with lime within 50 cm of the surface, before filling the rest of the pit with soil.

(2) It must be ensured that animals do not have any access to burial sites. Covers of galvanised iron or wire meshes may be used.

(3) On each occasion, when wastes are added to the pit, a layer of 10 cm of soil shall be added to cover the wastes.

(4) Burial must be performed under close and dedicated supervision.

(5) The deep burial site should be relatively impermeable and no shallow well should be close to the site.

(6) The pits should be distant from habitation, and located so as to ensure that no contamination occurs to surface water or ground water. The area should not be prone to flooding or erosion.

(7) The location of the deep burial site shall be authorised by the prescribed authority.

(8) The institution shall maintain a record of all pits used for deep burial.

(9) The ground water table level should be a minimum of six meters below the lower level of deep burial pit.

STANDARDS FOR LIQUID WASTE

(1) The effluent generated or treated from the premises of occupier or operator of a common bio medical waste treatment and disposal facility, before discharge into the sewer should conform to the following limits-

PARAMETERS PERMISSIBLE LIMITS :	pH 6.5-9.0
Suspended solids:	100 mg/l
Oil and grease:	10 mg/l
BOD :	30 mg/l
COD :	250 mg/l

Bio-assay test 90% survival of fish after 96 hours in 100% effluent.

MTP Act 1971 and MTP (Amendment) Act 2002, 2021.

Medical Termination of Pregnancy Act, 1971 provides for the termination of certain pregnancies by registered medical practitioners and for matter connected therewith or incidental thereto. In accordance with Act, a MTP may be carried out either in a hospital established or maintained by Government, or at a place for the time being approved for the purpose of this Act by Government. Under earlier provisions of the pregnancy could be terminated by a registered medical practitioner in the following conditions:-

I. Where the length of the pregnancy did not exceed twelve weeks, or

II. Where the length of the pregnancy exceeded twelve weeks but did not exceed twenty weeks, if not less than two registered medical practitioners were of opinion formed in good faith, that

    - the continuance of the pregnancy would involve a risk to the life of the pregnant woman or of grave injury to her physical or mental health, or
    - If there is a substantial risk that if the child was born, it would suffer from such physical or mental abnormalities to be seriously handicapped.

Under amendments to the act 2021

a pregnancy may be terminated by a registered medical practitioner,— (a) where the length of the pregnancy does not exceed twenty weeks, if such medical practitioner is, or

(b) where the length of the pregnancy exceeds twenty weeks but does not exceed twenty-four weeks in case of such category of woman as may be prescribed by rules made under this Act, if not less than two registered medical practitioners are, of the opinion, formed in good faith, that—

(i) the continuance of the pregnancy would involve a risk to the life of the pregnant woman or of grave injury to her physical or mental health; or

(ii) there is a substantial risk that if the child were born, it would suffer from any serious physical or mental abnormality.

The provisions of sub-section (2) relating to the length of the pregnancy shall not apply to the termination of pregnancy by the medical practitioner where such termination is necessitated by the diagnosis of any of the substantial foetal abnormalities diagnosed by a Medical Board. (2C)

Every State Government or Union territory, as the case may be, shall, by notification in the Official Gazette, constitute a Board to be called a Medical Board for the purposes of this Act to exercise such powers and functions as may be prescribed by rules made under this Act. (2D) The Medical Board shall consist of the following, namely:—

(a) a Gynaecologist;

(b) a Paediatrician;

(c) a Radiologist or Sonologist;

(d) such other number of members as may be notified in the Official Gazette by the State Government or Union territory, as the case may be".

No registered medical practitioner shall reveal the name and other particulars of a woman whose pregnancy has been terminated under this Act except to a person authorised by any law for the time being in force. Whoever contravenes the provisions of sub-section (1) shall be punishable with imprisonment which may extend to one year, or with fine, or with both.".

The Drugs & Cosmetics Act, 1940 with the Drugs, Cosmetics Act 1955,1960,1962,1964,1972,1982, 1986, 1995 and the Drugs & Cosmetics Rules, 1945 (as amended in 2006)

An act to regulate the import, manufacture, distribution and sale of drugs and cosmetics.

Few salient features of the Act are:

I. The main objective of the Act is to prevent sub-standards in drugs, presumably for maintaining high standards of medical treatment.

II. Enhancement of the quantum of punishment for offences relating to the manufacture or sale of adulterated, spurious drugs.

III. Substances governed by the act can nevertheless be applicable to narcotic or intoxicating liquor.

"Drug" includes—

(i) all medicines for internal or external use of human beings or animals and all substances intended to be used for or in the diagnosis, treatment, mitigation or prevention of any disease or disorder in human beings or animals, including preparations applied on human body for the purpose of repelling insects like mosquitoes;

(ii) such substances (other than food) intended to affect the structure or any function of human body or intended to be used for the destruction of vermin or insects which cause disease in human beings or animals, as may be specified from time to time by the Central Government by notification in the Official Gazette.

(iii) all substances intended for use as components of a drug including empty gelatin capsules; and

(iv) such devices intended for internal or external use in the diagnosis, treatment, mitigation or prevention of disease or disorder in human beings or animals, as may be specified from time to time by the Central Government by notification in the Official Gazette, after consultation with the Board.

Misbranded drugs; A drug shall be deemed to be misbranded if (a) it is so coloured, coated, powdered or polished that damage is concealed or if it is made to appear of better or greater therapeutic value than it really is; or (b) if it is not labelled in the prescribed manner; or (c) if its label or container or anything accompanying the drug bears any statement, design or device which makes any false claim for the drug or which is false or misleading.

Adulterated drugs; A drug shall be deemed to be adulterated if it consists, in whole or in part, of any filthy, putrid or decomposed substance; or (b) if it has been prepared, packed or stored under insanitary conditions whereby it may have been contaminated with filth or whereby it may have been rendered injurious to health; or (c) if its container is composed in whole or in part, of any poisonous or deleterious substance which may render the contents injurious to health; or (d) if it bears or contains, for purposes of colouring only, a colour other than one which is prescribed; or (e) if it contains any harmful or toxic substance which may render it injurious to health; or (f) if any substance has been mixed therewith so as to reduce its quality or strength.

Spurious drugs; A drug shall be deemed to be spurious— (a) if it is imported under a name which belongs to another drug; or (b) if it is an imitation of, or a substitute for, another drug or resembles another drug in a manner likely to deceive or bears upon it or upon its label or container the name of another drug unless it is plainly and conspicuously marked so as to reveal its true character and its lack of identity with such other drug ; or (c) if the label or the container bears the name of an individual or company purporting to be the manufacturer of the drug, which individual or company is fictitious or does not exist; or (d) if it has been substituted wholly or in part by another drug or substance; or (e) if it purports to be the product of a manufacturer of whom it is not truly a product .

The notable schedules of drugs are

Schedule G : Most of the drugs in this group are Hormonal preparations. The Drug Label must display the text "Caution". It is dangerous to take this preparation except under medical supervision. Examples of subtances under this schedule : Testolactone, Hydroxyurea, Carbutamide, Primidone etc.

Schedule H : The drug label must display the texts "Rx" and Schedule H drug. Warning : To be sold by retail on the prescription of a Registered Medical Practitioner only" prominently. It can only be supplied to licensed parties. It cannot be sold without a prescription and only the amount specified in the prescription should be sold. The time and date of prescription must be noted. If a schedule H drug also comes under the purview of Narcotic Drugs and Psychotropic Substances Act, 1985, it must carry the texts "NRx" and Schedule H drug. Examples : androgenic, anabolic, oestrogenic and progestational substances; Alprazolam, Hepatitis B vaccine, Ibuprofen, Vasopressin etc.

Schedule X : All the regulations of schedule H apply. The retailer must keep a copy of the prescription for two years. The drugs must be kept under lock and key. Examples : Amobarbital, Amphetamine, Barbital, Cyclobarbital, Dexamphetamine, Ethchlorvynol, Glutethimide, Ketamine etc

Schedule J : Contains a list of various diseases and conditions that cannot be treated under any drug currently in market. No drug may legally claim to treat these diseases. Examples AIDS, Blindness, Cancer etc

Penalty for manufacture, etc., of drugs or cosmetics in contravention of section 26A; Whoever himself or by any other person on his behalf manufactures or sells or distributes any drug or cosmetic in contravention of the provisions of any notification issued under section 26A, shall be punishable with imprisonment for a term which may extend to three years and shall also be liable to fine which may extend to five thousand rupees. Under section 26A, if the Central Government is satisfied, that the use of any drug or cosmetic is likely to involve any risk to human beings or animals or that any drug does not have the therapeutic value claimed or purported to be claimed for it or contains ingredients and in such quantity for which there is no therapeutic justification and that in the public interest it is necessary or expedient so to do, then, that Government may, by notification in the

Official Gazette, prohibit the manufacture, sale or distribution of such drug or cosmetic.

In case of licences for import of drugs manufactured by one manufacturer a single application may be made, and a single licence may be issued in respect of the import of more than one drug or class of drugs manufactured by the same manufacturer provided that the drugs or classes of drugs are manufactured at one factory or more than one factory functioning conjointly as a single manufacturing unit. Provided further that if a single manufacturer has two or more factories situated in different places manufacturing the same or different drugs a separate licence shall be required in respect of the drugs manufactured by each such factory.

Import of drugs by a Government Hospital or Autonomous Medical Institution for the treatment of patient. Small quantities of new drug, as defined in rule 122-E, the import of which is otherwise prohibited under this section 10 of the Act, may be imported for treatment of patients suffering from life threatening diseases, or diseases causing serious permanent disability, or such disease requiring therapies for unmet medical needs, by a Medical Officer of a Government Hospital or an Autonomous Medical Institution providing tertiary care, duly certified by the Medical Superintendent of the Government Hospital, or Head of the Autonomous Medical Institution, subject to the following conditions :- (a) no new drug shall be imported for the said purpose except under a licence in Form 11-A, and the said drug has been approved for marketing in the country of origin; (b) the licence shall use the substances or drugs imported under the licence exclusively for the purpose of treatment of patients suffering from life threatening diseases, or diseases causing serious permanent disability, or such diseases requiring therapies for unmet medical needs, under the supervision of its own Medical Officers at the place, specified in the licence or at such other places, as the licensing authority, may from time to time authorize; (c) the licencee shall allow an Inspector authorised by the licensing authority in this behalf to enter, with or without prior notice, the premises where the substances or drugs are stocked, and to inspect the premises and relevant records and investigate the manner in which the substances or drugs are being used and to take, if necessary, samples thereof ; (d) the licencee shall keep a record of, and shall submit the said report half yearly to the licensing authority, the substances or drugs imported under the licence, together with the quantities imported and issued to the patients, the date of importation, the name of the manufacturer, the name and address of the patient for whom the drug is prescribed and the name of disease. (e) the licencee shall comply with such other requirements, if any, applicable to the holders of import licences for import of new drugs for treatment of patients by Government Hospitals, as may be specified from time to time in any rule subsequently made under Chapter 111 of the Act and of which the licensing authority has given to him not less than one month's notice; (f) the drug shall be stocked under proper storage conditions and shall be dispensed under the supervision of a registered pharmacist; (g) the quantity of any single drug so imported shall not exceed 100 average dosages per patient.

Conditions of import licence: An import licence shall be subject to the following conditions:

(i) the manufacturer shall at all times observe the undertaking given by him or on his behalf in Form 9.

(ii) the licensee shall allow any Inspector authorized by the licensing authority in that behalf to enter with or without notice any premises where the imported substance is stocked, to inspect the means, if any, employed for testing the substance and to take samples.

(iii) the licensee shall on request furnish to the licensing authority from every batch of each substance or from such batch or batches as the licensing authority may from time to time specify a sample of such amount as the licensing authority may consider adequate for any examination required to be made, and the licensee shall, if so required, furnish full protocols of the tests, if any, which have been applied.

(iv) if the licensing authority so directs the licensee shall not sell or offer for sale any batch in respect of which a sample is or protocols are furnished under the last preceding subrule until a certificate authorizing the sale of the batch has been issued to him by or on behalf of the licensing authority;

(v) the licensee shall, on being informed by the licensing authority that any part of any batch of the substance has been found by the licensing authority not to conform with the standards of strength, quality and purity prescribed by Chapter III of the Act, or the Rules thereunder and on being directed so to do withdraw the remainder of that batch from sale and, so far as may in the particular circumstances of the case be practicable, recall the issues already made from that batch.

(vi) the licensee shall maintain a record of all sales by him of substances for the import of which a licence is required, showing particulars of the substance and of the person to whom sold and such further particulars, if any, as the licensing authority may specify and such record shall be open to the inspection of any Inspector authorised in that behalf by the licensing authority;

Provided that in respect of the sale or distribution of drugs specified in Schedule X, the licensee shall maintain separate record or register showing the following particulars, namely; 1. Name of the Drug, 2. Batch number, 3. Name and address of the manufacturer, 4. Date of transaction, 5. Opening stock on the business day, 6. Quantity of drug received, if any, and the source from which received, 7. Name of the purchaser, his address and licence number, 8. Balance quantity of drug at the end of the business day, 9. Signature of the person under whose supervision the drugs have been supplied.

(vii) the licensee shall comply with such further requirements, if any, applicable to the holders of import licenses, as may be specified in any Rules, subsequently made under Chapter III of the Act and of which the licensing authority has given to him not less than four months' notice.

Duration of import licence: A licence unless, it is sooner suspended or cancelled, shall be valid for a period of three years from the date of its issue.

Provided that if application for a fresh licence is made three months before the expiry of the existing licence the current licence shall be deemed to continue in force until orders are passed on the application.

Offences by Government departments. Where an offence under Chapter1V or Chapter 1VA has been committed by any department of Government, such authority as is specified by the Central Government to be in charge of manufacture, sale or distribution of drugs or where no authority is specified, the head of the department, shall be deemed to be guilty of the offence and shall be liable to be proceeded against and punished accordingly.

Qualification of a Licensing Authority;

No person shall be qualified to be a Licensing Authority under the Act unless(i) he is a graduate in Pharmacy or Pharmaceutical Chemistry or in Medicine with specialization in clinical pharmacology or microbiology from a University established in India by law; and (ii) he has experience in the manufacture or testing of drugs or enforcement of the provisions of the Act for a minimum period of five years.

Provided that the requirements as to the academic qualification shall not apply to those inspectors and the Government Analysts who were holding those positions on the 12th day of April, 1989.

Substances specified in Schedule H or Schedule X shall not be sold by retail except on and in accordance with the prescription of a Registered Medical Practitioner and in the case of substances specified in schedule X, the prescriptions shall be in duplicate, one copy of which shall be retained by the licensee for a period of two years.

(b)The supply of drugs specified in Schedule H or Schedule X to Registered Medical Practitioners, Hospitals, Dispensaries and Nursing Homes shall be made only against the signed order in writing which shall be preserved by the licensee for a period of two years.

For the purposes of clause (9) a prescription shall (a) be in writing and be signed by the person giving it with his usual signature and be dated by him. (b) specify the name and address of the person for whose treatment it is given, or the name and address of the owner of the animal if the drug is meant for veterinary use. (c) indicate the total amount of the medicine to be supplied and the dose to be taken.

The person dispensing a prescription containing a drug specified in Schedule H [and Schedule X] shall comply with the following requirements in addition to other requirements of these Rules

(a) the prescription must not be dispensed more than once unless the prescriber has stated thereon that it may be dispensed more than once; (b) if the prescription contains a direction that it may be dispensed a stated number of times or at stated intervals it must not be dispensed otherwise than in accordance with the directions. (c) at the time of dispensing there must be noted on the prescription above the signature of the prescriber the name and address of the seller and the date on which the prescription is dispensed.

No person dispensing a prescription containing substances specified in [Schedule H or X], may supply any other preparation, whether containing the same substance or not, in lieu thereof.

Substances specified in Schedule X kept in retail shop or premises used in connection therewith shall be stored—

(a) under lock and key in cupboard or drawer reserved solely for the storage of these substances ;or

(b) in a part of the premises separated from the remainder of the premises and to which only responsible persons have access

A licensee whose licence has been suspended or cancelled may, within three months of the date of order under sub-rule (1), prefer an appeal against that order to the State Government, which shall decided the same.

REQUIREMENTS FOR THE COLLECTION, STORAGE, PROCESSING AND DISTRIBUTION OF WHOLE HUMAN BLOOD, HUMAN BLOOD COMPONENTS BY BLOOD BANKS AND MANUFACTURE OF BLOOD PRODUCTS.

Application for the grant and/or renewal of licence for the operation of a Blood Bank/processing of human blood for components/ manufacture of blood products shall be made to the Licensing Authority appointed under Part VII and shall be accompanied by licence fee of rupees six thousand and an inspection fee of rupees one thousand and five hundred for every inspection thereof or for the purpose of renewal of licence. Provided that if the applicant applies for renewal of licence after its expiry but within six months of such expiry the fee payable for the renewal of the licence shall be rupees six thousand and inspection fee of rupees one thousand five hundred plus an additional fee at the rate of rupees one thousand per month or a part thereof in addition to the inspection fee. Provided further that a licensee holding a licence for operation of Blood Bank/processing of whole human blood components/manufacture of blood products shall apply for grant of licence before the expiry of the said licence and he shall continue to operate the same till the orders on his application are communicated to him.

On receipt of the application for the grant or renewal of such licence, the Licensing Authority shall (i) verify the statements made in the application form (ii) cause the manufacturing of the testing establishment to be inspected in accordance with the provision of Rule 122-I and (iii) in case the application is for renewal of licence, call for information of past performance of the licence. If the Licensing Authority is satisfied that the applicant is in a position to fulfil the requirements laid down in the rules, he shall prepare a report to that effect and forward it along with the application and the licence (in triplicate) to be granted or renewed, duly completed to the Central Licence Approving Authority.

Provided that if the Licensing Authority is of the opinion that the applicant is not in a position to fulfil the requirements laid down in these rules, he may, by order, for reasons to be recorded in writing, refuse to grant or renew the licence.

The operation of Blood Bank and/or processing of whole human blood for components shall be conducted under the active direction and personal supervision of competent technical staff consisting of at least one person who is whole-time employee and who is Medical Officer, and possessing- (a) Postgraduate degree in Medicine - M.D (Pathology/ Transfusion Medicines); or (b) Degree in Medicine (M.B.B.S.) with Diploma in Pathology or Transfusion Medicines having adequate knowledge in blood group serology, blood group methodology and medical principles involved in the procurement of blood and/or preparation of its components; or (c) Degree in Medicine (M.B.B.S.) having experience in Blood Bank for one year during regular service and also has adequate knowledge and experience in blood group serology, blood group methodology and medical principles involved in the procurement of blood and/or preparation of its components. the degree or diploma being from a University recognized by the Central Government.

(ii) The applicant shall provide adequate space, plant and equipment for any or all the operations of blood collection or blood processing. (ii) The applicant shall provide and maintain adequate technical staff as specified in Schedule F, Part XII-B and/or XII-C. (iv) The applicant shall provide adequate arrangements for storage of whole human blood, human blood components and blood products. (v) The applicant shall furnish to the Licensing Authority, if required to do so, data on the stability of whole human blood, its components or blood products which are likely to deteriorate, for fixing the date of expiry which shall be printed on the labels of such products on the basis of the data so furnished.

An original licence or a renewed licence unless sooner suspended or cancelled shall be valid for a period of five years on and from the date on which it is granted or renewed.

Before a licence is granted or a renewal of licence, as the case may be, the Licensing Authority or the Central Licence Approving authority, as the case may be, shall cause the establishment in which Blood Bank is proposed to be operated/whole human blood for components is processed/ blood products are manufactured to be inspected by one or more Inspectors, appointed under the Act and/or along with the Expert in the field concerned. The Inspector or Inspectors shall examine all portions of the premises and appliance/equipments and inspect the process of manufacture intend to be employed or being employed along with the means to be employed or being employed for operation of blood bank/processing of whole human blood for components/ manufacture of blood products together with their testing facilities and also enquire into the professional qualification of the expert staff and other technical staff to be employed.

Further application after rejection If within a period of six months from the rejection of application of a licence the applicant informs the Licensing Authority that the conditions laid down have been satisfied and deposits an inspection fee of rupees two hundred and fifty the Licensing Authority may, if after causing further inspection to be made is satisfied that the conditions for the grant or renewal of a licence have been complied with, shall grant or renew the licence .

The Central Licence Approving Authority may, with the approval of the Central Government, by notification delegate his powers of signing licences and any other power under rules to persons under his control having same qualifications as prescribed for Controlling Authority.

Cancellation and suspension of licences.- (1) The Licensing Authority or Central Licence Approving Authority may for such licences granted or renewed by him after giving the licensee an opportunity to show cause why such an order should not be passed by an order in writing stating the reason thereof, cancel a licence issued under this part or suspend it for such period as he thinks fit, either wholly or in respect of some of the substances to which it relates or direct the licensee to stop collection, storage, processing, manufacture and distribution of the said substances and thereupon order the destruction of substances and stocks thereof in the presence of an Inspector, if in his opinion, the licensee has failed to comply with any of the conditions of the licence or with any provision of the Act or Rules thereunder.

A licensee whose licence has been suspended or cancelled may, within three months of the date of the order under sub-rule(1) prefer an appeal against the order to the State Government or Central government, which shall decide the same.

The licensee shall from time to time report to the Licensing Authority any changes in the expert staff responsible for the operation of a Blood Bank/processing of whole human blood for components and/or manufacture of blood products and any material alterations in the premises or plant used for that purpose which have been made since the date of last inspection made on behalf of the Licensing Authority before the grant of the licence.

The consumer protection Act 1986 (Amended 2002, 2019)

An Act is to provide for protection of the interests of consumers and for the said purpose, to establish authorities for timely and effective administration and settlement of consumers' disputes and for matters connected therewith or incidental thereto.

The Central Consumer Protection Council

The Central Council consists of the following members, namely, (a) the Minister in-charge of the consumer affairs in the Central Government, who is the Chairman, and (b) such number of other official or non-official members representing such interests as may be prescribed. The council deals with cases involving more than ten crore rupees.

The Central Council shall meet as and when necessary, but at least one meeting of the Council shall be held every year.

The State Consumer Protection Council

The State Council consists of the following members, namely:-

(a) The Minister incharge of consumer affairs in the State Government who is the Chairman, (b) such number of other official or non-official members representing such interests as may be prescribed by the State Government, (c) such number of other official or non-official members, not exceeding ten, as may be nominated by the Central Government. The State Council shall meet as and when necessary but not less than two meetings shall be held every year. The council has role where compensation claims are between one crore and ten crore.

The District Consumer Protection Council

consists of the following members, namely:-

(a) The collector of the district, who is the Chairman, and (b) such number of other official and non-official members representing such interests as may be prescribed by the State Government. The council has a role where compensation claims are less than one crore.

As consumer protection applies to hospitals also, medical care given should be quality care. In addition to proving best possible care hospitals and doctors now need to have indemnity insurance to protect themselves from litigations and claims. Doctors in West now do not hesitate to file counter suits to protect themselves from over-zealous patients. An appeal filed before the State Commission or the National Commission, as the case may be, shall be heard as expeditiously as possible and every endeavour shall be made to dispose off the appeal within a period of ninety days from the date of its admission. Whoever fails to comply with any order made by the District Commission or the State Commission or the National Commission, as the case may be, shall be punishable with imprisonment for a term which shall not be less than one month, but which may extend to three years, or with fine, which shall not be less than twenty-five thousand rupees, but which may extend to one lakh rupees, or with both. Every appeal under this section shall be preferred within a period of thirty days from the date of order of a District Commission or a State Commission or the National Commission, as the case may be. Provided that the State Commission or the National Commission or the Supreme Court, as the case may be, may entertain an appeal after the expiry of the said period of thirty days, if it is satisfied that the appellant had sufficient cause for not preferring the appeal within the said period of thirty days.

For the purpose of mediation, the National Commission or the State Commission or the District Commission, as the case may be, shall prepare a panel of the mediators to be maintained by the consumer mediation cell attached to it, on the recommendation of a selection committee consisting of the President and a member of that Commission.

Disaster Management Act

Disaster management act was enacted in 2005. Disaster management involves capacity-building by identification of existing resources and the resources to be acquired or created, acquiring or creating resources identified, organizing training of personnel. Disaster management means a continuous and integrated process of planning, organizing, coordinating and implementing measures which are necessary or expedient for prevention of danger or threat of any disaster, mitigation or reduction of risk of any disaster and its consequences, capacity building, preparedness, prompt response, assessing the severity of effects, evacuation, resource and relief, rehabilitation and reconstruction. The act established a ("National Disaster Management Authority") which consists of Prime Minister of India as chairperson, and other members not exceeding nine nominated by chairperson of Authority. The national authority meets as and when necessary. The national authority has the responsibility for laying down the policies, plans and guidelines for disaster management. The national authority may constitute an advisory committee consisting of experts in the field of disaster management. The members of advisory committee are paid allowances as prescribed by central government. The central government constitutes a national executive committee to assist the National Authority in the performance of its functions. The members of national executive committee are Secretary to Govt. of India in-charge of Ministry having administrative control of disaster management (chair person) and secretaries to Govt. of India of few other departments. The National Authority lays down policies on disaster management, approve the national plan, lay down guidelines to be followed by the state authorities in drawing up the state plan, coordinate the enforcement and implementation of the policy and plan for disaster management, recommend provision of funds for the purpose of mitigation, provide such support to other countries as determined by central govt, take measures for prevention of disaster or the mitigation etc. The national plan is prepared by the National Executive committee having regard to the National policy and to be approved by National Authority. The National authority recommends guidelines for the minimum standards of relief to be provided to persons affected by disaster which includes; minimum requirements to be provided in the relief camps in relation to shelter, food, drinking water, medical cover and sanitation, special provisions to be made for widows and orphans, ex-gratia assistance on account of loss of life as also assistance on account of damage to houses and for restoration of means of livelihood etc. State Disaster Management Authority consists of following members; the chief minister of state as chair person, other members not exceeding eight to be nominated by chairman of state Authority, chairperson of state executive committee. State authority has responsibilities of laying down plans and policies for disaster management in the state. District disaster management authority has Deputy Commissioner as its chairperson, elected representative of the local authority is co-chairperson. In any district where Zila parishad exists, the chairperson thereof shall be the chairperson of the district Authority. The district plan shall be prepared by District Authority after consultation with local authorities and having regard to the National plan and the State plan to be approved by the State Authority.

The Act lays down for constitution of a “National Institute of Disaster Management.” The Institute functions within the broad policies and guidelines laid down by National Authority and is responsible for planning and promoting training and research in the area of disaster management, documentation and development of national level information base relating to disaster management policies, prevention and mitigation; formulation of comprehensive human resource development plan covering all aspects of disaster management, develop educational material for disaster management, promote awareness of stake holders.

The Disaster management Act 2005 also lays down for constitution of a National Disaster response force for the purpose of specialist response to a threatening disaster situation or disaster. The central govt. established a National Disaster response fund for meeting any threatening disaster situation or disaster. The National Disaster response fund is made available to the National executive committee for meeting the expenses for emergency response, relief and rehabilitation. The national disaster mitigation fund is constituted exclusively for the purpose of mitigation. States and districts also have State disaster response fund, District disaster response fund, State Disaster mitigation fund and District Disaster mitigation fund. Where the national, state or district authority is satisfied that immediate procurement of provisions or materials is necessary it may authorize the concerned department to make emergency procurement and standard procedure requiring inviting of tenders shall be deemed to be waived and a certificate of utilization of provisions or materials by the controlling officer authorized shall be deemed to be a valid document. Whoever obstructs any officer or employee in discharge of his functions under this act shall be liable for punishment with imprisonment which may extend to one year or with fine or both. If the obstruction or refusal to comply results in loss of lives or imminent danger punishment may extend to two years. Whoever knowingly makes claim which he knows or has reason to believe to be false for obtaining any relief shall on conviction be punishable with imprisonment for a term which may extend upto two years and also with fine. Whoever being entrusted with money or materials meant for disaster misappropriates shall be punished with imprisonment up to two years and also with fine.

THE SURROGACY (REGULATION) ACT, 2021 (NO. 47 OF 2021) [25th December, 2021.] came into effect from 25th January 2022. An Act to constitute National Assisted Reproductive Technology and Surrogacy Board, State Assisted Reproductive Technology and Surrogacy Boards and appointment of appropriate authorities for regulation of the practice and process of surrogacy and for matters connected therewith or incidental thereto. The act aims to prohibit commercial surrogacy and allows for altruistic surrogacy. This Act is called the Surrogacy (Regulation) Act, 2021. The Act received the assent of the President of India on the 25th December 2021. "Altruistic surrogacy" means the surrogacy in which no charges, expenses, fees, remuneration or monetary incentive of whatever nature, except the medical expenses and such other prescribed expenses incurred on surrogate mother and the insurance coverage for the surrogate mother, are given to the surrogate mother or her dependents or her representative. Surrogacy means a practice whereby one woman bears and gives birth to a child for an intending couple with the intention of handing over such child to the intending couple after the birth. No surrogacy clinic, unless registered under this Act, shall conduct or associate with, or help in any manner, in conducting activities relating to surrogacy and surrogacy procedures. No surrogacy clinic, paediatrician, gynaecologist, embryologist, registered medical practitioner or any person shall conduct, offer, undertake, promote or associate with or avail of commercial surrogacy in any form. No surrogacy clinic shall employ or cause to be employed or take services of any person, whether on honorary basis or on payment, who does not possess such qualifications as may be prescribed. No registered medical practitioner, gynaecologist, paediatrician, embryologist or any other person shall conduct or cause to be conducted or aid in conducting by himself or through any other person surrogacy or surrogacy procedures at a place other than a place registered under this Act. No surrogacy clinic, registered medical practitioner, gynaecologist, paediatrician, embryologist or any other person shall promote, publish, canvass, propagate or advertise or cause to be promoted, published, canvassed, propagated or advertised which:

(a) is aimed at inducing or is likely to induce a woman to act as a surrogate mother.

(b) is aimed at promoting a surrogacy clinic for commercial surrogacy or promoting commercial surrogacy in general.

(c) seeks or aimed at seeking a woman to act as a surrogate mother.

(d) states or implies that a woman is willing to become a surrogate mother.

(e) advertises commercial surrogacy in print or electronic media or in any other form.

No surrogacy clinic, registered medical practitioner, gynaecologist, paediatrician, embryologist, intending couple or any other person shall conduct or cause abortion during the period of surrogacy without the written consent of the surrogate mother and on authorisation of the same by the appropriate authority concerned, provided that the authorisation of the appropriate authority shall be subject to, and in compliance with, the provisions of the Medical Termination of Pregnancy Act, 1971. No surrogacy clinic, registered medical practitioner, gynaecologist, paediatrician, embryologist, intending couple or any other person shall store a human embryo or gamete for the purpose of surrogacy. No surrogacy clinic, registered medical practitioner, gynaecologist, paediatrician, embryologist, intending couple or any other person shall in any form conduct or cause to be conducted sex selection for surrogacy. No surrogacy or surrogacy procedures shall be conducted, undertaken, performed or availed of, except for the following purposes, namely: (a) when an intending couple has a medical indication necessitating gestational surrogacy. Provided that a couple of Indian origin or an intending woman who intends to avail surrogacy, shall obtain a certificate of recommendation from the Board on an application made by the said persons in such form and manner as may be prescribed. (Gestational surrogacy means a practice whereby a surrogate mother carries a child for the intending couple through implantation of embryo in her womb and the child is not genetically related to the surrogate mother). (b) when it is only for altruistic surrogacy purposes (c) when it is not for commercial purposes or for commercialization of surrogacy or surrogacy procedures (d) when it is not for producing children for sale, prostitution or any other form of exploitation and (e) any other condition or disease as may be specified by regulations made by the Board.

No surrogacy or surrogacy procedures shall be conducted, undertaken, performed or initiated, unless the Director or in-charge of the surrogacy clinic and the person qualified to do so are satisfied, for reasons to be recorded in writing, that the following conditions have been fulfilled, namely:

(a) the intending couple is in possession of a certificate of essentiality issued by the appropriate authority, after satisfying itself, for the reasons to be recorded in writing, about the fulfilment of the following conditions, namely:

(i) a certificate of a medical indication in favour of either or both members of the intending couple or intending woman necessitating gestational surrogacy from a District Medical Board. District Medical Board means a medical board under the Chairpersonship of Chief Medical Officer or Chief Civil Surgeon or Joint Director of Health Services of the district and comprising of at least two other specialists, namely, the chief gynaecologist or obstetrician and chief paediatrician of the district.

(ii) an order concerning the parentage and custody of the child to be born through surrogacy, has been passed by a court of the Magistrate.

(iii) an insurance coverage of such amount and in such manner as may be prescribed in favour of the surrogate mother for a period of thirty six months covering postpartum delivery complications from an insurance company or an agent recognised by the Insurance Regulatory and Development Authority established under the Insurance Regulatory and Development Authority Act, 1999.

(b) the surrogate mother is in possession of an eligibility certificate issued by the appropriate authority on fulfilment of the following conditions, namely:

(i) no woman, other than an ever married woman having a child of her own and between the age of 25 to 35 years on the day of implantation, shall be a surrogate mother or help in surrogacy by donating her egg or oocyte or otherwise.

(ii) a willing woman shall act as a surrogate mother and be permitted to undergo surrogacy procedures as per the provisions of this Act, provided that the intending couple or the intending woman shall approach the appropriate authority with a willing woman who agrees to act as a surrogate mother.

(iii) no woman shall act as a surrogate mother by providing her own gametes.

(iv) no woman shall act as a surrogate mother more than once in her lifetime provided that the number of attempts for surrogacy procedures on the surrogate mother shall be such as may be prescribed.

(v) a certificate of medical and psychological fitness for surrogacy and surrogacy procedures from a registered medical practitioner.

(c) An eligibility certificate for intending couple is issued separately by the appropriate authority on fulfilment of the following conditions, namely:

(i) the intending couple are married and between the age of 23 to 50 years in case of female and between 26 to 55 years in case of male on the day of certification.

(ii) the intending couple have not had any surviving child biologically or through adoption or through surrogacy earlier provided that nothing contained in this item shall affect the intending couple who have a child and who is mentally or physically challenged or suffers from life threatening disorder or fatal illness with no permanent cure and approved by the appropriate authority with due medical certificate from a District Medical Board.

(iii) such other conditions as may be specified by the regulations. No person including a relative or husband of a surrogate mother or intending couple or intending woman shall seek or encourage to conduct any surrogacy or surrogacy procedures on her except for the purpose specified in clause (ii) of section 4.

Prohibition of conducting surrogacy:

(1) No person shall seek or conduct surrogacy procedures unless he has—

(i) explained all known side effects and after effects of such procedures to the surrogate mother concerned.

(ii) obtained in the prescribed form, the written informed consent of the surrogate mother to undergo such procedures in the language she understands.

(2) Notwithstanding anything contained in sub-section (1), the surrogate mother shall have an option to withdraw her consent for surrogacy before the implantation of human embryo in her womb. The intending couple or intending woman shall not abandon the child, born out of a surrogacy procedure, whether within India or outside, for any reason whatsoever, including but not restricted to, any genetic defect, birth defect, any other medical condition, the defects developing subsequently, or conception of more than one baby and the like.

A child born out of surrogacy procedure, shall be deemed to be a biological child of the intending couple or intending woman and the said child shall be entitled to all the rights and privileges available to a natural child under any law for time being in force. No person, organisation, surrogacy clinic, laboratory or clinical establishment of any kind shall force the surrogate mother to abort at any stage of surrogacy except in such conditions as may be prescribed.

Registration of surrogacy clinics:

(1) No person shall establish any surrogacy clinic for undertaking surrogacy or to render surrogacy procedures in any form unless such clinic is duly registered under this Act.

(2) Every application for registration under sub-section (1) shall be made to the appropriate authority in such form, manner and shall be accompanied by such fees as may be prescribed.

(3) Every surrogacy clinic which is conducting surrogacy or surrogacy procedures, partly or exclusively, referred to in clause (ii) of section 4 shall, within a period of sixty days from the date of appointment of appropriate authority, apply for registration: Provided that such clinic shall cease to conduct any such counselling or procedures on the expiry of six months from the date of commencement of this Act, unless such clinic has applied for registration and is so registered separately or till such application is disposed of, whichever is earlier.

(4) No surrogacy clinic shall be registered under this Act, unless the appropriate authority is satisfied that such clinic is in a position to provide such facilities and maintain such equipment and standards including specialised manpower, physical infrastructure and diagnostic facilities as may be prescribed. The appropriate authority shall after holding an enquiry and after satisfying itself that the applicant has complied with all the requirements of this Act and the rules and regulations made thereunder, grant a certificate of registration to the surrogacy clinic, within a period of ninety days from the date of application received by it, in such form, on payment of such fees and in such manner, as may be prescribed. Every certificate of registration shall be valid for a period of three years and shall be renewed in such manner and on payment of such fees as may be prescribed. The certificate of registration shall be displayed by the surrogacy clinic at a conspicuous place. The appropriate authority may, suo motu or on receipt of a complaint, issue a notice to the surrogacy clinic to show cause as to why its registration should not be suspended or cancelled for the reasons mentioned in the notice. If after giving a reasonable opportunity of being heard to the surrogacy clinic, the appropriate authority is satisfied that there has been a breach of the provisions of the Act or the rules or regulations made thereunder, it may, without prejudice to any criminal action that it may take against such clinic, suspend its registration for such period as it may think fit or cancel its registration, as the case may be. Notwithstanding anything contained in sub-sections (1) and (2), if the appropriate authority is of the opinion that it is necessary or expedient to do so in the public interest, it may, for reasons to be recorded in writing, suspend the registration of any surrogacy clinic without issuing any notice under sub-section (1). The surrogacy clinic or the intending couple or the intending woman may, within a period of thirty days from the date of receipt of the communication relating to order of rejection of application, suspension or cancellation of registration passed by the appropriate authority under section 13 and communication relating to rejection of the certificates

under section 4, prefer an appeal against such order. There shall be established a Registry to be called the National Assisted Reproductive Technology and Surrogacy Registry for the purposes of registration of surrogacy clinics under this Act.

The Central Government shall, by notification, constitute a Board to be known as the National Assisted Reproductive Technology and Surrogacy Board to exercise the powers and perform the functions conferred on the Board under this Act. The Board shall consist of (a) the Minister in-charge of the Ministry of Health and Family Welfare, the Chairperson, ex officio (b) the Secretary to the Government of India in-charge of the Department dealing with the surrogacy matter, Vice-Chairperson, ex officio (c) three women Members of Parliament, of whom two shall be elected by the House of the People and one by the Council of States, Members, ex officio (d) three Members of the Ministries of the Central Government in-charge of Women and Child Development, Legislative Department in the Ministry of Law and Justice and the Ministry of Home Affairs, not below the rank of Joint Secretary, Members, ex officio (e) the Director General of Health Services of the Central Government, Member, ex officio (f) ten expert Members to be appointed by the Central Government in such manner as may be prescribed and two each from amongst (i) eminent medical geneticists or embryologists (ii) eminent gynaecologists and obstetricians (iii) eminent social scientists (iv) representatives of women welfare organisations and (v) representatives from civil society working on women's health and child issues, possessing such qualifications and experience as may be prescribed (g) four Chairpersons of the State Boards to be nominated by the Central Government by rotation to represent the States and the Union territories, two in the alphabetical order and two in the reverse alphabetical order, Member, ex officio and (h) an officer, not below the rank of a Joint Secretary to the Central Government, in-charge of Surrogacy Division in the Ministry of Health and Family Welfare, who shall be the Member-Secretary, ex officio. (1) The term of office of a Member, other than an ex officio Member, shall be three years provided that the term of such Member shall come to an end as soon as the Member becomes a Minister or Minister of State or Deputy Minister, or the Speaker or the Deputy Speaker of the House of the

People, or the Deputy Chairman of the Council of States or ceases to be a Member of the House from which she was elected. The Board shall discharge the following functions, namely: (a) to advise the Central Government on policy matters relating to surrogacy (b) to review and monitor the implementation of the Act, and the rules and regulations made thereunder and recommend to the Central Government, changes therein (c) to lay down the code of conduct to be observed by persons working at surrogacy clinics (d) to set the minimum standards of physical infrastructure, laboratory and diagnostic equipment and expert manpower to be employed by the surrogacy clinics (e) to oversee the performance of various bodies constituted under the Act and take appropriate steps to ensure their effective performance (f) to supervise the functioning of State Assisted Reproductive Technology and Surrogacy Boards and (g) such other functions as may be prescribed. Each State and Union territory having Legislature shall constitute a Board to be known as the State Assisted Reproductive Technology and Surrogacy Board or the Union territory Assisted Reproductive Technology and Surrogacy Board, as the case may be, which shall discharge the following functions, namely: (i) to review the activities of the appropriate authorities functioning in the State or Union territory and recommend appropriate action against them (ii) to monitor the implementation of the provisions of the Act, and the rules and regulations made thereunder and make suitable recommendations relating thereto, to the Board (iii) to send such consolidated reports as may be prescribed, in respect of the various activities undertaken in the State under the Act, to the Board and the Central Government and (iv) such other functions as may be prescribed. The State Board shall consist of— (a) the Minister in-charge of Health and Family Welfare in the State, Chairperson, ex officio (b) the Secretary in-charge of the Department of Health and Family Welfare, Vice-Chairperson, ex officio (c) Secretaries or Commissioners in-charge of the Departments of Women and Child Development, Social Welfare, Law and Justice and Home Affairs or their nominees, members, ex officio (d) Director-General of Health and Family Welfare of the State Government, member, ex officio (e) three women members of the State Legislative Assembly or Union territory Legislative Council, members, ex officio (f) ten expert members to be appointed by the State Government in such manner as may be prescribed, two each from amongst (i) eminent medical geneticists or embryologists (ii) eminent gynaecologists and obstetricians (iii) eminent social scientists (iv) representatives of women welfare organisations and (v) representatives from civil society working on women's health and child issues, possessing such qualifications and experiences as may be prescribed (g) an officer not below the rank of Joint Secretary to the State Government in-charge of Family Welfare, who shall be the Member-Secretary, ex officio.

The appropriate authority shall discharge the following functions, namely: (a) to grant, suspend or cancel registration of a surrogacy clinic (b) to enforce the standards to be fulfilled by the surrogacy clinics (c) to investigate complaints of breach of the provisions of this Act, rules and regulations made thereunder and take legal action as per provision of this Act (d) to take appropriate legal action against the use of surrogacy by any person at any place other than prescribed, suo motu or brought to its notice, and also to initiate independent investigations in such matter (e) to supervise the implementation of the provisions of this Act and rules and regulations made thereunder (f) to recommend to the Board and State Boards about the modifications required in the rules and regulations in accordance with changes in technology or social conditions (g) to take action after investigation of complaints received by it against the surrogacy clinics and (h) to consider and grant or reject any application under clause (vi) of section 3 and sub-clauses (a) to (c) of clause (iii) of section 4 within a period of ninety days.

The appropriate authority shall exercise the powers in respect of the following matters, namely: (a) summoning of any person who is in possession of any information relating to violation of the provisions of this Act, and rules and regulations made thereunder (b) production of any document or material object relating to clause (a) (c) search any place suspected to be violating the provisions of this Act, and the rules and regulations made thereunder and (d) such other powers as may be prescribed. (2) The appropriate authority shall maintain the details of registration of surrogacy clinics, cancellation of registration, renewal of registration, grant of certificates to the intending couple and surrogate mothers or any other matter pertaining to grant of license, etc., of the surrogacy clinics in such format as may be prescribed and submit the same to the National Assisted Reproductive Technology and Surrogacy Board.

No person, organisation, surrogacy clinic, laboratory or clinical establishment of any kind shall (a) undertake commercial surrogacy, provide commercial surrogacy or its related component procedures or services in any form or run a racket or an organised group to empanel or select surrogate mothers or use individual brokers or intermediaries to arrange for surrogate mothers and for surrogacy procedures, at such clinics, laboratories or at any other place (b) issue, publish, distribute, communicate or cause to be issued, published, distributed or communicated, any advertisement in any manner regarding commercial surrogacy by any means whatsoever, scientific or otherwise (c) abandon or disown or exploit or cause to be abandoned, disowned or exploited in any form, the child or children born through surrogacy (d) exploit or cause to be exploited the surrogate mother or the child born through surrogacy in any manner whatsoever (e) sell human embryo or gametes for the purpose of surrogacy and run an agency, a racket or an organisation for selling, purchasing or trading in human embryos or gametes for the purpose of surrogacy (f) import or shall help in getting imported in, whatsoever manner, the human embryo or human gametes for surrogacy or for surrogacy procedures and (g) conduct sex selection in any form for surrogacy.

Notwithstanding anything contained in the Indian Penal Code, contraventions of the provisions of clauses (a) to (g) of sub-section (1) by any person shall be an offence punishable with imprisonment for a term which may extend to ten years and with fine which may extend to ten lakh rupees. For the purposes of this section, the expression "advertisement" includes any notice, circular, label, wrapper or any other document including advertisement through internet or any other media, in electronic or print form and also includes any visible representation made by means of any hoarding, wall-painting, signal light, sound, smoke or gas. Any registered medical practitioner, gynaecologists, paediatrician, embryologists or any person who owns a surrogacy clinic or employed with such a clinic or centre or laboratory and renders his professional or technical services to or at such clinic or centre or laboratory, whether on an honorary basis or otherwise, and who contravenes any Powers of appropriate authorities and rules and regulations made thereunder shall be punishable with imprisonment for a term which may extend to five years and with fine which may extend to ten lakh rupees. In case of subsequent or continuation of the offence referred to in sub-section the name of the registered medical practitioner shall be reported by the appropriate authority to the State Medical Council concerned for taking necessary action including suspension of registration for a period of five years. Any intending couple or intending woman or any person who seeks the aid of any surrogacy clinic, laboratory or of a registered medical practitioner, gynaecologist, paediatrician, embryologist or any other person for not following the altruistic surrogacy or for conducting surrogacy procedures for commercial purposes shall be punishable with imprisonment for a term which may extend to five years and with fine which may extend to five lakh rupees for the first offence and for any subsequent offence with imprisonment which may extend to ten years and with fine which may extend to ten lakh rupees. Whoever contravenes any of the provisions of this Act, rules or regulations made thereunder for which no penalty has been provided in this Act, shall be punishable with imprisonment for a term which may extend to three years and with fine which may extend to five lakh rupees and in the case of continuing contravention with an additional fine which may extend to ten thousand rupees for every day during which such contravention continues after conviction for the first such contravention. Notwithstanding anything contained in the Indian Evidence Act, 1872, the court shall presume, unless the contrary is proved, that the women or surrogate mother was compelled by her husband, the intending couple or any other relative, as the case may be, to render surrogacy services, procedures or to donate gametes for the purpose other than those specified in clause (ii) of section 4 and such person shall be liable for abetment of such offence under section 40 and shall be punishable for the offence specified under that section. Notwithstanding anything contained in the Code of Criminal Procedure, 1973, every offence under this Act shall be cognizable, non-bailable and non-compoundable. No court shall take cognizance of any offence punishable under this Act except on a complaint in writing made by— (a) the appropriate authority concerned, or any officer or an agency authorised in this behalf by the Central Government or the State Government, as the case may be, or the appropriate authority or a person including a social organisation who has given notice of not less that fifteen days in the manner prescribed, to the appropriate authority, of the alleged offence and of his intention to make a complaint to the court. No court inferior to that of a Metropolitan Magistrate or a Judicial Magistrate of the first class shall try any offence punishable under this Act.

The surrogacy clinic shall maintain all records, charts, forms, reports, consent letters, agreements and all the documents under this Act and they shall be preserved for a period of twenty-five years or such period as may be prescribed provided that, if any criminal or other proceedings are instituted against any surrogacy clinic, the records and all other documents of such clinic shall be preserved till the final disposal of such proceedings. All such records shall, at all reasonable times, be made available for inspection to the appropriate authority or to any other person authorised by the appropriate authority in this behalf. If the appropriate authority has reason to believe that an offence under this Act has been or is being committed at any surrogacy clinic or any other place, such authority or any officer authorised in this behalf may, subject to such rules as may be prescribed, enter and search at all reasonable times with such assistance, if any, as such authority or officers considers necessary, such surrogacy clinic or any other place and examine any record, register, document, book, pamphlet, advertisement or any other material object found therein and seize and seal the same if such authority or officer has reason to believe that it may furnish evidence of the commission of an offence punishable under this Act. The provisions of the Code of Criminal Procedure, 1973 relating to search and seizure shall apply, as far as may be, to all action taken by the appropriate authority or any officer authorised by it under this Act.

The Central Government may, by notification and subject to the condition of pre-publication, make rules for carrying out the provisions of this Act. In particular, and without prejudice to the generality of the foregoing power, such rules may provide for— (a) the prescribed expenses under clauses (b), (f) and (q) of sub-section (1) of section 2 (b) the minimum qualifications for persons employed at a registered surrogacy clinic under clause (iii) of section 3 (c) the period and manner in which a person shall store human embryo or gamete under clause (vii) of section 3 (d) the form and manner of application for obtaining certificate of recommendation from the Board under provison to sub-clause (a) of clause (ii) of section 4 (e) the insurance coverage in favour of the surrogate mother from an insurance company and the manner of such coverage under item (III) of sub-clause (a) of clause (iii) of section 4 (f) the number of attempts of surrogacy or providing of gametes under the proviso to item (III) of sub-clause (b) of clause (iii) of section 4 (g) the form in which consent of a surrogate mother has to be obtained under clause (ii) of section 6 (h) the number of oocytes or embryos to be implanted in the uterus of the surrogate mother under section 9; 2 of 1974. (i) the conditions under which the surrogate mother may be allowed for abortion during the process of surrogacy under section 10 (j) the form and manner in which an application shall be made for registration and the fee payable thereof under sub-section (2) of section 11 (k) the facilities to be provided, equipment and other standards to be maintained by the surrogacy clinics under sub-section (4) of section 11 (l) the period, manner and form in which a certificate of registration shall be issued under sub-section (1) of section 12 (m) the manner in which the certificate of registration shall be renewed and the fee payable for such renewal under sub-section (3) of section 12 (n) the manner in which an appeal may be preferred under section 14 (o) the qualifications and experiences of the Members as admissible under clause (f) of sub-section (2) of section 17 (p) the procedures for conducting an inquiry against the Members under sub-section (2) of section 21 (q) the conditions under which a Member of the Board eligible for re-appointment under section 24 (r) the other functions of the Board under clause (g) of section 25 (s) the manner in which reports shall be furnished by the State Assisted Reproductive Technology and Surrogacy Board and the Union territory Assisted Reproductive Technology and Surrogacy Board to the Board and the Central Government under clause (iii) of section 26 (t) the other functions of the State Board under clause (iv) of section 26 (u) the qualifications and experiences of the members as admissible under clause (f) of section 27 (v) the age of the person to be appointed as a member, referred to in clause (f) of section 27, under the proviso to clause (b) of sub-section (1) of section 28 (w) the procedures for conducting an inquiry against the members under sub-section (2) of section 31 (x) the conditions under which the members of State Board eligible for re-appointment under section 34 (y) empowering the appropriate authority in any other matter under clause (d) of section 36 (z) the other powers of appropriate authority under clause (d) of sub-section (1) of section 37 (za) the particulars of the details of registration of surrogacy clinics, cancellation of registration, etc., in such format under sub-section (2) of section 37 (zb) the manner of giving notice by a person under clause (b) of sub-section (1) of section 44 (zc) the period up to which records, charts, etc., shall be preserved under sub-section (1) of section 46 (zd) the manner in which the seizure of documents, records, objects, etc., shall be made and the manner in which seizure list shall be prepared and delivered under sub-section (1) of section 47 and (ze) any other matter which is to be, or may be, or in respect of which provision is to be made by rules.

Assisted Reproductive Technology (Regulation) Act, 2021

Parliament on December 8, 2021 passed the *Assisted Reproductive Technology (Regulation) Act, 2021,* which received the assent of the President on December 18, 2021. The Act aims at the regulation and supervision of ART clinics and assisted reproductive technology banks, prevention of misuse, and safe and ethical practice of ART services.

- The Act seeks to regulate and supervise the assisted reproductive technology clinics and the assisted reproductive technology banks, prevention of misuse, safe and ethical practice of assisted reproductive technology services for addressing the issues of reproductive health where assisted reproductive technology is required for becoming a parent or for freezing gametes, embryos, embryonic tissues for further use due to infertility, disease or social or medical concerns and for regulation and supervision of research and development and for matters connected therewith or incidental thereto.
- Under the Act, every assisted reproductive technology (ART) clinic and bank must be registered under the National Registry of Banks and Clinics of India. The Registry is meant to act as a central database for all facilities providing ART services in India, with state governments appointing relevant authorities in their respective states to facilitate the registration process.
- The Registration must be renewed every five years and may be cancelled or suspended if an entity contravenes the provisions of the Act.

- The National Assisted Reproductive Technology and Surrogacy Board to be constituted under the National Board for the purposes of this Act.
- The Central Government may, within a period of ninety days from the date of commencement of this Act, by notification, establish for the purposes of this Act and Surrogacy Act, a Registry to be called the National Assisted Reproductive Technology and Surrogacy Registry.
- The National Registry shall consist of such scientific, technical, administrative and supportive staff and the terms and conditions of their service under the Act.
- The Act enumerates the procedure of registration of Assisted Technology Clinics and Banks, which includes provisions for grant of registration, renewal, suspension or cancellation. The National Board, the National Registry and the State Board shall have the power to, — (i) inspect, any premises relating to assisted reproductive technology or (ii) call for any document or material, in exercise of their powers and discharge of their functions.

The clinics and banks shall perform the following duties:

- the clinics and banks shall ensure that commissioning couple, woman and donors of gametes are eligible to avail the assisted reproductive technology procedures subject to such criteria as may be prescribed
- the clinics shall obtain donor gametes from the banks and such banks shall ensure that the donor has been medically tested for such diseases as may be prescribed
- the clinics shall make commissioning couple or woman, aware of the rights of a child born through the use of assisted reproductive technology
- every clinic and every bank shall maintain a grievance cell in respect of matters relating to such clinics and banks and the manner of making a compliant before such grievance cell shall be such as may be prescribed
- the clinics shall issue to the commissioning couple or woman a discharge certificate stating details of the assisted reproductive

technology procedure performed on the commissioning couple or woman.

Offences and Penalties

- The clinic, or bank or agent thereof, shall not issue, publish, distribute, communicate or cause to be issued, published, distributed or communicated any advertisement in any manner including internet, regarding facilities of sex selective assisted reproductive technology.
- Contravention of provisions shall be punishable with imprisonment for a term of five years, extendable to ten years or with fine which shall not be less than ten lakh rupees but may extend to twenty-five lakh rupees or with both.

Under the Act, any medical geneticist, gynaecologist, registered medical practitioner or any person shall not

- abandon, disown or exploit or cause to be abandoned, disowned or exploited in any form the child or children born through assisted reproductive technology.
- sell human embryos or gametes, run an agency, a racket or an organisation for selling, purchasing or trading in human embryos or gametes.
- import or help in getting imported in whatsoever manner, the human embryos or human gametes.
- exploit the commissioning couple, woman or the gamete donor in any form.
- transfer human embryo into a male person or an animal.
- sell any human embryo or gamete for the purpose of research.
- use any intermediates to obtain gamete donors or purchase gamete donors.

Any contravention of the provisions of clauses (a) to (g) shall be punishable with a fine which shall not be less than five lakh rupees but may extend to ten lakh rupees for the first contravention and for subsequent contravention, shall be punishable with imprisonment for a term which shall not be less than three years but may extend to eight years and with fine which shall not be less than ten lakh rupees but may extend to twenty lakh rupees.

While the Act is a decisive and considerable step towards curbing the menace of illegal and unregulated ART clinics and towards safeguarding donors and women undergoing ART from the health implications faced due to unsafe and illegal procedures, it falls short of addressing some serious concerns.

First and foremost, the Act excludes unmarried men, divorced men, widowed men, unmarried yet cohabiting heterosexual couples, transpersons and homosexual couples (whether married or cohabiting) from availing ART services. This exclusion is relevant as the Surrogacy Act also excludes above said persons from taking recourse to surrogacy as a method of reproduction.

The Act is also limited to those commissioning couples who are infertile - those who have been unable to conceive after one year of unprotected coitus. Thus, it is limited in its application and significantly reduces the reproductive choices of those excluded. Third, the prices of the services are not regulated; this can certainly be remedied with simple directives.

Licenses, permits and other legal documents required to open and operate a hospital

The laws applicable for commissioning and operating a hospital can be categorised as;

1. Laws for governing the commissioning of hospital:

- Municipality to Local Authority
- Society Registration Act –1960
- Delhi Fire Service Act-1956
- St. John Ambulance Association (India) Transfer of Funds Act – 1956
- Red Cross Society (Allocation of Property) Act- 1936
- Delhi Fire Service Act – 2007
- Karnataka Medical Registration (Amendment) Act – 2003
- Delhi Fire Prevention and Fire Safety Act – 1986
- Fire Safety Rules – 1987
- Government Buildings Act – 1899
- Electricity Rules – 1956

- The National Capital Territory of Delhi Laws (Special Provisions) Second Bill -2007
- Delhi Lift Act – 1942
- The Registration Act. – 1908
- Bombay Lifts Act – 1939
- Building and Other Construction Workers (Regulation of Employment and Conditions of Service) Act – 1908
- Delhi Nursing Home Registration Act – 1953
- Clinical Establishments Bill – 2010
- Bombay Nursing Homes Registration (Amendment) Act-2005
- Indian Telegraph Act – 1885
- Bombay Nursing Homes Registration (Extension and Amendment) Act -1959
- Atomic Energy (Safe disposal of Radioactive Waste) Rules -1987
- Bombay Nursing Homes Registration Act – 1949
- Radiation Protection Certificate for Radiology Department from BARC
- Atomic Energy Regulatory Body Approval for Radiology / Nuclear Medicine Services under the Atomic Energy Act – 1962

2. Laws/Regulations governing hospital business aspects:

- The Public Liability Insurance Act – 1991/1992
- The Public Liability Insurance Rules – 1991/1993
- Charitable and Religious Trust Act-1920
- Contract Act – 1982
- Income Tax ACT – 1961
- Copyright Act – 1982
- Customs Act – 1962
- Gift Tax Act – 1958
- Foreign Exchange Management Act-1999
- Cable Television Network ACT – 1995
- Wireless Operation Certificate from Post and Telegraphs

- Insurance Act – 1938
- Rules for display of Red Cross Insignia
- Vehicle Registration Certificate
- Sales of Good Act – 1930

3. Laws governing sales/storage of drugs and safe medication:

- Sales of Good Act – 1930
- Drugs and Cosmetic Act – 1940
- Central Excise Act (for permit to use and store sprit) – 1944
- The Drug and Cosmetics Rules (Amendment 2005) – 1945
- Pharmacy Act – 1948
- The Drugs Control Act – 1950
- Central Sales Tax Act -1956
- Homoeopathy Central Council Act – 1973
- Drug and Cosmetic Act Amendment – 1982
- Narcotics and Psychotropic Substances Act -1985
- Blood Bank Regulations under Drugs and Cosmetic (2nd amendment) rules – 1999
- Homoeopathy Central Council (Amendment) Act -2002
- License for Possession and use of Rectified / denatured spirit
- Retail Drug License
- VAT Act
- Adulteration of Drugs (IPC Sec 274)
- Sales of Adulterated Drugs (IPC Sec 275)
- Sales of Drug as Different Drug or Preparation (IPC Sec 276)
- Negligent Conduct with Regard to Poisonous Substances (IPC Sec 284)

4. Laws governing qualifications, practice and conduct of professionals:

- Indian Nursing Council Act -1947
- The Dentists Act – 1948
- Indian Medical Council Act – 1956

- Karnataka Anatomy Act – 1957
- Kerala Anatomy Act – 1957
- The Apprenticeship Act – 1961
- The Dentists (Code of Ethics Regulation) – 1976
- All India Council for Technical Education ACT – 1987
- Rehabilitation Council of India Act – 1992
- Delhi Nursing Council Act- 1997
- Kerala Co-operative Hospital Complex and the Academy of Medical Sciences (taking over the management) Act – 1997
- Rehabilitation Council of India (Amendment) Act – 2000
- Indian Medical Council (professional conduct, etiquette and ethics) regulations- 2002
- Dental Council of India Regulations – 2006
- Kerala Professional Colleges or Institutions (Prohibition of Capitation Fee, Regulation of Admission, Fixation of Non-exploitative Fee and Other Measures to Ensure Equity and Excellence in Professional Education) Amendment Act – 2007
- Indian Medical Degrees Act
- Registration of Medical Practitioners with State Medical Councils
- The ICN Code of Ethics for Nurses
- AICTE Rules of Physiotherapy Rules

5. Laws governing management of patients:

- Birth, Death and Marriage Registration Act – 1886
- Guardians and Wards Act – 1890
- The Epidemic Disease Act – 1897
- Indian Lunacy Act – 1912
- Drugs and Magic Remedies (objectionable) Advertisements Act 1954 – 1954
- Delhi Registration of Birth and Deaths Act – 1969
- MTP Rules – 1971

- Delhi Municipal Corporation (Malaria and other mosquito Borne disease) Bye Law – 1975
- Lepers Act – 1975
- Ear Drums and Ear Bones (Authority for Use for Therapeutic Purposes) Act – 1982
- Eyes (Authority for Use for Therapeutic Purposes) Act -1982
- The Mental Health Act – 1987
- Transplantation of Human Organ Act – 1994
- PNDT Act – 1994
- Transplantation of Human Organ Rule – 1995
- Pre Conception and Prenatal Diagnostic Techniques (prohibition of sex selection) Rules – 1996
- MTP Act – 1997
- Rules for Insurance Cover for the Sterilization Cases
- Laws of Contract Section 13 (Consent)
- National Guidelines for Clinical Management of HIV / AIDS, NACO, Govt. of India.
- Manual for Control of Hospital Associated Infections: SOPs, NACO, Govt. of India

6. Laws governing environmental protection/safety:

- DMC Sanitation and Public Health Bye Laws – 1959
- The Water (Prevention and Control of Pollution) Act – 1974/1988
- The Water (Prevention and Control of Pollution) Rules – 1975
- The Water (Prevention and Control of Pollution) Cess Rules – 1978
- Air (Prevention and Control of Pollution) Act – 1981/1987
- The Air (Prevention and Control of Pollution) Rules – 1982
- The Air (Prevention and Control of Pollution) (Union Territories) Rules – 1983
- Environment protection Rule – 1986
- Environment protection Act – 1996

- Biomedical waste management handling rules – 1998/2000
- The Noise Pollution (Regulation and Control) (Amendment) Rules – 2000
- Noise pollution control Rules – 2000
- The Noise Pollution (Regulation and Control) (Amendment) Rules – 2002
- The Water (Prevention and Control of Pollution) Cess (Amendment) Act- 2003
- The Noise Pollution (Regulation and Control) (Amendment) Rules – 2006
- The Noise Pollution (Regulation and Control) (Amendment) Rules – 2010
- Rules regarding the safe discharge of effluents in the public sewers / drains
- IPC sec 278 (making atmosphere noxious to health)
- IPC sec 269 (negligent act likely to spread infection or disease dangerous to life, unlawfully or negligently)

7. Laws governing employment of manpower:

- Negotiable Instrument Act – 1881
- Workmen's Compensation Act – 1923
- Official Secrets Act – 1923
- Indian Trade Union Act – 1926
- Payment of Wages Act – 1936
- Industrial Disputes Act – 1947
- Weekly Holidays Act – 1942
- ESI Act – 1948
- Minimum Wedge Act – 1948
- ESI (Central) Rules – 1950
- Employees Provident Fund and Misc. provision Act – 1952
- Citizenship Act – 1955
- Employment Exchange (Compulsory notification of vacancies) Act – 1959
- PPF Act – 1968
- Payment of Bonus Act – 1965

- Payment of Gratuity Act – 1972
- Equal Remuneration Act -1976
- SC and ST Act – 1989
- Persons with Disabilities Act – 1995
- Persons With Disabilities (Equal Opportunities, Protection of Rights and Full Participation) Act 1995
- Information Technology Act – 2000
- Maternity Benefit (Amendment) Act – 2008
- Information Technology (Amendment) Act – 2008
- Workmen's Compensation (Amendment) Act – 2009
- Karnataka Prohibition of Violence against Medicare Service Personnel and Damage to Property in Medicare Service Institutions Act – 2009
- Shops and Factories Act (for National Holidays)
- Child Labour Act
- TDS Act

8. Law governing the safety of patients, public and staff within the hospital premises:

- Vaccination Act – 1880
- Explosive Act 1884 (for diesel storage) – 1884
- Indian Boilers Act – 1923
- Arms Act – 1950
- Prevention of Food Adulteration Act -1954
- The Indian Fatal Accidents Act – 1955
- Insecticide Act – 1968
- Radiation Protection Rules – 1971
- The Radiation Surveillance Procedures for the Medical Application of Radiation – 1989
- Protection of Human Rights Act – 1993
- Vaccination (Repeal) Act – 2001
- AERB safety code no. AERB/SC/Med -2 (REV -1) – 2001
- Petroleum Act + Storage Rules – 2002

- The Cigarettes and other Tobacco products (prohibition of advertisement and regulation of trade, commerce, production, supply and distribution) Bill – 2003
- Gas Cylinder Rules -2004
- Disaster Management Act – 2005
- Prohibition of Smoking in Public Places Rules – 2008
- The Tamil Nadu Medicare Service Persons and Medicare Service Institutions (prevention of violence and damage or loss to property) Act – 2008
- IPC Sec 336 (act endangering life and personal safety of others)
- IPC Sec 337 (causing hurt by act endangering life and personal safety of others)
- IPC Sec 338 (causing grievous hurt by act endangering the life and personal safety of others.
- Rules for Provision of Safe Drinking Water
- Rules for Provision of Uninterrupted Power supply

9. Laws governing medico legal aspects:

- Consumer protection Act – 1986
- Law of privileged communication
- Protection of human rights Act
- IPC section 52
- IPC section 80
- IPC section 89
- IPC section 92
- IPC section 93
- IPC section 269
- Law of torts
- Indian Evidence act (disclosure of privileged / confidential patient related information before a court of law – under protest)

10. Law governing professional training and research:

- ICMR Rules Governing Medical Research
- MCI Rules for Internship Training

- Nursing Council of India Rules for starting School / College of Nursing
- National Board of Examinations Rules for DNB training

11. Law governing Biomedical research:

- Reconstitution of Committee for the Purpose of Control and Supervision of Experiments on Animals (CPCSEA).
- Breeding of and Experiments on Animals (Control and Supervision) Amendment Rules – 2005.

The Clinical Establishments (Registration and Regulation) Act, 2010

The Clinical Establishments (Registration and Regulation) Act, 2010 has been enacted by the Central Government to provide for registration and regulation of all clinical establishments in the country with a view to prescribe the minimum standards of facilities and services provided by them. The Ministry has notified the "National Council for Clinical Establishments" and 'The Clinical Establishments (Central Government) Rules, 2012" under this Act vide Gazette. This Act is applicable to all kinds of clinical establishments from the public and private sectors, of all recognized systems of medicine including single doctor clinics. The only exception will be establishments run by the Armed forces. The Clinical Establishments Act was passed by Parliament of India on 17th August 2010, to provide for registration and regulation of all clinical establishments in the country with a view to prescribing minimum standards of facilities and services which may be provided by them so that mandate of article 47 of the constitution for improvement in public health may be achieved. The Act was notified vide Gazette notification dated 28th February, 2012. The Ministry of Health and Family Welfare has notified the National Council for Clinical Establishments and the Clinical Establishments (Central Government) Rules, 2012 under this Act vide Gazette notifications dated 19th March, 2012 and 23rd May, 2012 respectively.

Clinical establishments not covered under the Act are:

1. Clinical establishments owned, controlled or managed by the Armed Forces .

2. Clinical Establishment in the States /UTs mentioned in the schedule of the Act; unless they repeal existing Act and adopt Clinical Establishments Act.
3. Also, Clinical Establishments of those categories and of those recognised systems of medicine for which date has not been appointed by the State Government, who has other wise adopted the Act.

Clinical Establishments Act aims to register and regulate clinical establishments based on minimum standards in order to improve quality of public health care in the country. To establish digital registry of Clinical Establishments at National, State and District level and to prevent quackery by unqualified practitioners by introducing registration system, which is mandatory.

Conditions to be fulfilled by every Clinical Establishment for Grant of Registration (Permanent) and continuation .

1. Minimum standards of facilities and services.
2. Minimum requirement of personnel.
3. Provision and maintenance of records and reports.
4. Every clinical establishment is required to provide treatment "with in the staff and facilities available" to stabilize the emergency medical condition of an individual who comes or is brought to the clinical establishment.
5. Other conditions (as prescribed under Central Govt. Rules)
    - Details of rates charged and facilities available to be prominently displayed at a conspicuous place in local and in English language
    - Maintain and provide Electronic medical records or Electronic Health records of every patient as may be determined and issued by Central/State Govt.
    - Clinical Establishments shall charge the rates for procedures and services within the range of rates determined by the Central Government from time to time in consultation with the State Governments.
    - Clinical Establishments shall ensure compliance to Standard Treatment guidelines as may be issued by Central/State Govt.

- Every Clinical Establishments shall maintain information and statistics in accordance with all applicable laws and rules.

Fee for registration, renewal and appeal

- Shall be specified by respective State Government/UT administration under section 54.
- State/UT may charge fee category wise.
- Enhanced fee may be charged if renewal not applied within the prescribed time.
- State Government/UT Administration may charge fee for appeal made to state/UT Council.

Time period to Apply for Renewal of Registration

- 30 days before expiry of the validity of certificate in case of provisional registration.
- 6 months before expiry of the validity of certificate in case of permanent registration.

Cancellation of registration of clinical establishment after registration is granted

- If conditions of registration are not being complied .
- Person who is responsible for management of the Clinical establishment has been convicted of offence under this Act.
- If there is imminent danger to the health and safety of patients, then after cancellation, the authority may immediately restrain the clinical establishment.

Penalties under the Act

- No imprisonment under this Act .
- Monetary penalties: Rs 10000 to 5 lakh; depends on size, category, type and local conditions.

Provisional Registration

The clinical establishment is expected to apply for provisional registration initially. However after notification of minimum standards, the clinical establishment may apply for direct permanent registration also. For purpose of provisional registration, an application form in the prescribed proforma along with the prescribed fee as determined by the State Government will be required. For provisional registration, the authority shall not undertake any inspection or make any enquiry prior to the grant of provisional registration and shall within a period of ten days from the date of receipt of such application, grant to the applicant a certificate of provisional registration containing particulars and information as per format of certificate of provisional registration either by post or electronically . Every provisional registration shall be valid to the last day of the twelfth month from the date of issue of the certificate of registration and such registration shall be renewable. The application for renewal of registration shall be made to the authority within thirty days before the expiry of the validity of the certificate of provisional registration. In case the application for renewal is made after the expiry of the provisional registration, the authority shall allow renewal of registration on payment of such enhanced fees, as may be prescribed by State Government.

Permanent Registration

A clinical establishment, applying for permanent registration, has to submit evidence of it having complied with the prescribed minimum standard.

The registering authority may authorise an inspection or an inquiry of any registered clinical establishment to be made by a multi-member inspection team. A show cause notice may be issued if the authority feels that a clinical establishment is not complying with the conditions of its registration. It may also cancel the registration. The authority may enter and search in the prescribed manner after giving notice of its intention to the clinical establishment, if it suspects that an establishment is operating without registration. Information pertaining to compliance with standards and conditions of registration by clinical establishments is to be displayed in the public domain. Every permanent registration shall be valid for a period of five years from the date of issue of the certificate of registration and such registration shall be renewable. The application for renewal of permanent registration shall be made six months before the expiry of the validity of the certificate of permanent registration and, in case the application of renewal is not submitted within the stipulated period, the authority may allow renewal of registration on payment of such enhanced fees and penalties as may be prescribed.

References

1. Indian legislation, Ministry of law and consumer affairs ,Govt. of India.
2. International Journal of Research Foundation of Hospital & Healthcare Administration, rfhha.org/index.php?option=com_content&view= article& id=1 &Itemid=51
3. Ministry of Health and Family Welfare . Govt of India. www.mohfw.gov.in.
4. Ministry of law and Justice . Govt of India.

17

Hospital Architecture

Rapid changes in medical technology in the twentieth century required changes in typical hospital environment in cycles of as few as 5 or 10 years. Because the process of design and construction is both long and expensive planners faced the challenge that many hospitals were out of date the moment they were commissioned. One of the challenges facing the architecture profession in the 21st century is how to design a flexible hospital to suit unpredictable future needs. Change over time is a constant feature of architecture, yet the pace of change and its intensity are much greater in hospitals than in any other type of building. There is a need to design the health care facilities to allow for change and adaptability and also there is a need of humanizing the healthcare environment for patients and staff. There is a perceived need to shift the emphasis from a system empowerment perspective where staff and clinical needs prevail to one that emphasized the empowerment of the patient and their family as part of the health care process. Humanizing the health care environment means an emphasis on achieving natural light and ventilation, outlook and views for patients, thus producing pleasant and non stress feel healing environment. We look for rooms and spaces that are interesting and pleasantly stimulating to be within, yet at the same time address the needs of patients. Patient empowerment is achieved but not at the expense of recognizing and responding to the reality of a health care facility as the primary work place for its staff. To remain competitive, facilities must be open to integrating new technologies. Despite its recent growth, introducing new technologies in hospitals is not a simple matter. New technologies are often not embraced by staff or they don't effectively mesh with existing systems. An engineering master plan goes beyond bricks and mortar to the heart of a building. Using variety of tools, an engineering master plan gauges compatibility of existing infrastructure with potential new technologies. It also sets the stage for facility growth.

Patient Focused Hospitals

Hospital should foster a connection to nature and should encourage care givers to be responsive to patients. Value needs to be attached to way finding devices, views and public spaces. To achieve patient and family centered facility, hospitals feature single occupancy rooms and sleeping accommodation for patient's families. Family zones are integrated within each room. Floor to ceiling windows and internal courtyards ensure increased day light. However providing single occupancy rooms do not guarantee the best patient care environment especially if other factors were sacrificed in order to achieve them. Studies have shown that team work and communication involving the patient's family contribute to patient's safety. The active process of involving the patient and family with the care of the patient helps catch errors, so care givers can recover potential adverse events. Each patient room in the facility is a private room allowing more space for staff to provide care and for family members who want to stay close to the patient. A small charting alcove adjacent to the room will allow nurses to observe without disturbing the patient's rest, creating a better healing environment. All rooms are truly standardized in layout and placement of equipment and supplies. A cabinet or nurse server in each alcove holds the patient's barcoded medication in a locked box along with other supplies needed for patient care. Noise reduction can be achieved through single rooms and the use of special noise absorbing ceiling tiles, structural systems designed to reduce vibrations, the elimination of over head paging and insulation between rooms. For added safety, patient rooms can be wired for the use of cameras, to assist with monitoring of high risk patients. The cameras connect directly to the nurses station or other appropriate location, and will only be used with the consent of the patient. Additional technologies such as the use of automatic lights that go on when the patient attempts to get out of bed are considered to reduce the potential for patient falls. Other design considerations to reduce patient falls are bathrooms at the head end of the bed with a handrail from bed to the bathroom, beds that lower to reduce the harm to patients falling and rubber flooring that is safer than traditional hard flooring alternatives. In Europe in many instances the balance tips away from the higher proportion of patient single rooms that are often regarded as non-negotiable by Americans. In Europe single rooms is seen as having a place but the provision of all single rooms may not be the most important factor under consideration in terms of planning a facility. Tight urban sites mean that if the whole of a building's perimeter is allocated to the windows required by single patient bedrooms, there will be very little left for staff offices and recreational areas. Longer narrow buildings, often a combination of double loaded single corridors and deeper internally planned linking spaces mean that more external walls are available for a variety of purposes. However to ensure that staff walking distances are kept to a reasonable dimension requires that something has to be conceded. The wider incidence of few two, three or more bed patient rooms positively impacts the issue of ever lengthening corridors in health care buildings, reduces the initial capital cost of these facilities and often allows the allocation of windows and outlook to staff spaces such as offices and tea rooms.

Hospital can be made accommodating to children with positive distractions. When a child enters a hospital there should be journey of discovery by having distraction around every corner.

Hospital Design and Safety

In hospital there are active failures or latent conditions. Active failures are errors made by those who provide care and latent conditions arise from decision made by management, architects, designers and include lack of standardization of equipment, poor visibility etc. Whereas a poorly designed and maintained hospital provides the conditions that precipitate accidents, a well-designed hospital has inbuilt safeguards that make it difficult for these accidents to occur or that may help stop the chain of events before they result in accidents. Aspects of hospital design such as air quality, lighting, patient room design and other interior design elements directly impact safety outcomes such as nosocomial infections, patient falls and medical errors. The traditional architect's brief given by a hospital consultant requires architects to be provided program objectives, room requirements and functional space requirements but safety aspects get a back seat. The management team, facility advisors and department design teams should meet routinely with architects during the design process and FMEA (Failure Mode and Effect Analysis) should be used. FMEA is conducted at each major stage of the design process, schematics and design development. Although the use of FMEA is very time consuming and often labour intensive, it is highly beneficial in identifying potential failures and developing innovative solutions associated with design considerations. A report by Joint Commission on Accreditation of Health care organizations cited physical environment as a root cause in 50% of patient falls. Studies have identified bedrails strongly linked with falls. Other studies have shown comprehensive multi-intervention strategies that include environmental modifications being effective in reducing falls. Among specific interior design elements, flooring can contribute to the incidence of falls and the severity of injuries upon impact. Healey reported patients suffer more injuries when they fall on vinyl floors compared with carpeted floors. Sampson et al reported that risk of fracture being lower for wooden subfloors compared with concrete subfloors.

Air borne infections are spread when dust and pathogens are released and are caused by contamination and malfunction of hospital ventilation systems. High-efficiency particulate air (HEPA) filters can be highly effective in preventing air borne infections in hospitals. Provision of single rooms reduces incidence of nosocomial infection. Mullin et al reported a decrease in Acinetobacter baumanii in mechanically ventilated patients from 28.1 to 5% after moving from a unit with both enclosed and open patient care areas to one with all private rooms. Psychological and physiological effects of lighting in hospitals has been shown in literature. ICU psychosis in adult patients is partly attributed to bright or constant lighting conditions in ICUs that lack night/day cues. Buchanan et al found errors in dispensing medication in a high volume out-patient pharmacy were significantly lower at an illumination level of 146 foot candles. Noise levels in most hospitals are higher than what WHO recommends. Common sources of noise include telephones, alarms, shift changes, trolleys, staff caring for other patients, door closings, staff conversations and patients crying or coughing. Noise can significantly be reduced by proper design and management measures in place. Nurses spend a lot of time walking which includes the time to locate and gather supplies and equipment and to find other staff members. One study found that 28.9% of nursing staff time was spent walking. Unnecessary walking leads to a waste of precious staff time and adds to fatigue and stress among staff. Studies suggest that bringing staff and supplies physically and visually closer to the patient help reduce walking. To take advantage of the idea many hospitals incorporate decentralized nurses stations and supplies servers next to patient rooms. This allows for increased time spent on direct patient care activities. One important way to avert adverse events related to patients is for the staff to have the ability to observe patients continuously and provide assistance as needed. Multiple decentralized nurse work areas and charting alcoves next to patient room help facilitate this activity. Hendrich showed that falls were cut by two thirds after a move from an old unit with a centralized nursing station to a new unit with decentralized observation units.

Design for Adaptability

Complexity of hospital operations and ever improving technology demands frequent alterations and expansion of buildings. The aim of hospital architect should be to design a building that inhibits change of function least and not that fits specific to facilitate the docking of mobile and plug-in modules. In future we may have specialized major diagnostic and therapeutic equipment manufactured in pre constructed modules intended for docking at strategic points. One should anticipate as far as possible where changes are most likely to occur, to provide maximum flexibility in design. Master planning remains a basic tool in planning for an unknown future, yet its success depends on the clients understanding of architectural ideas and willingness of successive hospital authorities to honor the architect's original vision. In terms of providing expansion possibilities horizontal expansion is preferred to vertical although it requires large areas of land and consideration of walking distances. A concern for maximizing flexibility continues to be achieved by modularity, full or partial interstitial spaces and the separation of functions. Some of the areas of the hospital can be left unfinished to accommodate inward growth.

Security Concerns

Security planning should proceed hand in hand with the architectural design process. The architect should acquaint himself with the range of security factors that affect design. Waiting until the last stages of the design process to begin thinking about security system requirements can spell trouble for budgets and construction schedules and is a sure way to guarantee that the system installed is less than optimal. Control of access has to be complemented by control of egress. Material property and information must be protected from harm. Connection between security and fire protection is obvious. Effective security is always an interplay of three elements: natural and architectural barriers, including anything from landscaping strategies that discourage access, to the number, location, size and type of doors and windows, human security including the protection provided by guards and other personnel and electronic security provided by any one of the array of systems available. Local building codes regarding ease of egress during fire and other emergency situations present another set of issues affecting building security. The design strategies that will ensure that a building is both secure and accessible to the disabled need to be carefully thought out, especially since this is new territory that remains relatively unexplored. Specialized functions within health care facilities also show how security needs are sometimes intimately linked to other aspects of facility management. This can be clearly seen in the containment and disposal of infectious and other hazardous wastes where physical spaces and procedures must be carefully monitored to prevent liability suits. Security engineers help architects optimize a building's security system. Interaction between the architect and a security consultant can help with the minor details of architectural specification and decision making e.g. if a client plans to begin with a system of mechanical locks but hopes to convert to electronic door locks at a later time the security engineer can ensure that adequate conduits, cables and spaces to ease that transition are installed at the beginning.

Green Building

Modern hospitals have earth friendly features which result in what we call Green building. Green building design features include cool roofs, low VOC materials and finishes, furniture and other contents built from recycled materials, high performance glazing, solar shading, and efficient ventilation that uses fresh outdoor air. Cool roofs reflect solar heat to reduce air conditioning costs. Polyvinyl chloride (PVC) is widely used in health care. PVC disintegrates to produce large volume of organochlorine which is a health hazard. VOCs are potentially harmful gases such as benzene, formaldehyde which are released into air by new interior finish materials.

Construction of building at an angle to sun is important. The major orientation of the building to face north and south maximizes use of natural light. Shades on south block unwanted direct sun light. Rain water can be harvested. Waterless or ultra low flush toilets and low flow shower heads minimize waste water. Digital devices can be used in place of mercury devices. Landscaping, plenty of greenery and scenic views can be soothing to the eyes of patients and staff. Natural sounds including those created by running water have a calming and relaxing effect. This is used in the form of fountains. Energy-efficient features help the health care industry spend less on energy consumption. Some of the energy efficient building options are reflective roofing or cool roofs which reduces AC charges by 20-70%, high efficiency glass block heat and keep out cold, natural lighting allow more sunlight and less electricity spent on lighting, alternative power sources such as solar or wind, high efficiency light fixtures with occupancy sensors, roof top gardens, buying organic foods, more efficient and alternative fuel vehicles, consider heat recovery systems, install lighting control system, install equipment to measure water and energy performance. In addition use rapidly renewable building materials such as bamboo flooring, strawboard, linoleum, etc. Use durable products and materials that require low maintenance track efforts to comply with recycling, think green during construction and comply with recycling, establish a team to monitor progress towards environmental goals.

Intelligent / Smart buildings successfully merge building management and IT systems that can dynamically optimize system performance and simplify facility operations. IBI, which is also known as the Intelligent Building Institute (IBI) of the United States, as well as the UK-based European Intelligent Building Group (EIBG), proposed that the most accepted definitions of the term can be summarized as: "one which provides a productive and cost-effective environment through optimization of its four basic elements including structures, systems, services and management and the interrelationships between them." It is safe to say that intelligent buildings mainly consist of ten 'Quality Environment Modules (QEM)' which are as follows:

M1: environmental friendliness – health and energy conservation;

M2: space utilization and flexibility;

M3: cost effectiveness – operation and maintenance with emphasis on effectiveness;

M4: human comfort;

M5: working efficiency;

M6: safety and security measures – fire, earthquake, disaster and structural damages, etc.

M7: culture;

M8: image of high technology;

M9: construction process and structure

M10: health and sanitation.

Rating of Buildings

GRIHA V2019 (Green Rating for Integrated Habitat Assessment)

Today, buildings have evolved into a diverse array of typologies designed to meet the highly specific requirements of the people who live and work in them. Over time, with growing technological skills, these buildings have also been increasingly designed and operated to place exorbitant demands on natural resources, such as land, water, and energy, to mention a few. Therefore, incorporation of sustainable practices in building design and operation is no longer a choice but a necessity for a sustainable future.

The GRIHA v.2015 has undergone an extensive revision to account for the ongoing advancements in the highly dynamic construction sector. This version (i.e. GRIHA v2019) integrates concepts like life cycle cost analysis, life cycle analysis, and water performance index to name a few. This version has taken into consideration the incorporation of user experience, market feedback, and enhanced ease of implementation and adoption.

All new construction projects with built up area more than 2500 m2 (excluding parking, basement area, and typical buildings) are eligible for certification under GRIHA v.2019.

Table 17.1: GRIHA v. 2019

Section	Criterion No.	Criterion Name	Maximum Points
1. Sustainable Site Planning	1 2 3	Green Infrastructure Low Impact Design Design to Mitigate UHIE	5 5 2
2. Construction Management	4 5 6	Air and Soil Pollution Control Top Soil Preservation Construction Management Practices	1 1 2
3. Energy Efficiency	7 8 9	Energy Optimization Renewable Energy Utilization Low ODP and GWP Materials	12 5 1
4. Occupant Comfort	10 11 12	Visual Comfort Thermal and Acoustic Comfort Maintaining Good IAQ	4 2 6
5. Water Management	13 14 15 16	Water Demand Reduction Wastewater Treatment Rainwater Management Water Quality and Self-Sufficiency	3 3 5 5
6. Solid Waste Management	17 18	Waste Management-Post Occupancy Organic Waste Treatment On-Site	4 2
7. Sustainable Building Materials	19 20 21	Utilization of Alternative Materials in Building Reduction in GWP through Life Cycle Assessment Alternative Materials for External Site Development	5 5 2
8. Life Cycle Costing	22	Life Cycle Cost Analysis	5
9. Socio-Economic Strategies	23 24 25 26	Safety and Sanitation for Construction Workers Universal Accessibility Dedicated Facilities for Service Staff Positive Social Impact	1 2 2 3
10. Performance Metering and Monitoring	27 28 29	Commissioning for Final Rating Smart Metering and Monitoring Operation and Maintenance Protocol	7 0 0
		Total Points 100	
11. Innovation 30 innovation 5			
Grand Total Points			100 + 5

Note: Adapted from : GRIHA V.2019 grihaindia.org/griha-rating.

Rating Threshold

25-40 : one Star.

41-55 : two Star.

56-70 : three Star.

71-85 : four Star.

86 or more : five Star.

Leed Rating System

The Leadership in Energy and Environmental Design (LEED) system was designed by the United States Green Building Council (USGBC) to evaluate the influence of building design and construction on the environment.

The LEED rating system has seven areas of concentration; Sustainable Sites, Water Efficiency, Energy and Atmosphere, Materials and Resources, Indoor Environmental Quality, Innovation in Design Process and Regional Priority. Projects obtain credits in these areas to achieve certification. A building becomes certified after receiving a minimum of 40 credits from the USGBC.

LEED certification Levels

LEED Certified : 40-49 points.

Silver Level : 50-59 points.

Gold Level : 60-79 points.

Platinum Level : 80 + points.

The point distribution over the seven categories are as follows:

Category	Available Points
Sustainable Sites	26
Water Efficiency	10
Energy and Atmosphere	35
Materials and Resources	14
Indoor Environmental Quality	15
Innovation in Design	6
Regional Priority	4
Total Possible Points	110

Note: Adapted from LEED RATING SYSTEM. Expanded Shale, Clay and Slate (ESCS) Institute.

SEISMIC DESIGN

The earthquake resistance of buildings depends upon three quite different processes in design. First is the overall layout of the building which determines the magnitude of the forces which come onto the building and their distribution, a distribution which is important in the vertical direction as well as in horizontal direction. Secondly there is the ability of the various parts of the building to resist these forces, the strength of individual members and the connection between them. Thirdly those aspects of construction which are rarely mentioned at all: non-structural or architectural aspects of building, non-load bearing walls and finishes. There behavior is quite independent from that of the main structural elements and is a serious danger to people or building.

There are three stages in ensuring adequate earth quake resistance. First there must be an adequate code to guide engineering designers. Secondly the provisions of the code need to be incorporated into designs and thirdly there must be a means of inspection to ensure that buildings are actually built according to appropriate designs and specifications. If met these three requirements cover the engineering aspects of buildings. They do nothing to ensure that architectural design is sensible and does not result in large forces with which the engineer has to cope, nor do they ensure that the non-structural components of the building are designed with earthquake effects in mind. Architects need to take care of the forces generated by earthquake and the effect they have on hospital structure. Architects also need to take care of those aspects of the building which do not come under engineering scrutiny e.g. suspended ceilings, non-load bearing partitions etc. The architectural aspects of the earthquake performance of buildings are those features that are decided by architect before the engineer makes his contribution. On the other hand the architect may select or design non-structural elements or decide upon their configuration without reference to the engineer. Earthquake resistance is a shared architectural and engineering responsibility. Proper utilization of metallic truss especially in vertical columns and corners help to withstand earthquakes. Architects have started using seismic dampers in the form of friction pendulum bearings in one of the most modern hospitals in northern California. The first base isolated hospital will be able to move up to 30 inches horizontally and 2 inches vertically without incurring major damage during an earthquake of at least a magnitude of 8.0. In the base isolation system, 176 bearings were positioned between the foundation and the columns in the building. When an earthquake hits, the building slides on the bearings in a gentle pendulum motion. The ground beneath may move vertically, but it is independent of the building. Earthquakes generate strong forces that show up as strong lateral acceleration of the building. The buildings need to be exceptionally strong. The strong lateral acceleration generated during earthquakes at ground can magnify the problem at the roof generating twice the acceleration at upper levels of the building. Health care design firms use building information modeling (BIM) technology to generate 3-D model of the entire project. The project firms are able to digitally model and integrate their respective systems into 3-D including mechanical, structural, electrical and plumbing system. The project team can use software to test various systems. The building information model can also enable the design team to simulate and create "halo" areas or clear zones around each of the base isolators to ensure that their movement during an earthquake would not cause them to collide with anything else.

Floor deflection and vibration is a major concern with steel floor system, especially under sensitive medical equipment. Concrete floor mass and monolithic construction can also address the design team's concern for deflection and vibration. Stair and elevator shafts are cast in place concrete and provide lateral force resistance and building stability. Higher strength concrete provides the added stiffness to control drift without additional shear walls.

Green Field and Brown Field Hospital Projects

The Greenfield project means that a work which is not following a prior work. In infrastructure the projects on the unused lands where there is no need to remodel or demolish an existing structure are called Green Field Projects. The projects which are modified or upgraded are called brownfield projects.

Reference

1. Shakti Gupta, Sunil Kant. Trends and Dimensions in Hospital Architecture. A Hospital Administrators Perspective. J K Science 2005 Vol. 7 No. 2.
2. Reason J Human Error. New York Cambridge University Press; 1990.

3. Reason J Human Error: Models and Management. BMJ 2000; 7237: 768 – 70.
4. Moray N. Error Reduction as a system Problem: In Bogner, MS Editor, Human Error in Medicine pp. 67 – 91. Hillsdale, N J: Lawrence Erlbaum Associates; 1994.
5. Nolan TW. System Changes to improve patient safety. BMJ 2000: 7237; 771 – 3.
6. General Motors co-operation. Potential failure Mode and Effects Analysis (FMEA), reference manual, 3rd ed. Detroit; 2001.
7. Joseph. A, Rashid M. The architecture of safety: Hospital design Current Opinion in Critical Care 2007. 13: 714 – 719.
8. Humphreys H, Johnson EM, Warnock DW. An outbreak of Aspergillosis in general ITU. J Hosp Infect 1991; 18: 167-177.
9. Mullin B, Rouget C, Clement C et al. Association of Private Rooms with ventilator associated Acinetobacter Baumanii Pneumonia in a surgical intensive care unit. Infect control Hosp Epidemiology 1997; 18: 499 – 503.
10. Buchanan TL, Barker KN, Gibson JT, et al. Illumination and errors in dispensing. Am J Hosp pharmacy 1991.
11. Busch- Vishniac. I, West J. Barnhill et al. Noise level in John Hopkins Hospital. J Accoust SOC America 2005: 118: 3629-3645.
12. Joint Commission on Accreditation of Health care organizations. Root causes of patient falls. Sentinel event statistics 2006. www.jointcommission.org.
13. Drahota A, Gai D, Windsor; J Flooring as an intervention to reduce injuries fram falls in health care settings. Quality ageing 2007; 8: 3-9.
14. Healay F.Does flooring type affect risk of injury in older in patients? Nursing times 1994:90: 40-41.
15. Shapley MM, Daviesk. Nursing unit configuration and its relationship to noise and nurse walking behavior: an AIDS/HIV unit case study. AIA Academy Journal 2003. www.aiaorg/aah
16. Zeidler, Eberhard H. Healing the Hospital. MC Master Health Science Centre: its conception and Evolution: Toronto; Zeidler partnership, 1974:7.
17. Homayoun Arabian. The role of architects in Seismic design. Paper presented in International conference on Seismic performance of Traditional buildings 2000.
18. Patrick M Building an earth friendly yet earth quake- resistant hospital. HCARE Design 2008. www.healthcaredesignmagazine.com.
19. Cooker W, De Grazio Robert. Building Security. An Architects Guide.
20. Shakti Gupta, sunil Kant. Hospital Architecture: Emerging issues and strategic options. Journal of Academy of Hospital Administration 2004 Vol. 16, No. 1.

21. Aurac Beidler. Hospitals Turn to Best Environmental Practices Using Green Building. Energy Efficient Health Care Centre. www.suite101.com
22. Building green hospital. Check list: Canadian Coalition for Green Health Care, 2002. www.greenhealthcare.com
23. Osama Omar. Intelligent building, definitions, factors and evaluation criteria of selection. Alexendria Engineering Journal. 2018 ; 57: 4: 2903-2910.
24. GRIHA V.2019 : grihaindia.org/griha-rating accessed on 11.07.2021
25. LEED RATING SYSTEM. Expanded Shale, Clay and Slate (ESCS) Institute. Rotary Kiln structural light weight aggregate.

18

Hospital Infection Control Measures

Nosocomial infections are infections that develop within a hospital or are produced by micro organisms acquired during hospitalization. Nosocomial infection can involve patients, staff, visitors, volunteers and delivery personnel. Nosocomial infections may become apparent while the patients are still hospitalized, however the onset of disease can occur after a patient has been discharged. Infections incubating at the time of the patient's admission to the hospital are not nosocomial, however they can serve as a ready source of infection for other patients or personnel. To determine whether a nosocomial infection problem exists in a particular hospital, one must relate the current frequency of cases to the past history of disease in that institution. To characterize the disease's frequency as sporadic, endemic or epidemic investigators must know something of the past occurrence of that disease in relation to time, place and person.

The center for Disease control and prevention (CDC) has estimated that 88,000 patients die as a direct or indirect result of nosocomial infections in US hospitals annually. Nosocomial infections result in additional suffering, prolong stay and increase the cost of care significantly. With prospective payment plans, about 95% of the excess costs due to nosocomial infections have not been reimbursed by third-party payers in the US. It is therefore to the hospitals advantage to prevent infections because this saves lives and also the hospital money. Surgical wound infections also cause prolongation of hospital stay and excess cost. Urinary tract infections, the least severe but most frequent nosocomial infection have been associated with prolongation of stay ranging from one to three days in different studies.

Hospital infection control programmes were introduced three decades ago to control nosocomial infections. Most effective programmes in a study were associated with a 32% relative reduction in nosocomial infections as compared with hospitals lacking infection control programmes. Health care organizations can demonstrate a commitment to preventing transmission of infectious agents by incorporating infection control into the objectives of the organization's "patient and occupational safety programs".

A key administrative measure is provision of fiscal and human resources for maintaining infection control and occupational health programs that are responsive to emerging needs. Specific components include:

- Bedside nurse.
- Infection prevention and control professional (ICP) staffing levels.
- Inclusion of ICPs in facility construction and design decisions.
- Clinical Microbiology laboratory support.
- Adequate supplies and equipment including facility ventilation systems.
- Adherence monitoring.
- Assessment and correction of system failures that contribute to transmission.
- Provision of feedback to health care personnel and senior administrators
- Institutional leadership.

Infection Control Committee

An infection control committee should be present in every hospital and should have representation from most hospital departments. Although infection control committee is often independent and decisions taken are binding through out the hospital they may require approval by top management. The committee has representation from the disciplines of medicine, surgery, obstetrics and gynecology, pediatrics, pathology, administration, nursing, microbiology section of the hospital laboratory etc. The committee meets regularly usually monthly to deal with current developments and problems. The multidisciplinary representation is important for at least three reasons: first, since infection problems and control measures often cross departmental lines, effective decision making requires regular participation of members from most departments. Second, to carry out the committee decision it is most effective to have committee members exert influence in their respective departments to ensure agreement and compliance. Third, multidepartmental representation acts as a advocate for the whole hospital and negates the interests of any individual departments.

Infection control physician: is a physician who has special training in epidemiology. The position of the chairperson of the infection control committee is either held by administrator or by the hospital epidemiologist. Most of the teaching hospitals now have a full time hospital epidemiologist.

Infection control practitioner (ICP) or infection control nurse occupies the key position in the infection control programme. There is agreement in the literature that one ICP per 250 acute care beds is no longer adequate to meet current infection control needs. A ration of 0.8 to 1.0 ICP per 100 occupied beds is an appropriate level of staffing. Infection control nurse holds a nursing position equivalent to nursing supervisor or higher and obtains advice and supervision from infection control physician. Infection control nurse should have had a training course in infection control. Infection control nurse should spend approximately half of her time on surveillance, one fourth on policy developments and the rest about equally divided between training, consulting and investigating potential outbreaks. Post of ICP can also be held by senior technologist with training in infection control.

Infection control Nurse liaison: The bedside nurse on a patient care unit is an infection control liaison nurse or link nurse who increases the awareness of infection control at the unit level, implements new policies or control interventions at unit level though maintaining the primary role as bedside care giver.

A CDC study found that the most important predictors for infection control programmes for covering infections were (in decreasing order of importance)

1. Intensity of surveillance
2. Intensity of control measures
3. The ratio of the number of infection control practitioners (ICPs) to the number of patient beds.
4. Having a trained hospital epidemiologist on staff
5. Providing surgical wound infection rates to surgeons.

There is an increasing evidence that the level of bed side nurse-staffing influences the quality of patient care. If there is adequate nursing staff it is more likely that infection control practices including hand hygiene and standard and transmission based precautions will be given appropriate attention and applied consistently. Over and hurried workers are likely to cut corners and this has resulted in epidemic infection in some situations.

Surveillance for Hospital associated infections

Surveillance is an essential tool for case finding of single patients or clusters of patients who are infected or colonized with epidemiologically important organisms such as S. aureus, S. pyogenes, C. difficile, influenza virus etc. Surveillance is defined as the ongoing systematic collection, analysis, interpretation, and dissemination of data regarding a health related event for use in public health action to reduce morbidity and mortality and to improve health. Surveillance of both the process measures and the infection rates to which they are linked are important for evaluating the effectiveness of infection prevention efforts and identifying indications for change. Surveillance is the only component of infection control programme that results in reduced rates of nosocomial surgical site infections, pneumonia, urinary tract infection and bacteremia in acute care hospitals. The essential elements of a surveillance system are (1) standardized definitions (2) identification of patient populations at risk for infection (3) statistical analysis (4) feedback to care givers.

It is of utmost importance to define carefully the events to be studied. For example it is necessary to define or establish criteria to decide what will be called a urinary tract infection and what will be considered urinary catheterization. CDC has published guidelines for determining the presence of nosocomial infections. These guidelines are not rigorous definitions of disease but instead serve as practical, operational definitions for most hospitals. Data gathering through surveillance of high risk populations, device use, procedures and facility locations are useful for detecting transmission trends. Identification of clusters of infection should be followed by a systematic epidemiologic investigation to determine commonalities in persons, places and time and guide implementation of interventions and evaluation of effectiveness of those interventions. Targeted surveillance based on the highest risk areas or patients has been preferred over facility-wide surveillance for the most effective use of resources however, surveillance for certain epidemiologically important organisms may need to be facility wide.

Some of the active and passive case finding methods used in surveillance in U.S hospitals are:

Active Techniques

- Culture reports other than blood cultures are routinely reviewed and cases of suspected infections are investigated further.
- Blood culture reports are routinely reviewed and cases of suspected sepsis are investigated further.
- Hospitalized patients and their charts are examined on ward rounds by the infection control personnel.
- Ward nurses, physicians and other personnel are contacted regularly for reports of newly infected patients.
- Nurses vital charts are screened regularly to find new cases of hospital acquired infection.

Passive Technique

- Special infection report forms are filled out by ward nurses or physicians to alert the IC staff to new cases of infection.
- Charts of discharged patients are reviewed by the infection control personnel.

- Charts of discharged patients are reviewed by the medical records librarian to detect hospital acquired infections.
- Discharged patients or their physicians are surveyed regularly to identify cases of infection with onset after discharge.

The active techniques of case finding are strongly preferred to the passive techniques. Periodic ward rounds by ICP are an integral part of an effective surveillance programs. New infections are identified and previously identified are followed up.

Clinical Microbiology laboratory support

Health care organizations need to ensure the availability of the recommended quality of laboratory services, a sufficient number of appropriately trained laboratory staff members and systems to promptly communicate epidemiologically important results to those who will take action i.e. Infection control committee members.

Adherence of health care personnel to recommended guidelines

Adherence to recommended infection control practices decreases transmission of infectious agents in health care settings. Health care personnel must use personal protective equipment (PPE). PPE refers to variety of barriers and respirators used alone or in combination to protect mucous membranes, air ways, skin and clothing from contact with infectious agents. The selection of PPE is based on the nature of the patient interaction and likely mode of transmission

Gloves: Gloves are used to prevent contamination of healthcare personnel hands when (1) anticipating direct contact with blood or body fluids, mucous membranes, non intact skin and other potentially infectious material (2) having direct contact with patients who are colonized or infected with pathogens transmitted by the contact route e.g. RSV (3) handling or touching visibly or potentially contaminated patient care equipment and environmental surfaces. The selection of glove type for non-surgical use is based on a number of factors including the task to be performed, anticipated contact with chemicals and chemotherapeutic agents, latex sensitivity, sizing and facility policies for creating a latex free environment. For contact with blood and body fluids during nonsurgical patient care, a single pair of gloves generally provides adequate barrier protection. However there is considerable variability among gloves, both the quality of the manufacturing process and type of material influence their barrier effectiveness. Vinyl gloves have higher failure rates than latex or nitrile gloves. Heavier reusable utility gloves are indicated for non-patient care activities such as cleaning surfaces. During patient care, transmission of infectious organisms can be reduced by adhering to the principles of working from clean to dirty and confining or limiting contamination to the surfaces that are directly needed for patient care. It is sometimes necessary to change gloves during the care of a single patient to prevent cross-contamination of body sites. When gloves are worn in combination with other PPE, they are put on last. Hand hygiene following gloves removal further ensures that the hands will not carry potentially infectious material that might have penetrated through unrecognized tears or that could contaminate the hands during glove removal.

Isolation gowns: Isolation gowns are always worn in combination with gloves and when other PPE are indicated. Gowns are usually the first piece of PPE to be donned. Isolation gowns should be removed before leaving the patient care area to prevent possible contamination of the environment outside the patient's room. Isolation gowns should be removed in a manner that prevents contamination of clothing or skin. The outer contaminated side of the gown is turned inward and rolled into a bundle and then discarded into a designated container to contain contamination.

Masks: Masks are used for three primary purposes in health care settings (1) placed on health care personnel to protect them from contact with infectious material from patients (2) placed on health care personnel when engaged in procedures requiring sterile technique to protect patients from exposure to infectious agents carried in health care worker's mouth or nose (3) placed on coughing patients to limit potential dissemination of infectious respiratory secretions from the patient to others. Wearing of masks, eye protection and face shield in specified circumstances when blood or body fluid exposures are likely to occur is mandated by the OSHA blood borne pathogens standard.

Goggles, face shields: Face shields provide protection to other facial areas in addition to eyes. Removal of a face shield, goggles and mask can be performed safely after gloves have been removed and hand hygiene performed. The ties, ear pieces and head band used to secure the equipment to the head are considered clean and therefore safe to touch with bare hands. The front of a mask, goggles and face shield are considered contaminated.

Respirator: Respiratory protection requires the use of a respirator with N95 or higher filtration to prevent inhalation of infectious particles. OSHA program components include medical clearance to wear a respirator, provision and use of appropriate respirators, education on respirator use and periodic reevaluation of the respiratory protection program when selecting particulate respirators. Models with inherently good fit characteristics are preferred and could theoretically relieve the need for fit testing. A user seal check should be performed by the wearer of a respirator each time a respirator is donned to minimize air leakage around the face piece. Retesting is indicated if there is change in facial features of the wearer, onset of a medical condition that would affect respiratory function in the wearer or change in the model or size of the initially assigned respirator, CDC currently recommends N95 or higher level respirators for personnel exposed to patients with suspected or confirmed tuberculosis, SARS, small pox, influenza etc. Respirators are also currently recommended to be worn during the performance of aerosol generating procedures (e.g. intubation, bronchoscopy, suctioning) on patients with SARS, avian influenza, pandemic influenza, HINI virus etc.

Prevention of needle and sharp related injuries

Injuries due to needles and other sharps have been associated with transmission of HBV, HCV and HIV to health care personnel. The prevention of sharp injuries has always been an essential element of universal and now standard precautions. Proper disposal of biomedical waste and sharps as per bio-medical waste management and handling rules is a legal binding on generators of such waste.

Visitors as sources of infection

Visitors can be a source of several types of hospital acquired infections. Such infections can be prevented by active and passive screening of visitors. Passive steps involve use of sign boards to alert family members and visitors with signs and symptoms of communicable diseases not to enter clinical area. More active screening tool or questionnaire which elicits information related to recent exposures or current symptoms. The information is reviewed by facility staff and the visitor is either permitted to visit or is excluded. Considering the experience of 2003 SARS outbreak and potential for pandemic influenza HINI out break, developing effective visitor screening will be beneficial. Barrier precautions can be used by family members and visitors depending on the level of interaction and organism suspected.

Respiratory Hygiene/cough etiquette

New elements have been added to standard precautions. These are respiratory Hygiene/cough Etiquette, and use of masks for insertion of catheters or injection of material into spinal or epidural spaces via lumber puncture procedures. While most elements of standard precautions evolved from universal precautions that were developed for protection of health care personnel, these new elements of standard precautions focus on protection of patients as well.

The Respiratory Hygiene/Cough Etiquette is targeted at patients and accompanying family members and friends with undiagnosed transmissible respiratory infections and applies to any person with signs of illness including cough, congestion, rhinorrhea or increased production of respiratory secretions when entering a health care facility. The elements include

1. Education of health care facility staff, patients and visitors.
2. Posted sing boards in local language about do's and do not's.
3. Covering mouth and nose when coughing.
4. Hand hygiene after contact with respirator secretions.
5. Spatial separation ideally > 3 feet of persons with respiratory infections in common waiting areas when possible.

Safe injection practices

The main reason for outbreaks related to injection practices have been:

- Reinsertion of used needles into a multiple dose vial or solution container

- Use of single needle/syringe to administer intravenous medication to multiple patients

A survey of US healthcare workers found that 1-3% reused the same needle/syringe on multiple patients.

Isolation Practices

Both positive and negative pressure rooms should be maintained in hospitals with specific engineering specifications.

Air borne infection isolation (AII): Every acute care inpatient facility should have at least one room equipped for patients with air borne infections. The number of such rooms will depend on the type of hospital and disease pattern in the population. Air borne infection isolation (AII) refers to the isolation of patients infected with organisms spread via airborne droplet nuclei < 5um in diameter. This isolation area receives numerous air changes per hour>12 ACH for new construction and >6ACH for constructions before 2001 and is under negative pressure such that the direction of air flow is from outside adjacent spaces into the room. The air in an AII room is preferably exhausted to outside but may be recirculated provided that the return air is filtered through a high efficiency particulate air filter. There has to be close monitoring of air flow direction using manometers or temporary or installed visual indicators (smoke tubes and flutter strips) placed in the room with the door closed. AII rooms are constructed either with or without an anteroom. When recirculation of air from AII rooms is unavoidable, HEPA fitters should be installed in the exhaust ducts leading from room to the general ventilation system. UVGI (ultra violet germicidal irradiation) can be placed in the ducts as an adjunct measure to HEPA filtration but cannot replace HEPA filter.

Protective Environment: is a specialized patient care area in the hospital with a positive air flow relative to the corridor (i.e. air flows from the room to the outside adjacent space). The combination of HEPA filtration, high number of air changes per hour (>12ACH) and minimal leakage of air into the room creates an environment that can safely accommodate patients who are immunocompromised e.g. who have undergone stem cell transplant. Self closing doors are mandatory for both of these areas to help maintain the correct pressure differential.

Hand-Hygiene Practices: Hand wash is important to reduce potential risks of transmission of micro organisms to patients, to reduce health care worker infection caused by organisms acquired from the patient, to reduce morbidity, mortality and costs associated with health care associated infections. Indications for hand hygiene are contact with patients intact skin, contact with environmental surfaces in the immediate vicinity of patients and after glove removal. Education is the corner stone in improving hand hygiene practices. When hands are visibly dirty or contaminated with blood or body fluids wash hands with soap and water. If hands are not visible soiled use an alcohol based hand scrub for routinely decontaminating hands. Washing hands with soap and water after each use of alcohol hand scrub is not necessary and not recommended because it may lead to dermatitis. However because personnel feel a build up of emollients on their hands after repeated use of alcohol hand gels, washing with soap and water after 5 to 10 applications of gel has been recommended. Pocket carriage of alcohol based hand rub solutions combined with availability of bed side dispensers has been associated with substantial improvement in adherence to hand hygiene. To avoid confusion between soap and alcohol hand rubs dispensers should not be placed adjacent to sinks. Do not add soap to a partially empty soap dispenser. This practice of topping up dispensers can lead to bacterial contamination of soap. The leading factor for non-compliance to hand hygiene is time constraint. Other reasons reported by health care workers for lack of adherence with hand hygiene recommendations include skin irritation by hand hygiene agents, inaccessibility of hand hygiene supplies, interference with health care worker patient relationship, patient needs perceived as a priority, wearing of gloves, forgetfulness, lack of knowledge of guidelines, high work load and under staffing and lack of scientific information showing a definitive impact of improved hand hygiene on hospital acquired infection rates. Guidelines for hand hygiene in health care settings have been revisited recently by an international group from the US Center for Disease Control and Prevention (CDC). Health care infection control practices advisory committee (HICPAC), the Society for Health Care Epidemiology of America (SHEA), the Association for professionals in Infection Control and Epidemiology (APIC) and the Infectious Diseases Society of America (IDSA).

Recommended indications for hand hygiene during patient care, classified according to their level of evidence are:

Table 18-1

CDC/HICPAC System for Categorising Recommendations

1A:	Strongly recommended for implementation and strongly supported by well-designed experimental, clinical or epidemiological studies.
1B:	Strongly recommended for implementation and supported by some experimental, clinical or epidemiological studies and a strong theoretical rationale.
1C:	Required for implementation as mandated by state regulation or standard.
II	Suggested for implementation and supported by suggestive clinical or epidemiological studies or a theoretical rationale.

(a) Wash hands with a non-antimicrobial soap and water or an antimicrobial soap and water when hands are visibly soiled or contaminated with proteinaceous material (1A)

(b) If hands are not visibly soiled, use an alcohol based hand rub for routinely decontaminating hands in all other clinical situations described in items listed below (1A)

- Before having direct contact with patients (1B)
- Before donning sterile gloves when inserting a central intravascular catheter (1B)
- Before inserting indwelling urinary catheters, peripheral venous catheters or other invasive devices that do not require a surgical procedure (1B)
- After contact with a patient's intact skin as in taking pulse or blood pressure or lifting a patient (1B)
- After contact with body fluids or excretions, mucous membranes, non-intact skin or wound dressings as long as hands are visibly soiled (1A)
- If moving from a contaminated body site during patient care (II)
- After removing gloves (1B)

(c) Wash hands with antimicrobial/non-antimicrobial soap and water if exposure to Bacillus anthracis is suspected or proven. The physical action of washing and rinsing hands under such circumstances is recommended because all antiseptics have poor activity against spores.

Disinfection

Medical equipment surfaces can become contaminated with infectious agents and contribute to the spread of health care associated infections. Environmental surfaces can also contribute to cross transmission by contamination of health care personnel from hand contact with contaminated surfaces, medical equipment or patients. In an investigation of the cleaning of hospital floors the use of soap and water was less effective (80%) in reducing number of bacteria than a phenolic disinfection (94%). However a few hours after floor disinfection, the bacterial count is nearly back to the pretreatment level. Reasons exist for using a detergent alone on floors because non critical surface contribute minimally to endemic health care associated infections and no difference has been found in health care-associated infection rates when floors are cleaned with detergent rather than disinfection. Spot decontamination on fabrics that remain in hospitals or clinic rooms while patients move in and out also should be considered. One study demonstrated the effectiveness of spraying the fabric with 3% hydrogen peroxide. Some hospitals have begun using a new mopping technique involving microfiber materials to clean floors. Microfibers are densely constructed polyester and polyamide fibers that are approximately 1/16th the thickness of human hair. The positively charged microfiber attract dust and are more absorbent than a conventional cotton loop mop.

Following measures need to be taken to reduce the frequency of bacterial growth in disinfectants and the threat of serious health care associated infections from the use of such contaminated products

- Some disinfectants should not be diluted
- Don't use contaminated containers for dilution if required
- Stock solutions of germicides must be stored as indicated on the product label.

Microorganisms may be protected from disinfectants by production of thick masses of cells and extracellular materials or biofims. Biofilms are microbial communities that are tightly attached to surfaces and cannot be easily removed. These biofilms make microbes resistant to disinfectants.

Ultraviolet radiation

U V light is used as a supplemental air cleaning measure in hospitals, but it has only a minimal inactivating effect on fungal spores.

UVGI (Ultra violet Germicidal irradiation) is also used in air handling units to prevent or limit the growth of bacteria and fungi. Most commercially available UV lamps used for germicidal effect are low pressure mercury vapor lamps that emit radiant energy predominantly at a wave length of 253.7nm which is near the maximum microbiological activity. Two systems of UVGI have been used in health care settings: duct irradiation and upper room air irradiation. In duct irradiation systems, UV lamps are placed inside ducts that remove air from rooms to disinfect the air before it is recirculated. When properly designed, installed and maintained high levels of UVGI can be attained in the ducts with little or no exposure of persons in the rooms. In upper room air irradiation UV lamps are either suspended from the ceiling or mounted on the wall. UVGI units have two basic designs (a) a pan fixture with UVGI unshielded above the unit to direct the irradiation upward (b) a fixture with a series of parallel plates to columinize the irradiation outward while preventing the light from getting to eyes of the room occupants.

Design considerations

Infection control has to be kept in mind when designing hospitals. Traffic flow has to be regulated so that there is no criss cross. Operating suite needs to be zoned with sterility increasing from protective zone to the sterile zone. Sterile supplies should be segregated from non sterile supplies. The corridors leading to OT and intensive care areas should not be used as thorough fare corridors. In wards the flow of supplies should be such that sterile supplies don't mix up with non-sterile supplies.

Sterilization

Proper sterilization of supplies and equipment is backbone of any infection control process. Sterilization by equipment like autoclave, ethylene oxide and plasma sterilizers has been recommended. Central sterile services departments (C.S.S.D) are established in hospitals to ensure proper sterilization of equipment and also its monitoring. In large hospitals separate sterilization facilities T.S.S.U (Theatre Sterile Services Unit) are recommended for theatres.

Reference

1. Farr. M.Barry. Prevention and control of Nasocomial infections. Business Briefing: Global health care 2002. (Issue 3). 37-42.
2. R W Haley, D H Culver, JW white, WM Morgan, TG Emori and VP Munn et al. The efficacy of infection surveillance and control programs in preventing nosocomial infections in U.S hospitals. Am. J. Epidemiol 121, 1985. 182-205.
3. S.K Fridkin, SM Pear, TH Williamson, J N Galgiani and W R Jarvis. The role of understanding in central venous catheter- associated blood stream infections. Infect control. Hospital Epidemiol, 17, 1996. 150-158.
4. Bennett. John.V, Brachmass.S. Philip. Hospital infections Lippincott – Raven 4th ed. 1998.
5. Mahander Nayak, Kala.S.Kulkarni. Modest measure with phenomenal effects. Alcohol based hand sanitizer. Medicine update 2003: 11(4), 41-44.
6. Weher DJ, Sickhelt- Bennelt E, Gergen M.f, Rutala WA. Efficacy of selected hand hygiene agents to remove Bacillus atrophacus (a surrogate of Bacillus anthrasis) from contaminated hands. JAMA 2003; 289 1274-1277.
7. Rutala WA, weher DJ. Guideline for disinfection and sterilization in health care facilities CDC 2008.
8. Boyce J, pittel D. Guideline for hand hygiene in health care setting- recommendations of the Health care infection control practices Advisory committee (HICPAC) and the HICPAC/SHEA/APIC/IDSA Hand Hygiene Task force. Infect control Hospital epidemiology 2002; 23: 53-540.
9. Boyce J, Pittel D. Guideline for hand hygiene in health care settings- recommendations of health care infection control practices advisory committee and the HICPAC/SHEA/APIC/IDSA. Hand Hygiene Task Force. AMJ Infection control 2002, 30: S1-S46.
10. Siegel JD, Rhimehart E, Jackson M, Chiarello L. Guideline for isolation precautions. Preventing transmission of Infection agents in Health care settings. 2007 www.cdc.gov/ncidod/dhqp/pdf/isolation2007.
11. Guideline for Environmental Infection Control in Health Care Facilities. Recommendations of CDC and Health Care Infection Control Practices Advisory committee (HICPAC) 2003.

19

Covid 19 and Hospital Preparedness

Coronaviruses are a large family of viruses that can cause illness in animals or humans. In humans there are several known coronaviruses that cause respiratory infections. These coronaviruses range from the common cold to more severe diseases such as severe acute respiratory syndrome (SARS), Middle East respiratory syndrome (MERS), and COVID-19. COVID-19 was identified in Wuhan, China in December 2019. COVID-19 is caused by the virus severe acute respiratory syndrome coronavirus 2 (SARS-CoV-2), a new virus in humans causing respiratory illness which can be spread from person-to-person. Early in the outbreak, many patients were reported to have a link to a large seafood and live animal market, however, later cases with no link to the market confirmed person-to-person transmission of the disease.

Transmission: Respiratory viruses are transmitted in three main ways. First, contact transmission, where someone comes into direct contact with an infected person or touches a surface that has been contaminated. Second, through droplet transmission of both large and small respiratory droplets that contain the virus, which would occur when near an infected person. Third, through airborne transmission of smaller droplets and particles that are suspended in the air over longer distances and time than droplet transmission. Infection control guidelines have stated that most respiratory virus transmission occurs from large infected droplets produced by coughing, sneezing, and breathing in close proximity to another person. This understanding has led to social distancing being the cornerstone of public health advice, but confusion exists as to the safe distance required between people to reduce transmission with the WHO suggesting 1 m and the CDC and NHS saying 2 m. For social distancing to be effective, infective respiratory particles would need to fall to the ground or be in low enough concentrations at 2 m from the source to not cause transmission. Studies and guidelines have historically used a threshold of 5 μm to differentiate between large and small particles, but researchers are now suggesting that a size threshold of 100 μm better differentiates aerodynamic behaviour of particles, and particles that would fall to the ground within 2 m are likely to be 60–100 μm in size. Investigators have also measured particle sizes of infectious aerosols and have shown that pathogens are most commonly found in small particle aerosols. There is growing evidence that COVID-19 infection can occur from airborne exposure to the virus under certain circumstances. Cases of transmission from people more than 2 m apart have occurred but in enclosed spaces with poor ventilation, and typically with extended exposure to an infected person of more than 30 min. The CDC have been clear to point out that most infections are spread through close contact and that airborne transmission is not the primary route of transmission. Whether droplet or airborne transmission is the main route, the risk of infection is known to be much lower outside where ventilation is better.

Symptoms

A wide range of symptoms for COVID-19 have been reported[4]. These include:

- Fever or chills
- Cough
- Shortness of breath or difficulty breathing
- Fatigue
- Headache
- Nasal congestion or runny nose
- Muscle or body aches
- Sore throat
- New loss of smell or taste

- Nausea or vomiting
- Diarrhea

The estimated incubation period is between 2 and 14 days with a median of 5 days. It is important to note that some people become infected and do not develop any symptoms or feel unwell.

Despite the important concerns about case fatality rates, most COVID-19 illnesses are – and we expect will continue to be – mild, and most patients will recover spontaneously with some supportive care, especially children and young adults. Data from several countries suggest that 14%-19% are hospitalized and 3%-5% will need intense care unit admission. Those admitted in ICUs have severe pneumonia, respiratory failure, septic shock, and/or multiple organ dysfunction or failure and death. Those of all ages with underlying medical conditions (including but not limited to heart disease, diabetes, or lung disease) appear to be at higher risk of developing severe COVID-19 compared to those without these conditions.

Infection Control Practices : Infection prevention and control (IPC) is the practice of preventing or stopping the spread of infections during healthcare delivery in facilities like hospitals, outpatient clinics, dialysis centers, long-term care facilities, or traditional practitioners. IPC is a critical part of health system strengthening and must be a priority to protect patients and healthcare workers. In the context of COVID-19, the IPC goal is to support the maintenance of essential healthcare services by containing and preventing COVID-19 transmission within healthcare facilities to keep patients and healthcare workers healthy and safe. CDC recommends using additional infection prevention and control practices during the COVID-19 pandemic, along with standard practices recommended as a part of routine healthcare delivery to all patients. These practices are intended to apply to all patients, not just those with suspected or confirmed SARS-CoV-2 infection.

These additional practices include:

Implement Telehealth and Nurse-Directed Triage Protocols

- Continue to use telehealth strategies to reduce the risk of SARS-CoV-2 transmission in healthcare settings while maintaining high quality patient care.

- When scheduling appointments for routine medical care (e.g., annual physical, elective surgery):
  - Advise patients that they should put on their own well-fitting form of source control (see Implement Universal Source Control Measures for more details) before entering the facility.
  - Instruct patients to call ahead and discuss the need to reschedule their appointment if they have symptoms of COVID-19 within the 10 days prior to their appointment, if they have been diagnosed with SARS-CoV-2 infection within the 10 days prior to their appointment, or if they have had close contact with someone with suspected or confirmed SARS-CoV-2 infection within 14 days prior to their scheduled appointment.
- When scheduling appointments for patients requesting evaluation for possible SARS-CoV-2 infection, use nurse-directed triage protocols to determine if an appointment is necessary or if the patient can be managed from home.
  - If the patient must come in for an appointment, instruct them (or their responsible party if they are unable to communicate) to take appropriate preventive actions (e.g., follow triage procedures, put on their own well-fitting form of source control before entry and throughout their visit or, if a well-fitting form of source control cannot be tolerated, hold a tissue against their mouth and nose to contain respiratory secretions) and immediately inform triage personnel upon arrival so they can be placed in an examination room.

Screen and Triage Everyone Entering a Healthcare Facility for Signs and Symptoms of COVID-19

Although screening for symptoms will not identify asymptomatic or pre-symptomatic individuals with SARS-CoV-2 infection, symptom screening remains an important strategy to identify those who could have COVID-19 so appropriate precautions can be implemented.

- Take steps to ensure that everyone adheres to source control measures and hand hygiene practices while in a healthcare facility

- Post visual alerts at the entrance and in strategic places (e.g., waiting areas, elevators, cafeterias) to provide instructions (in appropriate languages) about wearing a well-fitting form of source control and how and when to perform hand hygiene.
- Provide supplies for respiratory hygiene and cough etiquette, including alcohol-based hand sanitizer (ABHS) with 60-95% alcohol, tissues, and no-touch receptacles for disposal, at healthcare facility entrances, waiting rooms, and patient check-ins.

- Limit and monitor points of entry to the facility.
- Establish a process to ensure everyone (patients, healthcare personnel, and visitors) entering the facility is assessed for symptoms of COVID-19, or exposure to others with suspected or confirmed SARS-CoV-2 infection and that they are practicing source control.
  - Options could include : individual screening on arrival at the facility; or implementing an electronic monitoring system in which, prior to arrival at the facility, people report absence of fever and symptoms of COVID-19, absence of a diagnosis of SARS-CoV-2 infection in the prior 10 days, and confirm they have not been exposed to others with SARS-CoV-2 infection during the prior 14 days.
    - Fever can be either measured temperature $\geq$100.0°F or subjective fever. People might not notice symptoms of fever at the lower temperature threshold that is used for those entering a healthcare setting, so they should be encouraged to actively take their temperature at home or have their temperature taken upon arrival.
    - Obtaining reliable temperature readings is affected by multiple factors, including:
    - The ambient environment in which the temperature is measured. If the environment is extremely hot or cold, body temperature readings may be affected, regardless of the temperature-taking device that is used.

  - Proper calibration of the thermometers per manufacturer standards: Improper calibration can lead to incorrect temperature readings.
  - Proper usage and reading of the thermometers: Non-contact infrared thermometers frequently used for health screening must be held at an established distance from the temporal artery in the forehead to take the temperature correctly. Holding the device too far from or too close to the temporal artery affects the reading.

- Properly manage anyone with suspected or confirmed SARS-CoV-2 infection or who has had contact with someone with suspected or confirmed SARS-CoV-2 infection:
  - Healthcare personnel (HCP) should be excluded from work and should notify occupational health services to arrange for further evaluation.
  - Visitors should be restricted from entering the facility and be referred for proper evaluation.
- Patients should be isolated in an examination room with the door closed.
- If an examination room is not immediately available, such patients should not wait among other patients seeking care.
  - Identify a separate, well-ventilated space that allows waiting patients to be separated by 6 or more feet, with easy access to respiratory hygiene supplies.
  - In some settings, patients might opt to wait in a personal vehicle or outside the healthcare facility where they can be contacted by mobile phone when it is their turn to be evaluated.
  - Depending on the level of transmission in the community, facilities might also consider designating a separate area at the facility (e.g., an ancillary building or temporary structure) or nearby location as an evaluation area where patients with symptoms of COVID-19 can seek evaluation and care.

Re-evaluate admitted patients for signs and symptoms of COVID-19

Screening for fever and symptoms should also be incorporated into daily assessments of all admitted patients. All fevers and symptoms consistent with COVID-19 among admitted patients should be properly managed and evaluated.

Implement Universal Source Control Measures

Source control refers to use of well-fitting cloth masks, facemasks, or respirators to cover a person's mouth and nose to prevent spread of respiratory secretions when they are breathing, talking, sneezing, or coughing. In addition to providing source control, these devices also offer varying levels of protection for the wearer against exposure to infectious droplets and particles produced by infected people. Ensuring a proper fit is important to optimize both the source control and protection offered. Because of the potential for asymptomatic and pre-symptomatic transmission, source control measures are recommended for everyone in a healthcare facility, even if they do not have symptoms of COVID-19.

- Patients and visitors should wear their own well-fitting form of source control upon arrival to and throughout their stay in the facility. If they do not bring their own, they should be offered an option that is equivalent to what is recommended for people in the community
    - Patients may remove their source control when in their rooms but should put it back on when around others (e.g., when visitors enter their room) or leaving their room.
    - Cloth masks, facemasks and respirators should not be placed on young children under age 2, anyone who cannot wear one safely, such as someone who has a disability or an underlying medical condition that precludes wearing a mask safely, or anyone who is unconscious, incapacitated or otherwise unable to remove their cloth mask, facemask or respirator without assistance.
    - Visitors who are not able to wear source control should be encouraged to use alternatives to on-site visits with patients (e.g., telephone or internet communication), particularly

if the patient is at increased risk for severe illness from SARS-CoV-2 infection.

  - HCP should wear well-fitting source control at all times while they are in the healthcare facility.
  - To reduce the number of times HCP must touch their face and potential risk for self-contamination, when used for source control, HCP should consider continuing to wear the same respirator or well-fitting facemask throughout their entire work shift.
  - HCP should remove their respirator or facemask, perform hand hygiene, and put on their community source control when leaving the facility at the end of their shift.

- Educate patients, visitors, and HCP about the importance of performing hand hygiene, including immediately before and after any contact with their cloth mask, facemask, or respirator.

Encourage Physical Distancing

Healthcare delivery requires close physical contact between patients and HCP. However, when possible, physical distancing is an important strategy to prevent SARS-CoV-2 transmission. This can be achieved by

- Limiting visitors to the facility to those essential for the patient's physical or emotional well-being and care . Encourage use of alternative mechanisms for patient and visitor interactions such as video-call applications on cell phones or tablets.
- Scheduling appointments to limit the number of patients in waiting rooms, or creating a process so that patients can wait outside or in their vehicle while waiting for their appointment.
- Arranging seating in waiting rooms so patients can sit at least 6 feet apart.
- Modifying in-person group healthcare activities by implementing virtual methods or scheduling smaller in-person group sessions.
- In some circumstances, such as higher levels of community transmission or numbers of patients with

- COVID-19 being cared for at the facility, and when healthcare-associated transmission is occurring, facilities might cancel in-person group activities in favour of an exclusively virtual format.

For HCP, the potential for exposure to SARS-CoV-2 is not limited to direct patient care interactions. Transmission can also occur through unprotected exposures to asymptomatic or pre-symptomatic co-workers in breakrooms or co-workers or visitors in other common areas. Examples of how physical distancing can be implemented for HCP include:

- Reminding HCP that the potential for exposure to SARS-CoV-2 is not limited to direct patient care interactions.
- Emphasizing the importance of source control and physical distancing in non-patient care areas.
- Providing family meeting areas where all individuals (e.g., visitors, HCP) can remain at least 6 feet apart from each other.
- Designating areas and staggered schedules for HCP to take breaks, eat, and drink that allow them to remain at least 6 feet apart from each other.

Engineering control

Physical separation is efficient in reducing transmission of respiratory virus in hospital settings. The Australian, CDC, and WHO guidelines emphasize engineering control as an IPC measure. These guidelines recommend the following engineering control measures: spatial barriers or partitions to manage patients in triage areas, curtains around each bed in inpatient wards, closed suctioning systems for airway suctioning in intubated patients, and airflow management. The CDC guidelines also recommend installing physical barriers using glass or plastic windows in the hospital reception area.

Implement Universal Use of Personal Protective Equipment

Transmission from asymptomatic or pre-symptomatic patients with SARS-CoV-2 infection can occur in healthcare settings, particularly in areas with moderate to substantial community transmission.

The fit of the medical device used to cover the wearer's mouth and nose is a critical factor in the level of source control (preventing exposure of others) and level of the wearer's exposure to infectious particles. Respirators offer the highest level of both source control and protection against inhalation of infectious particles in the air. Facemasks that conform to the wearer's face so that more air moves through the material of the facemask rather than through gaps at the edges are more effective for source control than facemasks with gaps and can also reduce the wearer's exposure to particles in the air. Improving how a facemask fits can increase the facemask's effectiveness for decreasing particles emitted from the wearer and to which the wearer is exposed.

Consider if elective procedures, surgeries, and non-urgent outpatient visits should be postponed in certain circumstances.

Facilities must balance the need to provide necessary services while minimizing risk to patients and HCP. Facilities should consider the potential for patient harm if care is deferred when making decisions about providing elective procedures, surgeries, and non-urgent outpatient visits.

Patient Placement

- For patients with COVID-19 or other respiratory infections, evaluate need for hospitalization. If hospitalization is not medically necessary, home care is preferable if the individual's situation allows.
- If admitted, place a patient with suspected or confirmed SARS-CoV-2 infection in a single-person room with the door closed. The patient should have a dedicated bathroom.
    - Airborne Infection Isolation Rooms (AIIRs) should be prioritized for patients who will be undergoing aerosol generating procedures.
- Personnel entering the room should use PPE as described below.
- As a measure to limit HCP exposure and conserve PPE, facilities could consider designating entire units within the facility, with dedicated HCP, to care for patients with suspected or confirmed SARS-CoV-2 infection. Dedicated means that HCP are assigned to care only for these patients during their shifts.

- Determine how staffing needs will be met as the number of patients with suspected or confirmed SARS-CoV-2 infection increases and if HCP become ill and are excluded from work.
- It might not be possible to distinguish patients who have COVID-19 from patients with other respiratory viruses. As such, patients with different respiratory pathogens might be cohorted on the same unit. However, only patients with the same respiratory pathogen may be housed in the same room. For example, a patient with COVID-19 should not be housed in the same room as a patient with an undiagnosed respiratory infection or a respiratory infection caused by a different pathogen.

- To the extent possible, patients with suspected or confirmed SARS-CoV-2 infection should be housed in the same room for the duration of their stay in the facility (i.e., minimize room transfers).
- Limit transport and movement of the patient outside of the room to medically essential purposes.
  - Whenever possible, perform procedures/tests in the patient's room.
  - Consider providing portable x-ray equipment in patient cohort areas to reduce the need for patient transport.
- Communicate information about patients with suspected or confirmed SARS-CoV-2 infection to appropriate personnel before transferring them to other departments in the facility (e.g., radiology) and to other healthcare facilities.
- Patients should wear well-fitting source control to contain secretions during transport. If patients cannot tolerate a facemask or cloth mask or one is not available, they should use tissues to cover their mouth and nose while out of their room.
- Once the patient has been discharged or transferred, HCP, including environmental services personnel, should refrain from entering the vacated room until sufficient time has elapsed for enough air changes to remove potentially infectious particles. After this time has elapsed, the room

should undergo appropriate cleaning and surface disinfection before it is returned to routine use.

Personal Protective Equipment

- HCP who enter the room of a patient with suspected or confirmed SARS-CoV-2 infection should adhere to Standard Precautions and use a NIOSH-approved N95 or equivalent or higher-level respirator, gown, gloves, and eye protection.
- CDC has provided strategies for Optimizing Personal Protective Equipment (PPE) Supplies that include a hierarchy of strategies to implement when PPE are in short supply or unavailable (e.g., use of a respirator approved under standards used in other countries that are similar to NIOSH-approved N95 filtering facepiece respirators or a well-fitting facemask when NIOSH-approved N95 or equivalent or higher-level respirators are not available).
- NIOSH-approved N95 or equivalent or higher-level respirators are preferred; when shortages exist, they should be prioritized for situations where respiratory protection is most important and the care of patients with pathogens requiring Airborne Precautions (e.g., tuberculosis, measles, varicella).

Hand Hygiene

- HCP should perform hand hygiene before and after all patient contact, contact with potentially infectious material, and before putting on and after removing PPE, including gloves. Hand hygiene after removing PPE is particularly important to remove any pathogens that might have been transferred to bare hands during the removal process.
- HCP should perform hand hygiene by using ABHS with 60-95% alcohol or washing hands with soap and water for at least 20 seconds. If hands are visibly soiled, use soap and water before returning to ABHS.
- Healthcare facilities should ensure that hand hygiene supplies are readily available to all personnel in every care location.

How to Put On (Don) PPE Gear

More than one donning method may be acceptable. Training and practice using your healthcare facility's procedure is critical. Below is one example of donning.

1. **Identify and gather the proper PPE to don.** Ensure choice of gown size is correct (based on training).
2. **Perform hand hygiene using hand sanitizer.**
3. **Put on isolation gown.** Tie all of the ties on the gown. Assistance may be needed by other healthcare personnel.
4. **Put on NIOSH-approved N95 filtering facepiece respirator or higher (use a facemask if a respirator is not available).** If the respirator has a nosepiece, it should be fitted to the nose with both hands, not bent or tented. Do not pinch the nosepiece with one hand. Respirator/facemask should be extended under chin. Both your mouth and nose should be protected. Do not wear respirator/facemask under your chin or store in scrubs pocket between patients.
    - **Respirator:** Respirator straps should be placed on crown of head (top strap) and base of neck (bottom strap). Perform a user seal check each time you put on the respirator.
    - **Facemask:** Mask ties should be secured on crown of head (top tie) and base of neck (bottom tie). If mask has loops, hook them appropriately around your ears.
5. **Put on face shield or goggles.** When wearing an N95 respirator or half facepiece elastomeric respirator, select the proper eye protection to ensure that the respirator does not interfere with the correct positioning of the eye protection, and the eye protection does not affect the fit or seal of the respirator. Face shields provide full face coverage. Goggles also provide excellent protection for eyes, but fogging is common.
6. **Put on gloves.** Gloves should cover the cuff (wrist) of gown.
7. **Healthcare personnel may now enter patient room.**

How to Take Off (Doff) PPE Gear

More than one doffing method may be acceptable. Training and practice using your healthcare facility's procedure is critical. Below is one example of doffing.

1. **Remove gloves.** Ensure glove removal does not cause additional contamination of hands. Gloves can be removed using more than one technique (e.g., glove-in-glove or bird beak).
2. **Remove gown.** Untie all ties (or unsnap all buttons). Some gown ties can be broken rather than untied. Do so in gentle manner, avoiding a forceful movement. Reach up to the shoulders and carefully pull gown down and away from the body. Rolling the gown down is an acceptable approach. Dispose in trash receptacle.
3. **Healthcare personnel may now exit patient room.**
4. **Perform hand hygiene.**
5. **Remove face shield or goggles.** Carefully remove face shield or goggles by grabbing the strap and pulling upwards and away from head. Do not touch the front of face shield or goggles.
6. **Remove and discard respirator (or facemask if used instead of respirator).** Do not touch the front of the respirator or facemask.
    - **Respirator:** Remove the bottom strap by touching only the strap and bring it carefully over the head. Grasp the top strap and bring it carefully over the head, and then pull the respirator away from the face without touching the front of the respirator.
    - **Facemask:** Carefully untie (or unhook from the ears) and pull away from face without touching the front.
7. **Perform hand hygiene after removing the respirator/ facemask and before putting it on again if your workplace is practicing reuse.**

Long Covid

Multiorgan symptoms after COVID-19 are being reported by increasing numbers of patients. They range from cough and shortness of breath, to fatigue, headache, palpitations, chest pain, joint pain, physical limitations, depression, and insomnia, and affect people of varying ages. The occurrence of multiorgan complications is not unexpected, given that the SARS-CoV-2 entry receptor ACE2 is expressed in multiple tissues. There is a growing concern on long term effects of covid globally. Nevertheless, there is much that remains unknown, and the response to long COVID is still in its infancy. What are the diagnoses, definitions, and phenotypes of illness that are grouped under the term long COVID? How long does it last? Who is at risk of serious or prolonged sequelae? What are the underlying causes and mechanisms? How do we prevent or reduce the effects of such sequelae on patient health and wellbeing?

How do we address long COVID? First, health professionals must listen to patients to understand their concerns, validate their experiences, and manage their symptoms and comorbidities, referring patients as needed. Many patients already feel dismissed or overlooked. Second, discharged patients should have long term access to multidisciplinary health care, including rehabilitation services and telehealth. Third, long COVID affects even young adults, so effective public health messaging for such individuals about the risks of infection is warranted. Fourth, primary care services need the capacity to deal with patients with long COVID. Finally, health-care workers themselves are likely to have a high burden of long COVID and they must have adequate occupational health provision.

Standard Precautions to be followed by health care workers while handling dead bodies of COVID.

Standard infection prevention control practices should be followed at all times.

These include:

1. Hand hygiene.
2. Use of personal protective equipment (e.g., water resistant apron, gloves, masks, eyewear).
3. Safe handling of sharps.
4. Disinfect bag housing dead body; instruments and devices used on the patient.
5. Disinfect linen. Clean and disinfect environmental surfaces.
6. Training in infection and prevention control practices

All staff identified to handle dead bodies in the isolation area, mortuary, ambulance and those workers in the crematorium / burial ground should be trained in the infection prevention control practices.

7. Removal of the body from the isolation room or area
   - The health worker attending to the dead body should perform hand hygiene, ensure proper use of PPE (water resistant apron, goggles, N95 mask, gloves).
   - All tubes, drains and catheters on the dead body should be removed.
   - Any puncture holes or wounds (resulting from removal of catheter, drains, tubes, or otherwise) should be disinfected with 1% hypochlorite and dressed with impermeable material.
   - Apply caution while handling sharps such as intravenous catheters and other sharp devices. They should be disposed into a sharps container.
   - Plug Oral, nasal orifices of the dead body to prevent leakage of body fluids.
   - If the family of the patient wishes to view the body at the time of removal from the isolation room or area, they may be allowed to do so with the application of Standard Precautions.
   - Place the dead body in leak-proof plastic body bag. The exterior of the body bag can be decontaminated with 1% hypochlorite. The body bag can be wrapped with a mortuary sheet or sheet provided by the family members.
   - The body will be either handed over to the relatives or taken to mortuary.
   - All used/ soiled linen should be handled with standard precautions, put in biohazard bag and the outer surface of the bag disinfected with hypochlorite solution.
   - Used equipment should be autoclaved or decontaminated with disinfectant solutions in accordance with established infection prevention control practices.
   - All medical waste must be handled and disposed of in accordance with Biomedical waste management rules.

- The health staff who handled the body will remove personal protective equipment and will perform hand hygiene.
- Provide counselling to the family members and respect their sentiments.

8. Environmental cleaning and disinfection

   All surfaces of the isolation area (floors, bed, railings, side tables, IV stand, etc.) should be wiped with 1% Sodium Hypochlorite solution; allow a contact time of 30 minutes, and then allowed to air dry.

9. Handling of dead body in Mortuary
   - Mortuary staff handling COVID dead body should observe standard precautions.
   - Dead bodies should be stored in cold chambers maintained at approximately 4°C.
   - The mortuary must be kept clean. Environmental surfaces, instruments and transport trolleys should be properly disinfected with 1% Hypochlorite solution.
   - After removing the body, the chamber door, handles and floor should be cleaned with sodium hypochlorite 1% solution.

10. Embalming of dead body should not be allowed.

11. Autopsies on COVID-19 dead bodies

    Autopsies should be avoided. If autopsy is to be performed for special reasons, the following infection prevention control practices should be adopted:
    - The Team should be well trained in infection prevention control practices.
    - The number of forensic experts and support staff in the autopsy room should be limited.
    - The Team should use full complement of PPE (coveralls, head cover, shoe cover, N 95 mask, goggles / face shield).
    - Round ended scissors should be used.
    - PM40 or any other heavy duty blades with blunted points to be used to reduce prick injuries.

- Only one body cavity at a time should be dissected.
- Unfixed organs must be held firm on the table and sliced with a sponge – care should be taken to protect the hand
- Negative pressure to be maintained in mortuary. An oscillator saw with suction extraction of the bone aerosol into a removable chamber should be used for sawing skull, otherwise a hand saw with a chain-mail glove may be used.
- Needles should not be re-sheathed after fluid sampling – needles and syringes should be placed in a sharps bucket.
- Reduce aerosol generation during autopsy using appropriate techniques especially while handling lung tissue.
- After the procedure, body should be disinfected with 1% Sodium Hypochlorite and placed in a body bag, the exterior of which will again be decontaminated with 1% Sodium Hypochlorite solution.
- The body thereafter can be handed over to the relatives.
- Autopsy table to be disinfected as per standard protocol.

12. Transportation
    - The body, secured in a body bag, exterior of which is decontaminated poses no additional risk to the staff transporting the dead body.
    - The personnel handling the body may follow standard precautions (surgical mask, gloves).
    - The vehicle, after the transfer of the body to cremation/ burial staff, will be decontaminated with 1% Sodium Hypochlorite.
13. At the crematorium/ Burial Ground
    - The Crematorium/ burial Ground staff should be sensitized that COVID 19 does not pose additional risk.
    - The staff will practice standard precautions of hand hygiene, use of masks and gloves.
    - Viewing of the dead body by unzipping the face end of the body bag (by the staff using standard precautions)

may be allowed, for the relatives to see the body for one last time.

- Religious rituals such as reading from religious scripts, sprinkling holy water and any other last rites that does not require touching of the body can be allowed.
- Bathing, kissing, hugging, etc. of the dead body should not be allowed.
- The funeral/ burial staff and family members should perform hand hygiene after cremation/ burial.
- The ash does not pose any risk and can be collected to perform the last rites.
- Large gathering at the crematorium/ burial ground should be avoided as a social distancing measure as it is possible that close family contacts may be symptomatic and/ or shedding the virus

Covid Exit Strategy

Against all precedent, going into 2021, the world has several vaccines with demonstrated efficacy against symptomatic COVID-19 in its armamentarium. Numerous issues and uncertainties surround the existing COVID-19 vaccines. We do not yet know the quality or length of protection the vaccines will provide and how effectively they will stop viral transmission. New variants of SARS-CoV-2 with mutations in key proteins threaten vaccine efficacy. Certain countries that have relied on a suppression strategy for pandemic control, using non-pharmaceutical interventions to reduce cases, hospital admissions, and deaths to so-called acceptable levels before lifting restrictions, appear to be entirely dependent on population-level herd immunity generated through natural infection or immunization as an exit strategy. Public health messaging in these countries, which include most countries in Europe and the USA, is that we must both await the vaccines and become accustomed to living with the virus, as we have done with other viruses in the past. We should expect SARS-CoV-2 to become endemic and, potentially, seasonal. Another strategy in use—to eliminate—has been deployed by countries that have been arguably the most successful in their responses to the pandemic: New Zealand, Australia, Taiwan, South Korea, Vietnam, and China. This strategy, which is proactive rather than reactive, resembles an exit strategy to a far greater extent than does the suppression strategy. It has a clear goal: to reduce community transmission to near zero through a highly stringent, but short-term, lockdown, followed by implementation of a well sized, robust, and coordinated find, test, trace, isolate, and support system, with the aim to identify and end outbreaks before they become unmanageable. Key to the success of this strategy is removal of structural inequalities that might lead to resurgences of the virus in certain marginalized populations.

References

1. A Pandemic Era. Editorial. The Lancet Planetary Health . Jan 2021. Vol 5.
2. M. Saiful Islam, Kazi M. Rahman, Yanni Sun, Mohammed O. Qureshi, Ikram Abdi, Abrar A. Chughtai, Holly Seale. Current knowledge of COVID-19 and infection prevention and control strategies in healthcare settings: A global analysis. Infect Control Hosp Epidemiol. 2020 May 15: 1–11.
3. COVID-19 transmission—up in the air. The Editorial. The Lancet Respiratory Medicine. Dec 2020. Vol 8.
4. Interim Infection Prevention and Control Recommendations for Healthcare Personnel During the Coronavirus Disease 2019 (COVID-19) Pandemic. CDC. Feb 2021.
5. Using personnel Protective equipment (PPE). CDC. June 2020. www.cdc.gov/coronavirus.
6. Facing up to long COVID. Editorial. The Lancet. Dec 2020. Vol. 396.
7. Covid-19: Guidelines On Dead Body Management. Government of India Ministry of Health & Family Welfare Directorate General of Health Services. 2020.
8. The COVID-19 exit strategy—why we need to aim low. Editorial. The Lancet Infectious Diseases. March 2021. Vol 21.

20

Digital Hospital

Sky rocketing costs, reports of medical errors, consumers demanding better care and the ever-growing need to move away from paper charts are all restructuring the health system. For a while experts in information technology have been luring hospitals to slim down on the paper patient files and prescription slips and get into better digital shape. While many of the individual pieces of equipment in health care are now computerized, capturing data from these devices and storing in a centralized system which allows for an effective transmission of information to right people, at right time lag far behind. The concept of a digital hospital might evoke images of an impersonal facility but the reality is just the opposite. By definition the digital hospital is connected which leads to better efficiency and information flow laying the ground work for better patient care. One reason that hospitals have been slow to adopt such tools is that they are expensive. Now several big players in health care and data management are bringing their expertise and money to bear on the problem. It may include patient beds with information screens connected to a central data base, electronic medical records storage, digital imaging of X-ray films and wireless communication network that will permit doctors and nurses to update and access patients medical records using hand held devices. Data is available to every department, so prescription can be automatically checked for possible interactions and tests won't be repeated in different departments.

More and more hospitals across world are embracing health information technology and its benefits for quality of care and patient safety. Hospitals also reported dramatic increases in the use of computerized alerts to provide negative drug interactions. In 2006 51% of American hospitals were using real time drug interaction alerts.

The size of the hospital also plays considerable role in its IT use. The hospital with 500 beds or more show 74% use of moderate or high health IT in 2006 in U.S whereas only 23% of hospitals with 50 or fewer beds were in the top two levels of IT use. Hospitals in urban areas, teaching hospitals and with better financial health use more IT.

Digitally advanced hospitals experience greater reductions in the average length of patient stay and larger increases in operating revenues. Health care services productivity has risen about 2% annually since 2001. Recent developments in IT made the idea of a digital hospital seem logical and cost effective. Not only could electronic transmission help eliminate errors, it could also eliminate two or three hours a day that nurse spend charting patient data and dramatically improve communication between different departments. Experiences of hospitals in developed countries suggest that health care really is making its way into the digital age. Some of these hospitals have successfully put in place an electronic prescription drug system. IT (information technology) in hospitals is saving lives. Poor information kills some 7000 Americans each year just by missing drug interaction problems. Early evidence indicates that proper technology can reduce the toll. Hospitals that have begun using electronic prescription systems have seen up to 80% fewer prescription errors.

Nurses in these hospitals use wireless laptops on wheels to log in to this system to record patients symptoms and get all the information to shuttle patients through their stay. Doctors tap into the network via wireless laptops or PCs to order prescriptions and lab tests. Everything else is linked into the system from automated pharmacy to radiology. It means moving from scribbled notes and paperwork to networked software that accurately registers and quickly transmits patient records. With touch of a finger doctors and nurses have immediate access to high resolution digital images, laboratory results and medication histories that results in more informed decisions about diagnosis and treatment, which saves time, money and lives. By 2010 the European commission predicts that five percent of national health budgets will be invested in e-health systems and services.

Some of the problems encountered before the implementation of Digital hospital are:

- Too much time spent on tedious menial tasks.
- No access to critical information at patient's bedside.
- Slow retrieval or loss of critical information
- Disruption to patients rest.
- Illegible documentation by clinicians.
- Slower response time to unexpected abnormal vital signs readings.
- Human errors.
- Heavy usage of paper

Through the use of innovative technologies the expected outcomes include:

- Reduction in time spent on tedious menial tasks.
- Ability to have access to critical information at the patients bedside.
- Faster retrieval of critical information.
- Less disruption to patients rest, over all improvement for inpatient stay experience.
- Online documentation by clinicians.
- Fast response time to unexpected abnormal vital signs readings.
- Better reach and care for overseas and traveling patients.
- Reduction in human error.
- Reduced usage of paper.
- Automated tracking of door access data, staff attendance and staff immunization data.

Benefits of Digitalization

- Enables sharing of information which leads to better clinical decision making, leading to improved patient care, safety and management across clusters.

- IT empowers both clinicians and patients with the power of knowledge and information, anytime any where. Through telecare, the secure massaging provides a human touch through timely replies from clinicians to problems raised by patients.
- Digitalization improves patient doctor relationship and care provision. Clinicians have a convenient and efficient means to access patients medical information thereby improving patient dialogue and care provision.
- Digitalization results in time and cost savings. There are immense time savings which result from online access to complete information versus manual paper based reports and time spent making phone calls to laboratory and radiology departments for information. Nursing staff time to retrieve clinical information for review by clinicians is reduced significantly. There are cost savings for the patients by as much as $100 per patient as repeated laboratory tests and radiology procedures are avoided when a patient goes to another institution.
- There is improved quality of care and enhanced patient safety with quick online access to more complete, better quality and up-to-date clinical information and system alerts for abnormal results, duplicate medication orders and drug to allergy interactions.
- Clinical quality improvement: - Every hospital in America is thinking about quality. Employees are backing e-solutions for quality improvement.
- Care management: - The science of care management has been translated into care management protocols and electronic data analysis. In Baltimore specialists from John Hopkins University have developed an electronic ICU monitoring and telemedicine system that tele-monitors ICU patients on 24x7basis. They showed a 60% reduction in severity adjusted mortality, 40% fewer complication, 30% decrease in length of stay and a 28% reduction in cost per case.
- Reducing variation:- The use of benchmarks among top hospital is providing momentum to e-based initiatives to

reduce variation like clinical variation. Among the solucient top 100 hospitals, length of stay averaged 4.1days last year, which is seven percent lower than national average of 4.4 days. Longer inpatient stays and more intensive use of resources make a big difference in the financials.

- Physician networks:- Doctors are showing more interest in computer linkages as more physicians become regular internet users.
- Medication safety systems:- Medications safety systems like Bridge Medical, an Ameri source- Bergen Company based in Solano Beach, Calif use barcodes on unit- dose medication packages checked against a patients drug orders and drug allergies. The wireless computer assisted drug dispensing systems utilize sophisticated software and expert knowledge basis to attack the problem of a 1 to 3% estimate of medication errors in many U.S hospitals. Medication errors cost the nation an estimated $ 2billion in terms of cost, lost economic productivity, disability, legal and health care costs.
- Improved diagnostic accuracy: - Digital technology and diagnostic software can assist with problem of errors in diagnosis.

Process re-engineering:- The focus on costs in health organizations is leading to renewed initiatives in re-engineering and process improvement. Capital investments in electronic medical records will pay off because they address one of the greatest inefficiencies in health care because medical records are not mobile, the health system has always moved the patient rather than the information from location to location.

Online recruitment:- Internet access and interactive web sites are providing some solutions to health care's staffing crisis. Use of online recruitment is increasing rapidly among health care organizations.

Singapore health services believe there are three main pillars towards building a digital hospital. These are Digital ward, Digital clinic and Tele-care, Telemedicine and Home care. The digital ward was initiated by Singapore health services with the objective of transfering the way health care professionals capture and access clinical information. The digital ward project is made up of IT professionals from sing health ITAG (Innovative Technology Application Group). The project team works closely with users such as clinicians, nurses and operations colleagues of various sing health Institutions. Various wireless technologies and devices being implemented in the digital ward are:

1. Computer on wheels: Computer on wheels (COW) are WiFi note books on ergonomically designed mobile trolleys which enable clinicians to access patients medical records and digital radiology images as well as document patients progress anywhere anytime in the ward.
2. Mobile Electronic X-ray Computing (MERC): MERC is motorized WiFi enabled system with dual, triple or quadruple panel display screens which enable patient's electronic medical records and digital radiology images to be displayed across different screens. Clinicians can access these records and images wirelessly at the patient's bedside to explain various therapies and clinicians options to them. This innovation serves to enrich the face to face communication not only with patients but also with their family members.
3. VEGA:- The integrated wireless VEGA system enables remote automated monitoring of patients vital signs such as blood pressure, pulse rate, electrocardiogram (ECG), pulse oximetry, temperature and respiratory rate. The system also provides proximity contact tracing and location tracking. The patient's vital signs are captured automatically via customized monitoring devices (using WiFi and active RFID technologies) and clinicians can view the vital signs charts online. This reduces potential human errors and enhances patient safety. With this system nurses also spend less time on tedious menial tasks, enabling them to devote more time in delivering quality patient care. In addition patients can have an undisturbed rest without having their signs taken manually by the nurses.

   To enable proximity contact tracing specially designed wearable tags are issued to patients and hospital staff in the ward for the purpose of automatically and wirelessly recording and tracking people with whom to come into contact within the ward. The contact data captured in the tag is then automatically and periodically uploaded into the services using industry standard WiFi access points. Hospital staff can search, view and print records of the contact tracing details on line.

4. Patient Bed Side Terminal (PBT) : PBT is a touch screen integrated information system that provides both the clinic and patients an efficient and convenient means to access information within the hospital and globally. With PBT clinician can retrieve and display medical record and digital radiology images as well as their medical conditions at patient's bed side. Through the terminal patients can speak to the nurse on duty using a video nurse call function while nurses can order meals for patients electronically instead of ordering manually. In addition patients can also access a wide variety of entertainment and internet services.
5. Mobile clinical Assistant (MCA): MCA is a specially designed highly portable health care tablet PC equipped with an integrated camera for visual clinical documentation. The build in barcode/RFID reading is used to verify the patient's identification. MCA is also WiFi enabled empowering clinician with secured anywhere, any time access to hospitals EMR systems and other clinical information. Through the Bluetooth wireless technology it can interface with other medical devices e.g. vital signs monitors to obtain patient data from existing medical device and directly transmit captured patient data into hospital clinical application in real time.

   Such a mobile point of care solution helps in improving the quality of patient care and enhancing the production by enabling clinicians to quickly retrieve and document patient's information. This is especially critical in a fast environment.
6. Smart card: With smart card technology hospital staff carries only one card for multiple purposes. Besides door access control the same card can be used for tracking of attendance at staff events or trainings. Its tap and track method makes the whole process faster and easier. Staff immunization can be tracked by smart card.

Who Benefits from Hospital Information System

Hospital information systems can be characterized by their benefits; their functions; their types of processed information and their types of services offered. The following groups benefit from Hospital Information System:

(a) Physicians

- Introduces Computerized Provider Order Entry (CPOE).
- Improves accuracy & legibility of, and access to, the required patient medications.
- Improves clinicians' efficiency & effectiveness through provision of key patient information (e.g., allergies) at time of ordering, plus conflict checking, order checking and online access to best practice information.
- Improves care through the logging of all orders.
- Reduces medication error rates.

(b) Nurses

- Will allow immediate access to orders and results .
- Will provide immediate access to patient demographics, medication and test results.
- Will provide improved access to information on line (i.e.: suggested medications or drug alerts).
- Will decrease the need for paper, decrease errors and increase patient safety.

(c) Allied Health Professionals

- Will allow immediate access to orders and results .
- Will provide immediate access to patient demographics, medication and test results.
- Will provide improved access to information on line (i.e.: suggested medications or drug alerts).
- Will decrease the need for paper, decrease errors and increase patient safety.

(d) Ward and Registration Clerks

- Will provide a single point of contact for patient registration information and reduce duplication of effort.

(e) Clinical Benefits

- Provide a common source of information about person's health history.
- Enhance the ability of health care professionals to coordinate care by providing a person's health information and visit history at the place and time that it is needed.
- Link information from diagnostic information systems such as X-ray and laboratory into the EPR.
- Strengthen internal and external communication among health care providers.
- Eventually be accessible for use in all of Manitoba's academic and community hospitals, as well as long term care facilities.
- Allow care providers access to the patient's health history and results between facilities.
- Will provide improved access to information on line (ie: suggested medications or drug alerts).
- Will decrease the need for paper, decrease errors and increase patient safety.

(f) Administrative Benefits

- Will provide improved access to information on line (i.e. suggested medications or drug alerts) .
- Will decrease the need for paper, decrease errors and increase patient safety.
- Strengthen internal and external communication among health care providers.
- Will decrease the need for re-registrations of patients across multiple sites.

Components of Hospital Information System

Hospital Information System is a comprehensive, integrated computer system. Within this system, there are varieties of subsystems in medical specialties.

There are five key components or "modules" in the system, include:

1. Registration :The system captures and records patient demographics and visits at the point-of-care. Registration data will be displayed consistently and automatically on screens in the clinical system.
2. Order Entry and Results Reporting : All clinical orders will be listed with indications of what has been completed and what is pending. Electronic alerts will appear for orders duplication and errors and provide information to assist clinical decision-making. All test results in the patient's electronic chart will be filed with alerts for abnormal results.
3. Clinical Documentation: This module provides on-line documentation of clinical encounters such as flowcharts and structured notes.
4. Scheduling Patients: Schedules patients for appointments with clinicians or for tests and procedures.
5. Patient Billing: All billable health services will be accessible and processed in this system.

Subsystems of HIS

There are different types of HIS including routine and clinical HIS. Components of a hospital information system consist of two or more of the following:

1. Picture Archiving Communication System (PACS)

   Picture Archiving and Communication System (PACS): a PACS is a medical imaging technology which provides economical storage of, and convenient access to, images from multiple modalities (source machine types).[1] Electronic images and reports are transmitted digitally via PACS; this eliminates the need to manually file, retrieve, or transport film jackets. The universal format for PACS image storage and transfer is DICOM (Digital Imaging and Communications in Medicine). Non-image data, such as scanned documents, may be incorporated using consumer industry standard formats like PDF (Portable Document Format), once encapsulated in DICOM.

2. Radiology Information System (RIS)

   These systems are also popular for their ability to provide radiology billing services, appointment scheduling as well as reporting and patient database storage. The radiology practice has become more complex with advances in technology and more hospitals now turn to RIS to manage the business side of their practices

3. Clinical Information System (CIS)

   A Clinical Information System is a computer based system that is designed for collecting, storing, manipulating and making available clinical information important to the healthcare delivery process. Clinical Information System helps healthcare organizations improve the delivery of clinical services. Hospital information systems present clinical information and reports that enable clinicians to make more informed decisions at the point of care.

4. Physician Information Systems (PIS)

   Physician information systems are delivered through computers, servers, networks, and use widely deployed and popular applications such as, electronic medical records (EMRs), electronic health records (EHRs), and more. Most of these services have 24/7 remote support that allows hospital staff to troubleshoot problems occurring during system usage.

5. Financial Information System (FIS)

   Financial Information Systems are computer systems that manage the business aspect of a hospital. While healthcare organization's primary priority is to save lives and not making profits, they do acquire running costs from day to day operations; including purchase and staff payroll.

6. Laboratory Information System (LIS)

   A Laboratory Information Management System (LIMS), sometimes referred to as a Laboratory Information System (LIS) or Laboratory Management System (LMS), is a software-based laboratory and information management system that offers a set of key features that support a modern laboratory's operations.

7. Nursing Information Systems (NIS)

   A good Nursing Information Systems can perform a number of functions and deliver benefits such as improving staff schedules, accurate patient charting and improve clinical data integration. Patient charting applications allow users to enter details regarding patients' vital signs. Nurses also use it for admission information, care plan and all relevant nursing notes. All important data is securely stored and can be retrieved when required. It also allows nurses to collect, retrieve and analyze the clinical information and then integrate it to design patients care plan. All these features in NIS ultimately lead to a reduction in planning time and better assessments and evaluations. The chance of prescribing the wrong medication also decreases since there is always a reference for electronically prescribed drugs.

8. Pharmacy Information System (PIS)

   Designed to address the demands of a pharmacy department, PIS helps pharmacists monitor how medication is used in hospitals. PIS helps users supervise drug allergies and other medication-related complications. The system allows users to detect drug interactions and also helps administer proper drugs based on the patient's physiologic factors.

Important HIS Functions

(1) Display alerts for high risk medications (e.g. narcotics, sound-alike drugs, concentrated electrolytes) just prior to administration.

(2) Predict time to patient examination on admission.

(3) Record time to consultation after request from emergency department.

(4) Display real-time availability of patient beds.

(5) Flag and prioritize elderly and disabled patients.

(6) Provide electronic copy of patient records when requested (e.g. diagnosis list, lab test results, administered procedures, administered medications, discharge summary) .

(7) View all diagnostic test results including laboratory, radiology, pathology, nuclear medicine, endoscopy.

(8) Record times and performing staff of laboratory test samples throughout all laboratory phases i.e. sampling, accepting, analyzing, approving, and reporting.

(9) Display alerts for lab samples that do not meet acceptance criteria.

(10) Display alerts for laboratory tests that return panic values.

(11) Display reminders for internal and external lab quality control measures and keep their result for analyses.

(12) Record laboratory process problems (pre-analytic, analytic, and post-analytic).

(13) Provide digital radiology images within internal network i.e. Picture Archiving and Communication System (PACS).

(14) Monitor radiology appointment and reporting times.

(15) Support telemedicine applications.

(16) Monitor use of blood and blood products during order, preparation, acceptance, and implementation.

(17) Monitor blood and blood products stock and expiration date.

(18) Record disease severity as structured data (e.G. apache II, SAPS II, and PRISM).

(19) Integrate nursing care plans into medical record.

(20) Record and integrate all clinical orders into medical record including laboratory test orders, medication orders, nursing care orders, nutrition therapy orders, rehabilitation therapy orders.

(21) Record and integrate all diagnostic, clinical, and surgical procedures into medical record including endoscopy, cardiac catheterization, radiotherapy, CT, and ultrasound.

(22) Record usage and monitor complications of anesthetic agents and sedatives administered outside of anesthesiology (e.g. endoscopy, cardiac catheterization, and IVF units).

(23) Display clinical guidelines and provide alerts for deviations.

(24) Provide alerts for drug-drug interactions.

(25) Provide alerts for drug-food interactions.

(26) Provide alerts for drug-allergy interactions.

(27) Integrate Computerized Physician Order Entry.

(28) Provide alerts for patient education that is part of care plan or discharge plan.

(29) Record all patient education provided to patient.

(30) Record patient and staff safety events.

(31) Record emergency code alerts (e.g. Code Blue, Code White) and integrate with paging system.

(32) Record blood transfusion reactions as structured data.

(33) Monitor hospital key performance indicators automatically.

(34) Flag patients and warn staff of patients with risk of infection (e.g. HIV+, HepC+).

(35) Monitor nosocomial infections and transmit surveillance data to national or international networks.

(36) Monitor and record sterilization processes including procedure date and time and material expiration date.

(37) Display real-time information necessary for unit managers including bed occupancy, waiting list, surgeries scheduled.

(38) Report periodically on operational statistics including monthly admissions, income-expenditure, services delivered.

(39) Provide alerts for devices that require periodic maintenance or calibration.

(40) Provide alerts for medications and medical supplies near expiration or at critically low stock levels.

(41) Provide inventory of all medical devices including location and responsible staff.

(42) Monitor and provide reminders for routine health screening of clinical staff.

(43) Identify, flag, and, prohibit duplicate patient records.

(44) Monitor occupational accidents and injuries.

(45) Display current organizational policies and procedures and provide alerts of updated documents.

(46) Record clinical staff certification and licensing information.

(47) Integrate and update information with hospital external website.

(48) Provide online patient portal to view, download, and transmit lab results.

(49) Provide access control management for different staff groupings.

(50) Provide data security and protection for electronic health information.

Adapted from : Functionality of hospital information systems: results from a survey of quality directors at Turkish hospitals

Challenges for Healthcare Information Systems

New requirements and technological advances occurring in healthcare, information systems, and information technology have influenced the evolving role of healthcare information systems and related technology. Relevant aspects that took place in the evolution of systems and technology in order to appropriately support healthcare organizations are

- The diverse organizational healthcare environment of information systems which need to be adapted to multiple types of healthcare organizations.
- Dynamic changes in the required role of information systems, following changes in the role and dynamics of all levels of health care delivery and management.
- The need for integration of information systems within healthcare organizations, which are also organized as networks.
- Technological advances in systems structure and communications, facilitating the implementation of integrated healthcare networks.

How Secure is Digital Hospital

Biggest barrier to high technology is security of data. Wireless networks use shared radiofrequencies to move data, so security concerns about this method of information transmission have always been high. Wired Equivalent Privacy (WEP) protocol was meant to be a crack proof method of securing data that was being transmitted using wireless devices by encrypting the data. WEP has major security flaws. A cracker just needs some easily obtained equipment to be able to intercept the wireless transmission, change the data contained in those transmission and access the contents of wireless network. The flaw seriously undermines the security claims of the system. Hospitals use strong encryption and other methods to protect data but actual technology that will be used is under discussion and development. Hospitals make patient records available to doctors and patients via the internet and haven't had any security or privacy problems. Vital factors essential for making the jump from personal usage to clinical use include integrating technology into work flow at the point of care, addressing privacy and security concerns and demonstrating how online technologies will help physicians practice medicine more efficiently and effectively.

Hospitals must be prepared to offer medical services tailored to patients needs. It is essential for hospital management to conduct the assessment of HIS regularly by internal customers for incorporating continuous technology innovations and design requirements to satisfy external customers through seamless integration of HIS across all the departments in the hospital.

National Digital Health Mission

The National Digital Health Mission (NDHM) aims to develop the backbone necessary to support the integrated digital health infrastructure of the country. It will bridge the existing gap amongst different stakeholders of Healthcare ecosystem through digital highways. NDHM shall create a seamless online platform "through the provision of a wide-range of data, information and infrastructure services, duly leveraging open, interoperable, standards-based digital systems" while ensuring the security, confidentiality and privacy of health-related personal information. In a follow-up of the NHP's specific goals for adopting digital technologies, the Ministry of Health and Family Welfare constituted a committee headed by Shri J. Satyanarayana to develop an implementation framework for the National Health Stack. This committee produced the National Digital Health Blueprint (NDHB), laying out the building blocks and an action plan to comprehensively and holistically implement digital health. Since the implementation is envisioned to be in a mission mode, the initiative is referred to as the National Digital Health Mission (NDHM).

To strengthen the accessibility and equity of health services, including continuum of care with citizen as the owner of data, in a holistic healthcare programme approach leveraging IT & associated technologies and support the existing health systems in a 'citizen-centric' approach, the NDHM envisages the following specific objectives:

- To establish state-of-the-art digital health systems, to manage the core digital health data, and the infrastructure required for its seamless exchange;
- To establish registries at appropriate level to create single source of truth in respect of clinical establishments, healthcare professionals, health workers, drugs and pharmacies.
- To enforce adoption of open standards by all national digital health stakeholders.
- To create a system of personal health records, based on international standards, easily accessible to individuals and healthcare professionals and services providers, based on individual's informed consent.
- To promote development of enterprise-class health application systems with a special focus on achieving the Sustainable Development Goals for health.
- To adopt the best principles of cooperative federalism while working with the States and Union Territories for the realization of the vision.
- To ensure that the healthcare institutions and professionals in the private sector participate actively with public health authorities in the building of the NDHM, through a combination of prescription and promotion.
- To ensure national portability in the provision of health services.
- To promote the use of clinical decision support (CDS) systems by health professionals and practitioners.
- To promote a better management of the health sector leveraging health data analytics and medical research.
- To provide for enhancing the efficiency and effectiveness of governance at all levels.

- To support effective steps being taken for ensuring quality of healthcare and
- To strengthen existing health information systems, by ensuring their conformity with the defined standards and integration with the proposed NDHM. Patients are identified by "Ayushman Bharat Health Account" called ABHA and their whole medical history is stored in their digital locker, Health professionals have to get registered in Health Professional Registry and Health Institutes in the Repository of Health Care delivery providers.

The current strong public digital infrastructure—including that related to Aadhaar, Unified Payments Interface and wide reach of the Internet and mobile phones provides a strong platform for establishing the building blocks of NDHM. The existing ability to digitally identify people, doctors, and health facilities, facilitate electronic signatures, ensure non-repudiable contracts, make paperless payments, securely store digital records, and contact people provide opportunities to streamline healthcare information through digital management.

Opportunities

- The current strong public digital infrastructure provides opportunities to streamline healthcare information through digital management.
- Ayushman Bharat—Pradhan Mantri Jan Arogya Yojana (AB-PMJAY) has successfully used the available public digital infrastructure to provide end-to-end services through an information technology (IT) platform from identification of beneficiaries to their admission and treatment in hospitals to their discharge and paperless payment to hospitals. The experience of AB-PMJAY can be leveraged to expand the reach of digital health to all residents and develop an open and inter-operable health management system that empowers residents, healthcare providers, the Government and researchers.
- Emerging technologies such as artificial intelligence, the internet of things (IoT), Blockchain and cloud computing provide additional opportunities for facilitating a more holistic digital health ecosystem, that can increase the equitable access to health services, improve health outcomes and reduce costs.

Benefits

The implementation of NDHM is expected to significantly improve the efficiency, effectiveness, and transparency of health service delivery overall. Patients will be able to securely store and access their medical records (such as prescriptions, diagnostic reports and discharge summaries), and share them with health care providers to ensure appropriate treatment and follow-up. They will also have access to more accurate information on health facilities and service providers. Further, they will have the option to access health services remotely through tele-consultation and e-pharmacy. NDHM will empower individuals with accurate information to enable informed decision making and increase accountability of healthcare providers.

NDHM will provide choice to individuals to access both public and private health services, facilitate compliance with laid down guidelines and protocols, and ensure transparency in pricing of services and accountability for the health services being rendered.

Similarly, health care professionals across disciplines will have better access to patient's medical history (with the necessary informed consent) for prescribing more appropriate and effective health interventions. The integrated ecosystem will also enable better continuum of care. NDHM will help digitize the claims process and enable faster reimbursement. This will enhance the overall ease of providing services amongst the health care providers.

At the same time, policy makers and programme managers will have better access to data, enabling more informed decision making by the Government. Better quality of macro and micro-level data will enable advanced analytics, usage of health-biomarkers and better preventive healthcare. It will also enable geography and demography-based monitoring and appropriate decision making to inform design and strengthen implementation of health programmes and policies.

Finally, researchers will greatly benefit from the availability of such aggregated information as they will be able to study and evaluate the effectiveness of various programmes and interventions. NDHM would facilitate a comprehensive feedback loop between researchers, policymakers, and providers.

References

1. EU-European Health Strategy: "e-health-making health care better for European citizens: An action plan for a European e-Health care." April 30, 2004.
2. Naoh Tay chi Seng- Digital Hospital Sing Health's Journey towards Digitalization of health care. Sing Health Info Tech department.
3. Timothy J. Mullancy and Arlene Waintraub. Business week magazine cover storey, March 28, 2005.
4. David Allen, Malt Fenwick. New survey shows Information Technology use in hospitals continues to grow. High costs, lack of standards seen as major obstacles to greater adoption. AHA Feb 27 2007. www.aha.org
5. Susan Borden Digital Hospital. Technology Review July 2001.
6. Solucient "100 Top Hospitals: Benchmarks for success." Cited in Margaret Muckio, "Hospital vital signs lagging". On managed care. March 2001, 6(3): 1-2.
7. The New York times, " Naming hospitals, Good and Bad. " Online News storey. Nov 17 2000.
8. Business wire. "VISICU provides solution to leap frog Group Health care initiatives". Online news story. Nov 15 2000.
9. Friend D.B. Health care. Com Rx for reform. St. Lucie Press, Boca Raton, Fla, 2000.
10. Russel.C. collie. Managing the digital hospital-Next! Health Care Industry American College of Physician Executives 2003.
11. Yousef Mehdipour, Hamideh Zerehkafi. Hospital Information System (HIS): At a Glance. Asian Journal of Computer and Information System. 2013; 1 (2): 54-61.
12. Mehmet Saluvan, Al Ozonoff. Functionality of hospital information systems: results from a survey of quality directors at Turkish hospitals. BMC Medical Informatics and Decision . 2018: 18;6.
13. Acharyulu.G.V.R.K. Assessment of Hospital Information System Quality in Multi Speciality Hospitals. Internatiuonal Journal of Innovation, Management and Technology. 2012; 3(4): 349-352.
14. About NDHM. National Health Authority Govt Of India. nha.gov.in/NDHM.html. assessed on 5/6/2022.

21

Making Most Of Manpower

First and foremost responsibility of human resource manager is recruiting personnel. Most important functions in this respect are

1. Attraction
2. Selection
3. Retention.
4. Development
5. Assessment
6. Adjustment

Attraction involves activities of identifying the job requirements within an organization, determining the number of personnel required and qualities necessary to perform the job and making it public. Selection is the process of choosing the best fit for the job. Retention involves keeping the personnel motivated for performing effectively and ensuring safe and healthy work environment. Development involves enhancing the competence of personnel by improving their knowledge, skills and other abilities. Assessment involves observation and evaluation of performance of personnel. Adjustment involves discipline, promotions and transfers.

An occupation is a group of similar jobs found in different organizations at different times. The term job is used more narrowly and implies a within organization reference. The term occupation implies an across organization reference. The term job analysis describes the process of obtaining information about jobs. It includes information about the tasks to be done on the job and the personnel characteristics necessary to do the tasks.

An overall written summary of task requirements is called job description and overall written summary of worker requirements is called job specification. Together job description and job specification comprise job analysis.

Five popular job analysis methods are:

1. **JOB PERFORMANCE:** An analyst actually does the job under study to get first hand exposure to what it demands. This method is inappropriate for jobs that require extensive training or are hazardous to perform.
2. **OBSERVATION:** The analyst records information about a job by actually observing workers on job. Disadvantage of this method is that if the work in question is primarily mental observations alone may reveal little useful information.
3. **INTERVIEW:** The jobs which are not easy to perform or where observation is not possible information about jobs can be obtained by interview. Skills of interviewer and worker suspicion and motives are real concerns.
4. **CRITICAL INCIDENT:** Larger number of brief actual reports collected give a fairly clear description of jobs in question. It takes considerable time to gather, abstract and categorize the incidents.
5. **QUESTIONNAIRES:** The workers are subjected to a structured questionnaire. Questionnaires are often time consuming to develop but quicker to administer than other methods.

Human resource planning

Human resource planning is defined as an effort to anticipate future business and environmental demands on an organization and to provide the personnel to fulfill that business and satisfy those demands. Human resource planning can be strategic (Long term and general) or tactical (short term and specific).At the level of operational or tactical planning, HRP is concerned with detailed forecasts of employees supply and employee demand. Based on the forecasts specific action plans can be undertaken. These include recruitment, derecruitment, promotions, training or transfers. In labour market forces of supply interact with the forces of demand and thereby determine the price of labor. In a tight labour market reverse is true. One use of human resource information system is in the development of a personnel inventory for human resource planning. To estimate demand for manpower one must know conditions within the organization such as age, distribution of work force, terminations, retirements etc. This is done by management succession plan which includes setting a planning horizon, identifying replacement candidates for each key position, assessing performance and readiness for promotion, identifying career development needs and integrating the career goals of individual with institutions goal. Another approach that can be used to develop a forecast of the internal supply of human resources is Markov analysis. It tracks past patterns of personnel movements and uses them to project future patterns. A 5-10 years base period is used. The longer the base period the more meaningful will each past movement represent a probability of future movement. Demand forecasting on the other hand is beset with multiple uncertainties such as changes in technology, consumer attitudes and patterns of customer requirements and characteristics. Forecasts of human resource demand are often more subjective than quantitative. This can be done by Delphi technique and trend analysis. Delphi technique is an approach for reaching a consensus among experts about future development. In trend analysis we identify an appropriate business factor that relates to the work force in terms of size and constitution. Then we measure the past trends of this business factor in relation to the number of people employed and we project from that what the future trend will be and hence the future demand in terms of manpower.

Making most of health work force

A well performing work force is one that works in ways that are responsive, fair and efficient to achieve the best health outcomes possible given available resources and circumstances. The performance of manpower depends on availability, competence, responsiveness and productivity. Human resource indicators to assess health work force performance are shown in Table 19-1

Table 21.1: Human resource indicators to assess health workforce performance

Dimension	Possible Indicators
Availability	Staff ratios Absence rates Waiting time
Competence	Individual: prescribing practices Institutional: readmission rates; live births, cross- infections
Responsiveness	Patient satisfaction; assessment of responsiveness
Productivity	Occupied beds, out patient visits, interventions delivered per worker or facility.

Adopted from human resource indicators to monitor health service performance keele University

The instruments that influence personnel performance include clear job descriptions, professional norms and code of conduct, the proper matching of skills to the tasks in hand and supervision. Job descriptions that clearly set out objectives, responsibilities and lines of accountability are consistently associated with improved achievement of work goals for all sorts of workers. Health workers are expected to conduct themselves with integrity, selflessly to apply know how and to put the interests of the patients above their own. Professional codes of conduct are often instilled through unwritten channels and take time to develop, but can become a significant source of internal motivation. Many employers are now introducing written codes of conduct for all their employees. To have the desired effect such rules and regulations need to be well publicized and actions taken when they are broken. Tasks to be performed must match an individual workers skills. Workers are not always at work at the times when work load is highest. Shift patterns and time flexibility provide a way to increase workers productivity. Delegation is another way to increase over all worker productivity. Supervision especially coupled with audit and feedback to staff, has been consistently found to improve the performance of many types of health workers from providers to managers. Supervision is not effective if it is used as a fault finding and punitive tool. Supervision that is supportive, educational and consistent and helps to solve problems can improve performance, job satisfaction and motivation. Every health worker needs some key supports to perform his or her job: remuneration, information and infrastructure including equipment and supplies. Three aspects of remuneration influence the behavior of health workers: the level and regularity of pay, the way people are paid and other incentives. Health workers must be paid reasonably for the work they do. They need to receive a living wage, they also need to believe that the wage is commensurate with their responsibilities and that it is fair when compared with others in the same or equivalent jobs. Salary increases alone are not enough to change performance. These must be combined with other strategies to create significant change. Any efforts to improve overall work force productivity need to be based on reliable data about work force level, distribution and skill mix, coupled with information on the factors thought to be constraining better health worker performance and intelligence on potential policy options. No matter how motivated and skilled health workers are, they cannot do their jobs properly in facilities that lack clean water, adequate lighting, heating, vehicles, drugs, working equipment and other supplies. The physical environment needs to be safe. Health workers require up-to date knowledge to perform well. Rapid increases in knowledge and changing health systems make this need even more essential today. Off site training courses have a poor track record for changing the actual practice of health workers. In service training is most likely to change worker behavior when it is interactive, based on real life problems and coupled with continuing, intermittent support.

An extremely important part of professional treatment lies in the manager's leadership style. Authoritarian approaches are less likely to work with professional employees than with non professionals. On the other hand, consultative and participative approaches are far more appropriate to professional employees. Frequent conflicts arise as managers and professionals collide in matters of professional versus managerial judgment. In some such conflicts it is all too common for the authoritarian manager to wield the authority of the boss and overrule the professional. In an industry such as hospitals in which many judgments involves patient safety however both the parties have equal responsibility for making judgments. The leader has to keep his manpower motivated to produce the best results. The motivation to work is not present to an equivalent degree in all persons. The importance of work as part of one's life varies from top priority to last place. Popular theories of motivation work well with some people and combination of these theories work well with most people. Abraham Maslow's theory (1943) of motivation says that people in their drive to advance themselves and improve the quality of their lives, tend to move upward through a hierarchy of needs. When a given level of a need is met, an individual aspires to meet the next level in the hierarchy. The needs proceed from lower to higher levels in this manner: physiological needs (food, thirst, sex etc), safety needs, affiliation needs (acceptance needs, social needs), esteem needs (recognition), and need for self actualization (personal fulfillment). Frederick Herzberg concluded that true motivators are inherent in the work and he called them hygiene factors i.e. those things making up the environment surrounding the work are not motivators but rather potential dissatisfiers. Herzberg classified factors having a bearing on individuals relationship with their work into environmental factors and motivating factors. Environmental factors even if present do not necessarily motivate but if not acceptable have a strong potential to act as dissatisfiers. Some of the environmental factors which act as dissatisfiers when absent are; appreciation of one's efforts, tactful discipline and reasonable privacy, opportunity for growth and advancement, feeling of security, working conditions etc. True motivation factors are opportunities to learn, achieve, assume responsibility, work that is interesting and challenging etc. A manager has lot of opportunities to keep his staff motivated provided he has full knowledge and understanding of different motivational theories. Frequently managers in pursuit of their ego and authoritarian behavior make a mess of things. The primary reason is their lack of knowledge and understanding of vital organizational issues. Here comes a need for a qualified hospital administrator who can use his skills and tools appropriately. He has to use different leadership styles and skills at different times and with different class of employees. There is need to attract meritorious students into the specialty of hospital administration who when trained can utilize resources provided to them in an optimal manner. The manager can influence both motivating factors and environmental factors. However it also depends on the job and partly on the organization and in particular on how much latitude the individual managers are allowed. Managers must conduct exit interviews to study the factors that led employees to leave the job.

Mc Gregor gave theory X and Y of leadership in his work "The human side of enterprise". Theory X says that people have an inherent dislike for work and they need to be directed and controlled actively to achieve the goals. This theory believes in pure autocratic leadership. In health care organizations this applies to lower class employees like sanitary workers etc. Theory Y on the other hand believes that people are not naturally passive or resistant to work. If they appear to have become so, the reason lies in the management of organization. The management must organize conditions and methods of operation in a way that people are motivated to achieve the best.

Performance appraisal: Performance appraisal's which were the least favorite tasks for most managers are becoming more common now. The primary purpose of performance appraisal is to encourage improved performance for employee in job and to provide opportunity for those employees who wish to expand their knowledge and pursue promotion and growth. The performance appraisals should not be negatively oriented focusing primarily on criticism and fault finding. To start with each employee is given a chance of self appraisal and is asked to access his performance in the organization himself. He writes the appraisal and then appraisal interview is conducted. In performance appraisal systematic description of an employee's job-relevant strengths and weaknesses is done. Feed back is provided to the employees. Those who are outstanding performers are promoted. Performance appraisals interfere with more constructive supervisor-subordinate coaching relationships. Appraisal tend to encourage the superior position of the supervisor thus countering his vital role of a coach. The appraisal system should be relevant, sensitive, reliable, acceptable and practical. Formal appraisal should be done once or best twice a year. Many rating formats focus on employee behaviors either by comparing the performance of employees to each other (relative rating systems) or by evaluating each employee in terms of performance standards without reference to others (absolute rating systems). Other rating formats place primary emphasis on what an employee produces, so called results oriented systems.

Commonly used methods of performance appraisal are:

1. Ranking: Simple ranking requires a rater to order all employees from best to the worst. In alternate ranking the rater chooses the first best and the first worst, then second best and the second worst and keeps on alternating like this till all are ranked. In paired comparisons each employee is compared

with every other employee. These comparisons are based on the overall performance i.e. present value to organization.

2. Forced distribution: Over all distribution of ratings is forced into a normal or bell shaped curve. Some of the employees are outstanding, some average and some unsatisfactory. Most of the employees are average performers.

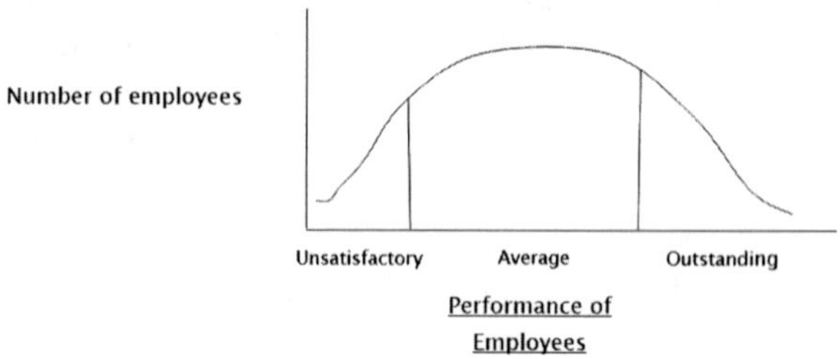

Fig. 21.1

3. Checklists: The rater here is provided with a series of statements that describe job-related behavior. The task is simply to check which statements best describe the employee behavior. In forced-choice system checklist items are arranged in groups from which the rater chooses statements that are most and least descriptive of each employee. Weights are assigned to all statements and these weight are kept secret from rater. An overall rating for each employee is then derived by applying a special scoring key to the rater's descriptions.
4. Critical incident: The critical incident approach to appraisal requires that manager keeps a running log of interesting events narrated by each employees. All critical incidents that fall outside the realm of so called normal performance are recorded as they occur. At the time of formal review the manager simply assembles the series of anecdotal notes into a picture of the employee's over all performance for the year.

Career ladder

Career ladder is the series of internal advancements available to an employee who remains within a particular occupational field. The advancement possibilities are limited by the number of levels on the career ladder and the number of positions available at each level. The biggest problem in health care organizations is when specialists reach the top in their career ladder and remain there for sometime they begin to feel the effects of limited opportunity and feeling of lack of expanding challenge. This is called topping out. These specialists then aspire for the post of chief executive. These specialists although trained in their field of specialization are not necessarily suited to top management. The result is poor or marginally effective managers. Not only is a specialist lost but resources at hand are also not effectively used. If this position is given to a trained, competent hospital administrator, effective utilization of resource and quality health care can be ensured. Some organizations have established a parallel growth paths (parallel path progression) such that more senior and more accomplished employees can acquire pay and benefits equivalent to those associated with top managerial positions. This can ensure advancement in chosen fields of specialists without pursuing movement into management.

Developing pay Systems

Pay systems assign monetary value to each job in the organization and an orderly procedure for increasing the same based on merit and seniority. To start with job analysis is done for identifying the relative worth of the job to the organization. Job evaluation is done to rank jobs in terms of relative worth to the organization. E.N Hay developed one of the popular methods of job evaluation. He compared those aspects of jobs that were common to all jobs rather than comparing whole jobs. Three factors identified were know-how, problem solving and accountability. Evaluation committee develops a point profile of each job on each factor. Evaluation is done to start with for "Bench mark" jobs i.e. those which have clear job content, represent large number of in-house jobs. Total point totals are translated into pay structure after surveying the relevant labour market in industry.

Johari Window

Johari Window is a technique for improving self-awareness within an individual. It helps in understanding your relationship with yourself and others. Johari Window model can be a useful tool if you want to improve your communication skills. It was developed by American psychologists Joseph Luft and Harry Ingham in 1955, hence the name Johari. Johari Window is generally used in Self-help groups in exercises which help a person to learn and discover things about themselves, like heuristic exercise. Johari Window is a method used for self-discovery. To improve communication in a group it is important to develop the perception of an individual in the group. Johari window model is based upon two things – to acquire the trust of others by revealing your information to them and by learning about yourself through feedback by others. here are four questions in the model just like panes in a window and each person fits into one of this pane. Each window in Johari window model signifies feelings, personal information, and motivation.

Also, the important point to know here is that through window panes one must determine whether one is known or unknown to oneself as well as the others.

	Known to Self	**Not Known to Self**
Known to Others	**Arena** "Open Self"	**Blindspot** "Blind Self"
Not Known to Others	**Facade** "Hidden Self"	**Unknown Self**

Johari Window

Here as you can see in the photo there are four different panes and each signifies one crucial idea behind it. Further, the panes are in the horizontal axis as well as the vertical axis. So, you have to determine in which window you fall and based on that your personality can be known.

In this model, the main focus is on feedback. Accepting of feedback and conveying of this feedback is done through this model. The panes given in the vertical direction represents part that is known and unknown to others. While the horizontal part represents the known and unknown part to your self. That is two windows represent your true self while the other two windows represent the part that is known to others but unknown to self. This information which is known to self and unknown to others can be transferred through socializing with others. While the part that is known to others but unknown to self is conveyed through feedback that you get through other members in the group. This model works on the basis of communication happening in the group and how to improve yourself. The model is very simple to understand and as a result, it is used in various organizations.

1. **Open/self-area or arena** – Here the information about the person his attitudes, behaviour, emotions, feelings, skills and views will be known by the person as well as by others. This is mainly the area where all the communications occur and the larger the arena becomes the more effectual and dynamic the relationship will be. 'Feedback solicitation' is a process which occurs by understanding and listening to the feedback from another person. Through this way the open area can be increased horizontally decreasing the blind spot. The size of the arena can also be increased downwards and thus by reducing the hidden and unknown areas through revealing one's feelings to other person.
2. **Blind self or blind spot** – Information about yourselves that others know in a group but you will be unaware of it. Others may interpret yourselves differently than you expect. The blind spot is reduced for an efficient communication through seeking feedback from others.
3. **Hidden area or façade** – Information that is known to you but will be kept unknown from others. This can be any personal information which you feel reluctant to reveal. This includes feelings, past experiences, fears, secrets etc. we keep some of our feelings and information as private as it affects the relationships and thus the hidden area must be reduced by moving the information to the open areas.
4. **Unknown area** – The Information which are unaware to yourselves as well as others. This includes the information, feelings, capabilities, talents etc. This can be due to traumatic past experiences or events which can be unknown for a

lifetime. The person will be unaware till he discovers his hidden qualities and capabilities or through observation of others. Open communication is also an effective way to decrease the unknown area and thus to communicate effectively.

Reference

1. Casio. W.F. Managing Human Resources. 1st Edition MC Graw-Hill Book Company :1986.
2. Mc Connell. R. Charles. Managing the Health Care professional. Jones and Bartlett Publishers: 2004.
3. Working together for Health. The World Health Report 2006.
4. Casio. W.F. Applied Psychology in personnel management (2nd ed). Reston, VA: Reston, 1982
5. Chamberlain, N.W. Cullen, D.E and Lewin D. The labor Sector (3rd ed) New York Mc Graw-Hill 1980
6. Perham. J. Management succession: A hard game to play. Dun's Review 1981, 117, 54-55, 58.
7. Rowland. K. M, and Sovereign. M.G. Markov Chain Analysis of internal manpower supply. Industrial relations 1969, 9, 88-89
8. Vroom.V and Mac Crimmon. K. Toward a stochastic model of managerial careers. Administrative Science quarterly, 1968, 12, 26-36
9. Walker, J. W. Models in Manpower planning. In E.H Burack and J.W Walker (eds) Man Power planning and programming. Boston: Allyn and Bacon, 1972
10. A.H. Maslow. A theory of Human Motivation Psychological Review 50 (1943): 370-96
11. F. Herzberg et al. The Motivation to work (New York: John Wiley and sons, Inc 1969)
12. Hornby P, Forte P. Human resource indicators to monitor health service performance. Keele, Keele University, Centre for Health planning and Management, 2002
13. Dieleman M, Cuong PV, Anh LV, Martineau T. Identifying factors for Job motivation of rural health workers in North vietman. Human Resources for Health, 2003, 1:10
14. Rowe Ak, de Savigny D, Lanata CF, Victoria CG. How can we achieve and maintain high- quality performance of health workers in low resource settings? Lancet, 2005, 366: 1026-1035
15. Mathever I, Imhoff I. Staff Motivation in Africa. The role of non-financial incentives and quality management tools. Eschborn, Germany Agency for Technical cooperation. 2005

16. Franco LM, Benett S, Kanfer R. Health sector reform and public sector health worker motivation: A conceptual framework, 2002, Social Science and Medicine, 54, 1255-1266
17. Blumenthal D. Doctors in wired world: Can professionalism survive connectivity? The Milbank quarterly, 2002, 80: 525-546
18. Mieltinen OS. Ideas and Ideals in medicine: fruits of reason or props of power? Journal of Evaluation in clinical Practice, 1999, 5: 107-116
19. Casicio. W.F. Scientific, legal and operational imperatives of work place Performance appraisal systems. Public personnel Management, 1982, 11, 367-375
20. Cummings L.L A field experimental study of the effects of two performance appraisal systems. Personnel psychology, 1973, 26, 489-502.
21. Sisson. D.E. Forced Choice, the new Army rating. Personnel Psychology, 1984, 1, 365-381

22

Managing organizations

Leadership Skills

There are three types of skills which a manager should have. Technical skills i.e. knowledge of the Job, Human skills i.e. skill needed in dealing with people and conceptual skills i.e. Vision and Mission and understanding of organization. Technical skills are important for lower level managers. Human skills are needed at all the three levels of managers i.e. lower level managers, middle levels managers and top level managers but are most important for middle level managers. Conceptual skills are most important for top managers who have to make Policy decisions for the organizations.

Leadership styles

In autocratic style of leadership decisions are taken by the leader and subordinates have to carry them out. In participative management the leader presents a tentative decision that is subject to change gets suggestions and makes the final decision. The area of decision freedom to subordinates here is much greater. In democratic style of leadership subordinates have a wide range of decision freedom within the boundaries of activity set by the leader.

Delegation

Delegation is a key management function through which a manager gets work done through subordinates. Delegation is important because it means lower management cost as jobs are done by lower level supervisors who are paid less and top level manager gets more time to plan and do those things for which he only has skill, knowledge and authority to handle. Delegation also provides an opportunity for lower level managers to grow. First step in the process of delegation is to select and define the task to do. The tasks usually delegated are technical in nature. The pure managerial tasks such as planning, decision making, budgeting etc are not delegated. The tasks should be of repeated occurrence in the organization so that time of manager is saved. Second step is to select the person to whom to delegate a task. The person should be ready to accept the challenge. He should be reasonably qualified to do the Job. He should be motivated to do the Job and results expected from him need to be made clear. Sufficient authority needs to be provided for accomplishing the task however the manager continues to retain the responsibility for the task in question. Another step in process of delegation is establishing controls and check points. Since manager remains accountable for the work he delegates, it is essential to follow through by way of formal and informal meetings, written reports or by walking out. Delegation has been proven to improve effectiveness of managers. Decentralization differs from delegation in that in former both accountability and responsibility is shifted to subordinate manager and it is more useful where greater geographical area is involved.

Management by objectives (MBO)

Management by objectives has been defined as continual process whereby superior and subordinate managers periodically define their common goals, define each individuals major areas of responsibility in terms of results expected and use agreed upon measures as guides for each operating department and for assessing the contribution of each manager to the work of the entire institution. Basic ingredients of management by objectives are establishing specific goals and objectives which have to be communicated properly to subordinate managers. MBO is not simply getting results done but achieving them within a times frame. There has to be a calendar when specific elements are to be achieved and when goal as a whole is to be completed. Quantifiable mile stones towards an objective can be effective in positive and negative feed back. There has to be coordination between individual managers and they have to be motivated towards achieving common goals established.

Unionization

Unionization is result of unfulfilled needs of employees in terms of conditions of employment, fairness in work setting and content of employees. Content employees do not unionize. The ability of individuals, and work groups, to have greater responsibility, particularly for professional employees to have some control over the parameters of one's Job and organization change and to be able to obtain satisfaction from employment are important to employees. The hospital manager should be aware of the many factors that cause employee dissatisfaction and individual and group behavior outcomes; one could be joining a union. If the hospital employees perceive their needs, aspirations and expectations are not being met, they will probably seek for a mechanism to correct them. Unionization has serious impacts on management not in terms of higher costs due to higher wages but most importantly due to restriction on management to manage. Collective bargaining limits managements flexibility in terms of promotions, demotions, discipline and bring about organizational change. The best strategy is to create an environment which is progressive and constructive with balancing interests of patients, employees and management.

Top management groups of health care organizations have paid dearly for operating under the assumption that all supervisors and middle managers are philosophically opposed to collective arrangements and thus guaranteed to be on sides of management. Much of what can be said about middle management is the same as what many are saying about professional employees. Specifically middle management frustration and discontent are increasing particularly because of prevailing working conditions, decreasing economies, job security and a declining sense of personal realization and achievement in their jobs. Top managements long term behavior has great deal to do with whether the organization is a fertile ground for union organizing activity, and the manager's conduct and actions during a union organizing campaign exert a significant influence on the employee's reaction to the organizing drive. When initially the organizing activity begins the management may know nothing about it. Outside agencies may exploit the situation in the organization by looking for inside organizers, who are active, influential, popular, articulate and discontent with top management. If union organizers feel that ground is not fertile for unionization they simply withdraw without ever making their presence known. If the ground is fertile the organizers step up their activities and attempt to uncover issues to be used for employee support and sympathy. They play on emotions of employees by highlighting instances of unfair treatment and discriminations. Management has to counter such moves by appropriate counter -organizing activities without making any commitments but listening to employees patiently.

Collective bargaining is process of joint decision making and basically represents a democratic way of life in hospital. It is the process of negotiation between hospital's and workers representatives for the purpose of establishing mutually agreeable conditions of employment. It is a technique adopted by two parties to reach an understanding acceptable to both through the process of discussion and negotiation. International labor organization has defined collective bargaining as negotiation about working conditions and terms of employment between an employer and a group of employees or one or more employee, with a view to reaching an agreement wherein the terms serve a code of defining the rights and obligations of each party in their employment with one another. Collective bargaining involves discussion and negotiations between two groups as to the terms and conditions of employment. It is called "collective" because both the employer and the employee act as a group rather than as individuals. It is known as 'bargaining' because the method of reaching an agreement involves proposals and counter proposals, offers and counter offers and other negotiations.

Management of change

There are two types of leadership in organizations. Transformational management which binds the employees as a group for achievement of objectives and goals which are laid by leader and transactional which keeps the organization on track once direction is decided. Transformational management may mean that people have to change their behavior or acquire new skills or develop different attitudes. Ideally the aim is to achieve absolute commitment to the proposed direction and objectives. However the ideal cannot always be achieved. The next best thing would be for compliance to the changes. This is where there is an acceptance by staff of the need for change and the approaches to achieving it. The least desirable state of mind is brought about when coercion has to be used to make people change. Transactional leadership deals with day to day business.

Change management entails thoughtful planning and sensitive implementation and above all consultation with and involvement of the people affected by the changes. If you force change on people problems arise. Change must be achievable, realistic and measurable. Change needs to be understood and managed in a way that people can cope effectively with. Change can be unsettling and managers need to have a settling influence. Check that people affected by the change agree with or at least understand the need for change and have a chance to decide how the change will be managed. Change should be steady as quick change prevents proper consultation and involvement which leads to difficulties that take time to resolve. Consulting with people and helping them to understand does not weaken your position, it strengthens it. Leaders who fail to consult and involve there people in managing challenges are perceived as weak and lacking in integrity. Responsibility for managing change is with management and executives of the organization, they must manage the change in a way that employees can cope with. Manager's role is to interpret, communicate and enable – not to instruct and impose which nobody really responds to well. If people are not approaching their tasks or the organization effectively then system in the organization is wrong and not the people. Change such as new structures, policies, targets, acquisitions, disposals, relocations etc create new systems and environments which need to be explained to people as early as possible so that people's involvement in change process is obtained. Whenever change is brought there are some people who are in loss. Treat these people with respect and avoid keeping them in dark. They must know what is happening and why. Strong resistance to change is often rooted in deeply conditioned or historically reinforced feelings. Patience and tolerance are required to help people in these situations to see things differently.

The transformational leader can use following approaches:

Integration approach: The aim is to facilitate the integration of individual goals and needs with those of organization. People should understand what has to be done and they must to participate in bringing in change.

Educational approach: People must be educated about the need for change and the reason for it.

Contextual change approach: Forced changes in relationships created by changed organizational positions will lead to behavioral change. This would mean organizational restructuring.

Negotiating approach: Managers negotiate with the employees putting up resistance. The essence of this approach is doing deals. They may agree to the changes on the understanding that they gain some benefits to themselves either from changes or something else.

Political approach: The manager develops a power base and then use this power to force change. Resistance can develop to this approach.

Threat approach: This approach is the least desirable and works in short term. The employees should feel that there is threat against them and to the existence of the organization if change is not implemented, however threat cannot be effective if the threat is constant.

Behavioral science approach: This approach is based on amalgam of approaches described above.

Typology of change

Change interventions fall into three main typologies

- Top down change management: is based on the assumption that if managers plan things properly change can be executed smoothly. The focus should be on changing the culture of an organization.
- Transformation change Management: Transformational leaders innovate and think outside the routine and provide safe environment for change.
- Strategic change management: The leader introduces new behaviours at work allowing people to witness the benefit for the organization and thus based on evidence internalize the change in their ways of working. All approaches highlight the importance of leadership, communications and involving people in the change process.

Managing the environment of change

Creating the momentum: Includes making the case, visioning, empowerment and voicing activities; by definition this is step for leadership to principally act upon. The employees can be motivated for change by advocacy activities i.e. sharing the rationales for change openly and transparently with key stake holders mainly employees. There has to be vision for the future. Visioning seeks to create consensus and commitment among all stake holders to a vision for the future. Defining a vision and having a broad consensus on goals and values to guide organizational change is an essential step in systems change. It is critical to building support for change among stake holders and within the organization itself. There should be empowerment of stake holders who may be discriminated against or are other wise disadvantaged.

Analysis of the change context

There has to be stake holder analysis to identify their knowledge, attitudes and practices in regard to the underlying issues. The main idea is to identify who are the net gainers and net losers in the process. For the losers not to put resistance to change, it is important to find areas where win-wins for all can be demonstrated. A SWOT analysis of change would be helpful. Operations research is necessary to support decision making and to know the potential impact of proposed changes or the actual impact of changes as they are implemented.

Facilitation of Change

Process consultation:- This is engaging of individuals to facilitate change processes. A process consultant enables "learning by doing" and thereby facilitates organizational learning. They start with whatever problem the organization is addressing at the time in order to gain experience and built trust. They identify, endorse and promote leadership in the various stake holder organizations that will own as well as lead the change process. Change that is locally owned is sustainable and the change which has been prescribed by outsiders usually is not. The process consultants sequence activities so as to logically lead to decisions, ensuring open processes to maximize the flow of new ideas and engender commitment from stakeholders.

Consensus building exercises: Consensus building facilitates change process and help in overcoming resistance to change.

Leadership: leadership is key component of successful change and leaders can increase performance by changes in organizational culture.

Communications about change

Multimedia communication activities**:** Factual information and stake holder positions should be communicated widely to all concerned parties. Information dissemination should include mass media such as newspapers, radio, television, Internet etc.

Inter active communications and public outreach**:** This is done by report cards, TV and radio discussions, web sites, Internet chat rooms, work shops etc.

Measuring progress: Measuring progress, seeking feed back and continuing to adjust and improve are all important for following through on change programmes.

Stress Management

Stress is epidemic in the work place. Stress is the manifestly uncomfortable feeling that an individual experiences when he or she is forced to deviate from normal or desired patterns of functioning. The signs of stress are short temper, lassitude or fidgeting. Stress results in significant organizational losses therefore managers have to develop strategies to minimize stress. Several studies have linked stress to decreased productivity, increased absenteeism, increased turnover, decreased employee health and decreased organizational commitment. Accumulation of job related stress results in burn out where mental and physical exhaustion usually coexist. Manages should be able to recognize signs and symptoms of stress. Determination of sources of stress is important so that treatment can focus on underlying problems rather than on symptoms. The diagnosis of stress is made only by proper communication with employees. Nature of the Job also results in stress. Jobs which are routine or too complex or involve physical strain create stress. Other factors leading to stress are long working hours, unhealthy environment, inadequate equipment, equipment break downs, lack of respect at work place, role ambiguity, role conflict, inadequate salary, lack of opportunity for advancement, inadequate staff, inadequate supervision, lack of recognition for good work, responsibility with out authority etc.

Most important strategy to ease stress is eliminating stressors and creating a warm, supportive and welcoming work place. Coping is the adaptive effort that individuals make to manage the demands that cause stress. Problem focused coping consists of taking action to change peoples behavior or change the environment. Emotion focused coping consists of attempts to decrease the emotional distress caused by stressors which may include not thinking about stress inducing situations.

Individuals can cope with stress by acknowledging stress is good i.e. use stress to push yourself little bit harder when it counts most, avoid stress sneezers i.e. limiting your contact with people in whom you recognize stress, learn from best stress managers, practice socially avertable heavy breathing (Breathe in Slowly for a count of 7 then breath out for a count of 11), don't worry needlessly about stressors, know your trigger points and hot spots (knowing what causes you stress is powerful information, so that action can be taken to make it less stressful) and have adequate sleep, diet and proper exercise.

Decision Making

Decision making is at the core of planning and involves choosing the appropriate course of action. First step in decision making is to have clear planning about what is to be achieved. Second step would be development of alternatives in the light of resources available. Third step is evaluating alternatives in terms of the goals sought and fourth is choosing an alternative.

Alternatives are always available in any situation and it is the responsibility of a manager to identify them. If a manager has only one way of achieving a result then the manager probably has not worked for development of alternatives. The ability to develop alternatives is as important as selecting correctly from amongst them.

There are two approaches for making a decision. The first is concerned with development and application of normative decision rules based on formal logic based on economics and statistics. The second involves descriptive accounts of how people actually go about making judgments and choices.

Normative analysis

A distinction is made between riskless choices and risky choices.

The riskless choices are called certain outcomes and risky choices are called uncertain outcomes.

Certain outcomes

MAU (Multi attribute utility) involves obtaining a utility value for each decision alternative and then selecting the alternative with the highest value. The utility for an alternative is derived from a weighed sum of separate part utilities for various attributes. Linear models are based on multiple regression analyses.

Uncertain outcomes

A decision tree is a graphical model that displays the sequence of decisions and the events that comprise a sequential decision situation. As adequate information is seldom available to make a confidential accurate decision at a given time, the tree depicts future decision points and possible chance events usually with a notation of the probabilities of the various uncertain events happening. The tree shows the manager in what direction the chance events are. There is a need for assessment of the probabilities of each course of possible events. As chance events increase the decision tree becomes more complicated and the compounding of various probabilities makes the solution much more difficult. In real life situations a computer may be necessary to calculate them. The Decision tree makes it possible for managers to see the major alternative available to them and by incorporating probabilities of various events in the tree, it is possible to comprehend the tree probability of a decision leading to results desired. Decision tree has been used to guide risky decision making such as marketing strategy, policy planning etc.

Descriptive analysis

Descriptive analysis is concerned with accounting for the discrepancies between normative rules and actual behavior.

All approaches of decision making reflect the importance of Ben Franklin's original insight into the problem decomposition: i.e. breaking a problem into parts, working on them and then combining them to make a final decision.

References

1. MC Connell, R. Charles. Managing the Health care professional. Jones and Bartlett Publishers: 2004
2. Casio. W.F. Managing Human Resources. 1st Edition. Mc Graw- Hill Book Company: 1986
3. Jonathan S Rakich and Kurt Darr. Hospital Organization and Management. SP Medical and Scientific books 3rd Ed. 1983
4. Robin Gourlay. The Management of change in Management for Hospital Doctors. Butter worth –Heinemann Ltd. 1994: 151-155
5. Institutional reform and change Management. Managing change in Public sector organization, AUNDP Capacity Development Resource. Working Draft Nov.06
6. Timothy P. Summers, Thomas A. Dacotis and Angelo S. Denisi, " A Field study of some Antecedent and Consequences of Felt Job stress, " in Rick Crandall and Pamela L. Perreive, eds. Occupational Stress: A Handbook (Washington, DC: Taylor & Francis 1995)
7. Charles D. Spielberger and Eric C. Reheiser, "Measuring Occupational stress: The stress survey, "in Rick Crandall and Pamela L. Perreive eds. Occupational stress. A Hand book (Washington, Dc: Taylor and Francis, 1995).
8. Burke J, "sources of Managerial and Professional stress in large organization," in Cary L. cooper and Roy Payne, eds., Causes, coping and consequences of stress at work (chichester, UK: John Wiley and sons 1988).
9. R.S. Lazarus, "Psychological stress in the work place, "in Rick Crandall and Perreive L eds. Occupational stress: A Hand book (Washington, Dc: Taylor Francis, 1995).
10. Stress: Anxiety and Depression. The Health care practitioners' Hand Book of Management 293-319
11. Lyndsay swinton. The 7 best stress management techniques! Know! Management for the rest of us. www.mftrou. com.
12. Shanteau. J. Encyclopedia of psychology and behavioral Science (3rded) Craig head, W.E & Nemeroff, C.B (Eds.). NY: Wiley. (PP 913-915)
13. Koontz, O'Donnell, Weihrich Decision Making In Management Seventh Ed. Mc graw-hill kogakusha Ltd. 1972. (PP 237-272).

23

Violence in Hospitals

For any given person in any job at any given work site, working entails interactions which permutations of peers, subordinates and superiors and in some jobs interacting with external clients or customers including the public at large. National Institute for Occupational Safety and Health (NIOSH) U.S defines work place violence as violent acts directed toward persons at work or on duty. These can range from verbal threats to physical assaults ranging from slapping and beating to rape, homicide, muggings and use of firearms. Violence is a significant concern for health care workers and risk managers. Considering violent and abusive behavior of patients, visitors or staff to be "part of the Job" is not acceptable nor is it safe as facilities find themselves confronted with more and more dangerous situations every day. Violence in health care industry is endemic and it is increasing in severity and frequency. According to estimates of the Bureau of Labor statistics (BLS), U.S, 2637 nonfatal assaults on hospital workers occured in 1999- a rate of 8.3 assaults per 10,000 workers. The rate is much higher than the rate of non-fatal assaults for all private sector industries which is 2 per 10,000 workers. In an American Management Association Survey about 52% of human resource managers reported at least one violent incident involving their companies since 1990. Fox et al (1994) found that in 1993 nurses in several agencies had the highest rate of injury from workplace violence in a group of twenty six Federal government agencies studied for injury rates. Assaults on health care workers are found in all areas of practice and constitute a serious hazard.

RISK FACTORS

Risk factors may be viewed under following headings.

1. Environmental factors.
2. Work practices.
3. Perpetrator and victims.

Environmental factors:- Violence in hospitals occurs more frequently in Psychiatric areas, emergency rooms, waiting rooms and is often precipitated by long wait for services, overcrowded and uncomfortable waiting rooms, patients under influence of drugs or alcohol, inadequate security, access to fire arms, poorly lit corridors, parking lots, and unrestricted movement of public.

Work practices:- Many studies and reports have implicated staffing patterns as a major contributor to the problem of violence. Other work practices which place health care workers at increased risk include: isolated work with clients in examination or treatment activities, working alone or in remote locations in high crime areas, long waiting times, inadequate security and poorly lit campus.

Perpetrator and victims: Perpetrators of violence in health care settings are more often male, with a wide age range. Drug and alcohol abuse may contribute to violent behavior due to the lowering of inhibitions and the problems associated with addiction. The California Department of Industrial relations Division of Occupational Safety and Health divides events of work place violence into three categories.

Type I :the perpetrator has no legitimate relationship to workplace.

Type II: is committed by someone who is the recipient of a service provided by the work place or the victim.

Type III: perpetrator has an employee related involvement with the workplace such as current or former staff member.

Jan FA et al found that in a study 83.5% of employees faced type II violence, 15% Type III and 1.4% faced Type I violence. Although any one working in a hospital may become a victim of violence, nurses and nursing aides who have the most direct contact with patients are at higher risk. Other hospital personnel at increased risk of violence include emergency response personnel, hospital safety officers. Jan

F.A et al found that eighty percent of employees working in accident and emergency faced violence, 40.5% employees working in wards faced violence and 27% employees in laboratories faced violence. 100% medical postgraduates and security attendants faced violence. 85% of the senior residents faced violence.

Hospital staff is untrained in recognizing and controlling escalating hostile behavior and management of assaultive people. Often they have no protective equipment such as communication devices or alarm system.

Violence Prevention Program

Management Commitment:- Management has to show commitment and involvement in violence prevention programs. It should be placed in the priority lists and at the same level as patient safety. Violence prevention programs should be integrated with diagnostic and therapeutic services so that it is a part of hospital daily activities. Management has to assign and communicate the responsibility for various aspects of safety and security to managers, supervisor, doctors and all other categories of staff. Management has to show zero tolerance for violence in hospitals. Managers and supervisors have to be held accountable.

Employee Involvement:- An effective program includes a commitment by the employer to provide for and encourage employee participation by encouraging reports from them regarding any incidents which should be analyzed and effective corrections then recommended. These incident reports may help to identify violent patients and to develop safe methods of managing difficult cases.

Record Review: - There has to be periodic review of the reports of incidents and near incidents of violent behavior. This will help identify and analyze trends in injuries by area of work, employee category, time of the day and perpetrator characteristics.

Identification of Risk Factors:- Based on the analysis of incident reports and investigations carried out risk factors can be identified and addressed while reviewing the violence prevention program. Use a check list to identify high risk factors that includes type of client, physical risk factors of the building, isolated locations, job activities, lighting problems, lack of communication devices, areas with uncontrolled access and areas of previous security problems.

Written Program:- In large organizations effective implementation requires a written program for job safety, health and security that is endorsed and advocated by the highest level of management. The program should establish goals and objectives. The written program should be suitable for the anticipated hazards and for the size type and complexity of the facility and its operations.

Prevention Strategies:- Although risk factors for violence are specific for each hospital and its scenarios, employees can follow general prevention strategies.

Engineering Controls

- Develop emergency signaling, alarms and monitoring systems.
- Install security devices such as metal detectors to prevent armed persons from entering the hospital.
- Install other security devices such as cameras and good lighting in hallways.
- Provide security escorts to the parking lots at night.
- Design waiting areas to accommodate and assist visitors and patients who may have a delay in service.
- Provide staff restrooms and emergency exits.
- Provide enclosed nurses stations.
- Arrange furniture and other objects to minimize their use as weapons.
- Curved mirrors should be installed at hallway intersections and concealed areas.

Administrative Controls:-

- Design staffing patterns to prevent personnel from working alone and to minimize patient waiting time.
- Restrict the movement of the public in hospital by card controlled access.
- Develop a system for alerting security personnel when violence is threatened.

- When there is a well established risk, there should be a trained response team which can provide transport or escort services or respond to emergencies without leaving another unit's staff at risk.
- Manager should be available to assist in emergencies, provide advice, make decision, and help in difficult situations.
- Administrator should work with local police to establish liaison and response mechanisms for police assistance and facilitate the hospital's assistance to local police in handling emergency cases.

Behavior Modifications:- Hospital should train all workers in recognizing and managing assaults. Training for all employees should encompass recognizing assaults, resolving conflicts and maintaining hazard awareness.

Post Incident Response

The employees who have been attacked should be given due medical and psychological support. "Critical Incident Debriefing" program should be established and provided whenever staff is victim of assaults. Counsellers should be well trained with a understanding of the issues of assault and its consequences.

Safety Tips for Hospital Workers

Watch for signals that may be associated with impending violence:-

- Verbally expressed anger and frustration
- Body language such as threatening gestures.
- Signs of drug or alcohol use.
- Presence of a weapon.

Maintain behavior that helps diffuse anger

- Present a calm, caring attitude.
- Don't match the threats.
- Don't give orders.
- Acknowledge the person's feelings.
- Avoid any behavior that may be interpreted as aggressive.
- Be alert.

- Evaluate each situation for potential violence.
- Be vigilant.

Proactive Security Departments

According to one definition the role of health care security is and always will be the protection of people and property with a secondary role to provide other specifically defined services to the hospital community.

One Program Approach to Security:-

- Effective screening (visitations and identification policy and procedures).
- Effective use of security technology.
- Appropriate security staffing (numbers, training, skill mix and deployment.)
- An informed and involved hospital staff.
- Continuous quality improvement.
- Effective communication with staff.

Important function of security program

Access control maintenance, administrative escorts, alarm monitoring, bomb threat investigation, crime prevention, currency escorts, domestic violence issues investigated, door openings, disaster committee participation, elevator entrapment assists, fire safety, gunshot wound evidence, hazardous material spills protection, helipad responders, key control, liaison with law enforcement agencies, media assists, missing person searches, motor vehicle assists including parking, patients valuable assists, store luggage for visitors, incident reporting.

O.W. Wilson one of the greatest police executives has defined preliminary investigation as.

P → Proceed to scene with safety

R → Render assistance to injured

E → Effect arrest of perpetrator

L → Locate and Identify witness

I → Interview complainant and witness

M → Maintain scene and protect evidence.

I → Interrogate suspects.

N → Note all conditions, events and remarks.

A → Arrange for collection of evidence.

R→ Report freely and accurately.

Y → Yield responsibility to investigators or higher authority.

Post Assignments

Fixed Post Assignment:- The individual assigned to a post generally has no discretionary autonomy in terms of geographical location and cannot leave the post unless relieved by another individual.

Modified Post Assignment:- In this deployment the officer is mandated to be in a rather close geographical area such as emergency department, lobby, or staff entrance.

Sectored or zone Post Assignment:- In this type persons are assigned to a specific geographical area of patrol and are generally dispatched to calls for service. These persons may also be dispatched out of their zone to provide back up a support to another zone officer.

Full time Equivalent:-The number of full time equivalent persons required for any staffing plan is the total weekly hours of scheduled coverage divided by 40.

References

1. California State Dept of Industrial Relations 1994, CAL/OSHA Guideline for work place security. Divisia of occupational safety and Health, San Francisco.
2. Fox, S, Freeman C, Bair B, et al. (1994) Identifying reported cases of workplace violence in Federal agencies, Washington DC.
3. Goodman, R, Jenkin's L, Mercy J (1994) Work place related Homicide Among Health Care works in the United States, 1980 through 1990. Journal of American Medical Association, 272(21): 1686-88.
4. Novello, A. (1992). A Medical Response to Violence. Journal of the American Medical Association 267:2007.
5. Department of labor, Bureau of Labor statistics (1994). Violence in the workplace comes under closer scrutiny. Issues in Labor Statistics. August.

6. Florence Kavaler, Allen D Spiegel. Assuring Safety and Security in Health care Institutions in Risk Management in Health care Institutions 2nd Ed. Jones and Bartlett Publishes (8) 187-214.
7. Occupational Hazards in Hospitals. Violence. DHHS (NIOSH) Publication No 2002-101
8. Russell. L. Colling. Development of Security Staff in Hospital and Health care Security 4th Ed 2001: (9) 215-246
9. O.W. Wilson, Police Administration, Mc Graw Hill Book Co, 1963 P 282.

24

Utilization of Operation Theatre

The term "hospital utilization" denotes the manner in which a certain community makes use of its hospital resources. Various indices are commonly used in the assessment of hospital utilization, but no one of them alone can give a full picture of the utilization pattern. The different indices may be calculated on gross or specific basis. A gross index is an index expressing the overall average utilization for all types of hospital in the area. The specific index, on the other hand, expresses the utilization of a certain type of hospital or of a certain service within the hospital. Lot of literature is available on utilization of various hospital services such as out-patient services, accident and emergency services, radiological services etc. but very few studies have been conducted on utilization of operating services.

Operating room utilization is noted by using formula

N

Σ

URJ=n= 1(room clean 1-open sterile supply1)

(RA stop – RA start)

(adapted from American Hospital Association)

Where

URJ = room utilization

J = room number

Room clean = time room is ready for next usage.

Open sterile supply =time first supply package is opened for that patients care.

1 = number of patients served.

N = total number of patients in room J/day.

RA stop =expected conclusion of surgery and end of day clean up.

RA start = expected time at which first case setup may begin.

UTILIZATION ANALYSIS

Utilization analysis involves surgical scheduling methods, instrument sterilization techniques, storage space utilization, equipment utilization and anesthetic procedures. Planning of surgical suite directly influences utilization of operation theatre. Operating room utilization is calculated for the normal day starting and stopping hours. Utilization is measured on week days as night and weekend cases represent a separate issue. One hundred % utilization/day for particular operating room would be 8 hours/day. Few hospitals regularly achieve 100% operating room utilization. For hospitals performing a representative diversity of cases 80% utilization is considered acceptable. If the average case length is short, acceptable utilization may be 50%. Therefore utilization has to be viewed in context of other information available such as the average case length for the institution. The longer the average case length the higher the expected utilization. Researchers found operating room utilization rates (operating time as a proportion of a notional 8 hours working day) to be low overall approximately 40-60% in widely varying settings including Chicago, Columbia and the United States department of Veterans affairs. A study of 76 operating rooms in Columbia conducted in 1974 showed that utilization was only 41.6%. In another study classic utilization for each block-day by surgical subspecialty ranged from 44-113%. Average daily block-specific underutilization ranged from 16 to 60% whereas overutilization ranged from 4 to 49%. A study by Jan. F.A et al showed theatre utilization of 64.3%. Underutilization and overutilization are important measures because they may be used to evaluate the quality of OR schedules and the efficiency of OR utilization. In a study, time utilization of operating rooms in a large teaching hospital, the maximum utilization was found to be between 10 a.m. and 1.p.m. Delay was caused by surgeons resulting in the operating rooms remaining idle to the extent of 105 minutes on an average. Jan. F. A showed idle time of 128 minutes per day in O.T. Unplanned scheduling of operations and late arrival of surgeons were the main causes.

The classic definition of OR utilization needs to be improved. As encountered in the literature, classic utilization is defined as the ration of the total OR time used to the total OR time allocated or budgeted. This definition of utilization is inadequate because it fails to differentiate the quality of utilization. Consider a simple example: a single OR is budgeted for 8 hours with two surgeries scheduled each of 4 hours duration. If the surgeries are performed consecutively within the budgeted work day, classic utilization is measured as 100% with no wasted resources. By contrast, consider the same OR when one 4 hour surgery is performed during regular hours and the other is performed entirely after regular hours. In the latter scenario there are 4 hours in which an expensive OR remains unused and 4 additional for which personnel must be recalled and overtime costs apply. Each scenario is an example of 100% classic utilization, but in the latter there is both under and over utilization, with penalties to the staff and institution inherent in each. Under utilization and over utilization as defined herein, are important measures because they may be used to evaluate the quality of OR schedules and the efficiency of OR utilization.

In one study it was shown that out of the available time, 54% of time was spent on actual surgery, 31% for supportive services and 15% waiting while the operating room was being made ready for operation. Jan.F.A found 66.02% was spent on actual surgery, 21% on supportive services, and 12.9% on making room ready for surgery out of the utilized time.

In a study at University of California for each patient undergoing operation following times were recorded: OR (operating room) ready, patient enters OR, anesthesia induction complete, surgery start, surgery end, patient leaves OR. It was observed that patients were brought into the OR just before the scheduled start time. Surgical incision was made 21 to 49 minutes after the patient was brought into the OR. Room turnover time (time from patient in to patient out) was almost uniformly 36 minutes. Patient turnover time (time from end of surgery in one patient to end of induction of next patient) was generally 1 hour. The time between cases when no surgery was occurring was significantly longer than room turnover time because of the need to wake up one patient and induce the following patient.

With a well co-ordinated team minimal turnover time between operations can be accomplished; in an average time of 15-20 minutes the room will be ready for the next patient.

SCHEDULING STRATEGY

(a) **Schedule efficiency:-** It is not a trivial matter to achieve a high level of utilization in the operation room(OR). The surgeon must give attention to schedule efficiency to contain costs. Surgeons should be aware that 100% utilization of OR time is unrealistic except when there are repetitive, uniform – length procedures. A regular utilization rate below 50% should suggest overstaffing, overbuilding or poor schedule management. Lessons from scheduling computer use can help make OR utilization more efficient. If a selective effective algorithm is used in scheduling, norms of utilization should be above 60% and peaks should exceed 75%. For efficiency of scheduling, all ORs should be completely modular and should be large enough to accommodate any type of surgery.

(b) **Block OR Scheduling:-**Operating rooms in hospitals represent big investments and must be utilized efficiently. Sequencing procedures for operations within an operating room is important in this regard. Before managed care all available operating rooms were essentially staffed 8 hours a day and procedures were booked on a first come, first served basis. Hospital collections for OR exceeded five times hospital costs, so there was little concern over how efficiently the ORs were scheduled. The primary goal was to provide as much care and surgical convenience as possible. As available ORs became filled with cases and surgeons experienced difficulty in booking elective cases, blocks of OR time were given to busy surgeons or surgical services. Because rewarding block time greatly increased surgeon satisfaction, hospital administrators felt pressure to grant it, especially if competing hospitals provided it. OR utilization is maximized by filling block time with as many hours of cases as possible. The key to maximizing OR utilization then is to determine (i) the appropriate amount of block time to allocate to each surgeon and (ii) how to choose which day to schedule a patient for surgery.

(c) Estimating case Duration:- Accurate predictions of operating room times for surgical procedures are probably a prerequisite for matching operating room suite workload to capacity. Wright and colleagues showed that the use of surgeons estimates can increase the accuracy of the commercial scheduling software to predict duration of surgery. Improvements in predicting case duration are of interest to hospitals because they may be able to produce cost swings. Improved operating room scheduling could reduce costs by reducing underutilization (operating rooms empty earlier than expected) and /or by reducing unplanned extension of the work day (operating rooms occupied later then predicted). The benefits of better scheduling would also extend to patients. (i.e. reduce unnecessary waiting time). When no historical time data are available for a surgeon scheduling a procedure, the mean of the duration of cases of the same scheduled procedure performed by other surgeons is as accurate a method to predict case duration as are more sophisticated analysis.

The goal of estimating case duration is to determine whether a case can fit into a "hole" (gap) in the OR schedule or whether an add on case will be completed within available time, then the maximum amount of time that a case is likely to require needs to be determined. The "upper predictive bound" specifies with a certain probability (e.g. 90%) that the duration of new case will be less than or equal to the bound. Upper predictive bounds measure the risk of an unusual and undesired event occurring (e.g. case runs over).

(d) Sequencing Cases:- The OR manager can use statistical decision theory to sequence cases to decrease the impact of limitations in equipment or personnel on case scheduling. One study recommends that a surgical suite manager should consider a probability of 80% to 90% of no overlap being an acceptable risk in scheduling of cases.

(e) **Predicting Surgical Groups Needs of Block Time:-** Block OR scheduling requires accurate forecasting of each surgical groups future need for OR time. A common approach to forecasting OR needs is to use the average of a surgical groups recent total hours of elective cases. Forecasting surgical groups need for OR time is necessary to ensure there is adequate staff available either to complete the work in a manner that minimizes labour costs or during regularly scheduled OR hours. It was found that total hours of elective cases over 4 weeks period can be normally distributed and unchanging over time. Consequently an OR manager can use equations based on normal distributions to calculate the upper prediction bounds (upper limit) for total hours of elective cases. The average of the most recent 2 to 4 weeks period can be used to predict surgical groups future use of block time.

Effect of waiting time on Utilization

How patients are scheduled into OR block time varies among surgical suites. Patient requests to be scheduled varies among surgical suits. Usually a patient needing surgery is given the first available surgical date for which the surgeon has open block time. Patient then wait to have surgery from the time they are given a surgical date until their day of surgery. Increasing the mean length of this waiting period (e.g. for 1 to 3 weeks) decreases the week to week variability in the surgical groups work load. Surgical suites with longer average length of time that patients wait to have elective surgery are more likely to have accurate forecasts of workload. This is because surgical suits with longer average patient waiting periods will have more flexibility in finding the best date to schedule a case to match the expected case duration with the open block time that day.

Optimizing OR Utilization

The results of one study suggest that to optimize OR utilizations add on cases should be considered simultaneously at a cut-off time (e.g. 4 p.m. the day before surgery) and then scheduled based on scheduled duration from longest to shortest. In a study it was shown that staffing costs were lowest when the operating room manager did not incorporate surgeon and patient preferences when scheduling cases into over flow block time. Over flow block time is operating room time for a surgical groups cases that cannot be completed in the regular block time allocated to each surgeon in the surgical group.

Cost of Canceling a Case

A study showed that cost of postponing a late day case is always greater than that of proceeding regardless of whether the costs were absorbed by patient, society or the hospital. It was concluded that a "zero tolerance for over time" policy may be too rigid to be consistently cost effective. In any event every effort should be made to publish next day's operating list by 14.00 hour on day before surgery.

Factors affecting Utilization of Operating room

A number of factors affect utilization of operation theatre. Most important ones of them are:

1. Theatre layout: Theatre lay out directly affects utilization of operation theatre. A centralized operation theatre suite has many advantages in this regard as there is efficient use of staff and facilities, better supervision, flexibility in scheduling operations and problem of supplies is simplified.
2. Operation list scheduling- Operating scheduling after the case duration has been estimated for every surgeon and for every type of surgery will prevent idle time and also over runs thus improving utilization.
3. Level of care- The utilization will also depend on the level of the care a hospital is providing. In secondary care hospitals, the utilization may be less and the turn over of cases will be more as compared to tertiary care medical centers where the complexity of the case will affect the utilization (which will be more) whereas the turnover will be less e.g., neurological, cardiovascular and plastic surgery cases consume more time.
4. Anaesthetic practice –If anaesthesia is given in separate room, the operating room can be used for more number of cases and number of the cases done will increase; increasing utilization.

5. Timing – The starting time of theatre has direct effect on utilization. If there is any delay in starting a case utilization is going to be affected.
6. Turn over times – Room turn over time i.e. the time between one patient out and second in also affects utilization. Longer turn over time means decreased utilization.
7. Case duration – If case length is short utilization is less because, more time is wasted between cases than if case length is long.
8. Type of surgeries – In an institution where similar type of surgeries are performed utilization is expected to be more then in an institution where diversity of cases are done.
9. Cancelling of surgeries – Canceling a case means no work for scheduled hours decreasing utilization. Therefore cancellation of cases needs to be avoided by fully preparing the cases and by proper scheduling.
10. Supportive services- There should be no electric breaks, no faults in supply of anaesthetic gases. Proper suction, equipment and sterilization facilities should be available.
11. Motivation of staff – There needs to be proper motivation of staff to do the job, they are expected to do. Co-operation between different staff members is a must for utilization of any facility.
12. Adequate Staff – The number of surgeons, anesthetists, nurses and nursing aides also affects the utilization. The number of different staff members should be optimal.

Utilization of Emergency Operation Theatre

Emergency surgery is a major component of every surgical specialty. It makes up a substantial volume of workload of surgeons in many hospitals and is relatively source intensive. A significant amount of emergency surgery activity relates to the treatment of injuries. A key determinant in emergency surgery is to identify that which surgery should be performed urgently. Adequate OT access must always be available to enable this proportion of emergency surgical work to be performed without delay or compromise. Time of day or day of week should present no limitation in hospitals designated to provide 24 hour access to emergency surgery. Emergency Operation theatre utilization is not quantified in terms of percentage utilization only but more importantly in terms of availability of OT and workload. Utilization of emergency operation theatre is found out for standard hours and after hours separately . Standard hours are usually from 8.00 hours up to 20.00 hours or even 22.00 hours and after hours 20.00 hours or 22.00 hours up to 8.00 hours. Some hospitals include weekend day time also in after hours.

Elective patients are the patients who are scheduled in advance, so they can be planned accordingly, while emergency patients just arrive at any moment and must be helped. Most patients have so called dedicated operating rooms ie separate operating rooms/suite for emergency patients only. An advantage of this is that the emergency patients do not affect elective schedule in other operating rooms.

Emergency or acute care surgery requires punctual evaluation and early intervention usually for diseases of short duration. The notion that expeditious management of acute surgical diseases is the appropriate strategy is based on the knowledge that delaying treatment may increase risks of adverse outcomes. Whereas deferring surgery to daytime hours is appropriate in certain situations.

NCEPOD (National Confidential Enquiry into Perioperative Deaths) classification of 2004 is used to categorize patients requiring emergency surgery. This classification replaced the categories of Emergent, Urgent, Scheduled and Elective previously used by NCEPOD.

Immediate : Immediate life, limb or organ-saving intervention-resuscitation simultaneous with intervention. Normally within minutes of decision to operate A) Life saving B) other eg limb or Organ Saving.

Urgent : Intervention for acute onset or clinical deterioration of potentially life threatening conditions, for those conditions that may threaten the survival of limb or organ, for fixation of many fractures and for relief of pain or other distressing symptoms. Normally within hours of decision to operate.

Expedited : Patient requiring early treatment where the condition is not an immediate threat to life, limb or organ survival. Normally within days of decision to operate.

Immediate and Urgent surgeries are time critical and need to be performed immediately (day or night). The majority of emergency procedures should be performed during daytime but very often theatre space is unavailable meaning that surgeons are faced with the choice of delaying an emergency surgical treatment or disrupting an elective list. There is evidence that delaying surgery for sick patients is detrimental both in terms of patient outcome and the immediate and longer term costs to the hospitals and society in general. It is therefore recommended that emergency surgical patients are prioritized according to their clinical need and this will usually mean prioritizing above elective patients. Studies have shown that expedited category if operated during after hours have relatively poor results if same cases are performed during daytime. Most after hour surgeries have been found to be performed by junior staff for need to gain experience and also because senior colleagues were not around. It has been seen that one third of operations currently performed at night could be postponed with better results.

It is important to note that NCEPOD classification does not describe the type of theatre session in which the intervention needs to be performed. "Patient urgency" and " type of list" are independent variables. Managers need to monitor data. NCEPOD recommends that the consultant who will perform the surgery should assign the category. The outcomes of emergency surgical cases are variable and poorly measured. They require greater ongoing scrutiny via clinical audits.

References

1. Jan FA, Tabish Amin, Qazi Shegufta. Utilization of main operation theatre at a large teaching hospital (thesis for M.D Hospital Administration)
2. Tabish Amin. Planning patient focused surgical suite system Journal of Acadamy of hospital Amdinistration 10(1) : 49-58, 1998
3. SakharKar BM. Operation theatre suite. Principles of hospital administration and planning. First edition 14: 197-207, 1998
4. Davies, R Llewelyn, Macaulay HMC. The technical medical services: Hospital planning and administration 10: 145-174.
5. Eric J Grigsby, Roy F Cucchiaria. Operating room management. Ronald D Miller. Anesthesia Fourth edition 2(82): 2603-2614.
6. Atkinson JO and Kohn Louise Mary. Division of duties: Set up, procedure, cleanup: Introduction to operating room technique. Fifth edition 8: 134-159.

7. Mc Quarrie DG. Limits to efficient operating room scheduling: lessons from computer use models. Arch Surg 116: 1065-1071, 1981
8. Gil AV, Galarza MT, Guerrero R, Develeez GP, Peterson OL, Bloom BL. Surgeons and operating rooms: under utilized resources. Am J public Health 73: 1361-1365, 1983.
9. Strum P David, Vargas G Luis, May H Jerrold. A minimal cost analysis model: Surgical subspecialty block utilization and capacity planning. Anesthesiology APV 90(4): 1176-1185, 1999.
10. Mazzei WJ. Operating room start times and turn over times in a University hospital. J clin Anesth 6(5): 405-408, 1994
11. Ozkarhan I. Allocation of surgical procedures to operating rooms. J Med syst. 19(4) : 333-352, 1995
12. Mazzei WJ. Maximizing operating room utilization: A land mark study. Anesth Analg 89: 1-2, 1999
13. Dexter Franklin, Macario Alex. Application of information systems to operating room scheduling. Anesthesiology 85(6) : 1996
14. Wright IH, kooperburg E, Bonar BA, Bashein G. Statistical modeling to predict elective surgery time: Comparison with a computer scheduling system and surgeon provided estimates. Anesthesiology 85: 1235-1245, 1996.
15. Macario A, Dexter F. Estimating the duration of a case when the surgeon has not recently scheduled the procedure at the surgical suit. Anesth Analg 89: 1241-1245, 1999
16. Dexter F. Application of prediction levels to OR Scheduling. AORN J 63: 607-615, 1996
17. Zhou J, Dexter F. Method to assist in the scheduling of add on surgical cases: Upper Predication bounds for surgical case durations based on log normal distribution. Anesthesiology 89: 1228-1232, 1998
18. Dexter F, Luharsky DA. Managing with information: Using surgical services information systems to increase operating room utilization. ASA Newsletter 62: 6-8, 1998.
19. Dexter F, Traub D Rodney Sequencing cases in the operating room: predicting whether one surgical case will last longer than another. Anesth analg 90: 975-979, 2000
20. Dexter F, Macario Aklex, Qian Fang, Traub DR. Forecasting surgical groups total hours of elective cases for allocation of block time: Application of time series analysis to operating room management. Anesthesiology 91(5): 1999.
21. Dexter F, Macario A, Traub DR, Hopwood M, Luharsky AD. An operating room strategy to maximize the use of operating room block time: computer simulation of patient scheduling and survey of patients preferences for surgical waiting time. Anesth Analg 89: 7-20, 1999

22. Dexter F, Macario, A, Rodney DT. Which algorithm for scheduling Add on elective cases maximizes operating room utilization: Use of Bin Packing Algorithm's and Fuzzy constraints in Operating Room Management. Anesthesiology 91 (5): 1999
23. Dexter F, Macario A, O. Nell Voim. Scheduling surgical cases into overflow block time- computer simulation of the effects of scheduling strategies on operating room labor costs. Anesth Analg 90: 980-988, 2000.
24. Bevan R.D The cost of cancelling surgery. Can J Anesthesiology 44(10): 1033-1035, 1997
25. Tessler JM, Kleiman JS Huherman MM. Reports of investigation: A "zero tolerance for overtime" increases surgical per case costs. Can J Anaesth 44(10): 1036-1041, 1997.
26. Skoyles RJ, Bowbotham JD. Operating department and recovery room management and design. Anesthesia 2nd Edt. 32: 625-640
27. American Hospital Association. Operating room utilization. Technical Bulletin Chicago 1983.
28. Jabeen Rukhsana, Jan Farooq, Naqash Imtiyaz. Utilization of Emergency Operation Theatre at a tertiary care hospital. (unpublished thesis for M.D Hospital Administration).
29. Deane SA, et al ANZ J Surg. 2010 March 80(3). 139-44.
30. Yoram Kluger, Offir Ben-Ishay, Masssimo Sartelli, et al. World Society of emergency surgery study group initiative on Timing of acute care surgery classification . World J Emerg Surg .2013: 8;17.
31. NCEPOD report 2004.
32. The Royal College of surgeons of England (M. Riuchard Collin, Dr Shuba Allan et al). Standards of unscheduled surgical care. Published in Feb 2013.

25

Crisis Management in Hospital

Crisis in hospital has a wide spectrum. The reasons can be external or internal. The external factors are those which interfere in the normal functioning of hospitals or those which put additional burden on hospitals in meeting demand for delivery or provision of services for which infrastructure is inadequate. Some of the external causes are wars, natural calamities (earth quake, floods), epidemics, blasts, bioterrorism etc. Internal factors can be fire, equipment breakdown, electric failure, collapse of building, strikes, increased rate of nosocomial infectious, breakdown of supply etc. Crisis puts the hospital and its management to test.

Every hospital must have a crisis management programme and a crisis management committee. A written crisis management committee is called as "Incident command Group" and its composition is as follows.

1. Chief executive
2. Chief of human resources'
3. Chief of Finances
4. Medical superintendent
5. Chiefs of Pharmacy, house keeping and sanitation, Security, Laboratory services, materials management, dietetics, laundry, telecommunication.
6. Chief of engineering services.

If there is no organized command structure in place, it is impossible to efficiently manage the response, the information and the resources. The primary responsibility of the group is establishment of a "First Incident action plan."

Incident action plan should take into consideration the different events and their implications on hospitals. Incident action plan should identify the place in the hospital from where the plan can be operated at the time of crisis. This room is called incident command room or control room. The roles and responsibilities are decided and distributed among members. Over all command will depend on

- What resources are available ?
- Which resources need to be mobilized ?
- Capacity to respond.
- Coordination with external agencies.
- Management information.
- Anticipation to take proactive decision.

Incident action plan lays down SOP's (standard operating procedures) to avoid chaos and confusion. Incident command group should meet every 3 hours or earlier depending on how the situation demands. Incident action plan identifies the capacity and capability of the hospital and probable evolution over time. Assess risks and consequences of event on functioning of hospital. Some of the priority issues which must be addressed are

Human Resources: Medical surge capacity of the hospital largely depends on the availability of staff necessary to deliver services. Availability of the staff is assessed and following points addressed

- If any staff needs to be called.
- How they can access hospital.
- Ensuring their safety.
- Where they will receive briefing and information.
- Additional staff needed.
- Providing any training to staff.

Logistics and supplies: logistics and supplies need to be ensured. Identify

- What you have (critical equipment and essential supplies).
- Consider the possibility of being isolated from outside sources and the possibility to evacuate the hospital.
- Develop action plan for resupply of critical items; for enhancing continuity of operations
- Identify the sources.
- Prioritize resource that need to be acquired
- Maintain record.
- Centralize logistic management.

Communication:- Incident command room should have time tested methods of communication which can be useful in linking with external agencies as well as internal departments in difficult circumstances. Back up systems must be available, the adequacy and resilience of which has been tested. Information Management aims not only at responding to the event but also at anticipating and recovering from the event. Information sharing within the hospital should be given high priority. At early stages of response one needs to identify the core data that must be collected and main processes for information management. The data which are needed in crisis are:

- The data for assessing the possible damages to the hospital and or the consequences on delivery of essential services.
- The data for assessing the probable demand for services.
- The data on availability of resources.
- The data concerning the dead and the missing.
- Data pertaining to health information.

Standard operating procedures: Standard operating procedure define how, when, what must be done and by whom for ensuring the provision of services from a particular unit or for a specific procedure.

They include also how information must be shared, what has to be recorded and how; whom to report, how and when. The issues to be addressed is

- Activity to be done.

- Description and sequence of activities
- Methodology
- Sequence of activities
- Safety rules and checking procedures
- Control and quality
- Time frame.
- Co-ordination with other stakeholders
- Reporting and recording.
- Persons involved.
- Monitoring.
- What to record and to whom to report how and when.
- Who can assist in case of major problems or doubts.
- Where to find phone numbers or addresses of people needed.
- Safety and security issues.
- Time frame for performing the activities.

Maintenance: electricity, water supply, roads and transport are life lines of hospital. Continuous supply and provision of these are important.

Security: of buildings, staff, visitors, patients, equipment and data is essential.

Food supply: Administration must ensure supply of clean food to patients and staff.

Waste management: What ever the circumstances hospital needs to be kept clean and nosocomial infection kept under control. Both internal and external constraints along with limited capacity for storing and managing hospital waste can be major challenges.

Laundry: the main challenges for laundry services are sudden increase in consumption of linen, sudden increase of workload for cleaning linen and limitation in hospital capacity to manage laundry overload.

Laboratory services and Blood bank: guidelines for infection control and prevention have to be strictly adhered to in addition to quality control. Universal and standard precautions are to be followed.

Pharmacy: guidelines to ensure continuity of supplies, means for assessing suppliers and transporting items.

Epidemics: The basic measures which should be in place to stop patient transmitting infection are

- Limit the number of staff in patients environment to a minimum.
- Encourage the patient to maintain a distance of at least 1 meter from others.
- Provide personnel protective equipment to patients and staff.
- Instruct on respiratory/ cough etiquette and hand hygiene.
- Make infection control supplies available.

Psychosocial support: Psychological counseling is most important at the time of crisis especially for victims and their attendants

Joint action sheets: Job action sheets (JAS) is a simple method for assigning and identifying roles and responsibilities and actions to be taken in a logical and sequential manner. Joint action sheets must be stored in a secured box, and be accessible at any time. A full set must also be kept in incident command room.

Services provided: What ever the crisis the hospital has to provide quality services and maintain its image in the public. Severe crisis may sometimes force administration to cut back on less important activities and augment some of the activities. Cold and elective cases may have to be discharged, out patient services minimized and more stress given on emergency services and ensuring optimal utilization of meager resources.

Crisis drills: The organization has to be in a state of preparedness and need to conduct drills at least twice a year.

Disaster Management in Hospitals

One of the important components of crisis management in hospitals is disaster management. WHO defines DISASTER as any occurrence that causes damage, economic disruption, loss of human life and deterioration of health and health services on a scale sufficient to warrant an extraordinary response from outside of the affected community or area.

140,000 deaths occur annually due to disasters and estimates of loss equal to 50000 million USD each year (Asian Development Bank). 2/3rd of the estimate cost is the direct cost of damage and rest 1/3rd is the cost of prevention, mitigation and preparedness. Asia – Pacific region witnesses a large number (about 60%) of natural disasters. Frequent distribution of disasters in Asia region showed that Indian subcontinent is one of the most disaster prone area and faced the largest number of disaster events. (U.N.O)

The High Power Committee on Disaster Management, constituted in 1999, has identified 31 various disasters categorized into five major sub-groups which are given below

List of various Disasters

(i) Water and climate related disasters
- (a) Floods and drainage management
- (b) Cyclones
- (c) Tornadoes and hurricanes
- (d) Hailstorm
- (e) Cloud burst
- (f) Heat wave and cold wave
- (g) Snow avalanches
- (h) Droughts
- (i) Sea erosion
- (j) Thunder and lightening
- (k) Tsunami

(ii) Geological related disasters
- (a) Landslides and mudflows
- (b) Earthquakes
- (c) Dam failures/ Dam bursts
- (d) Minor fires

(iii) Chemical, industrial and nuclear related disasters
- (a) Chemical and industrial disasters
- (b) Nuclear disasters

(iv) Accident related disasters
- (a) Forest fires

(b) Urban fires
(c) Mine flooding
(d) Oil spills
(e) Major building collapse
(f) Serial bomb blasts
(g) Festival related disasters
(h) Electrical disasters and fires
(i) Air, road and rail accidents
(j) Boat capsizing
(k) Village fire

(v) Biological related disasters
(a) Biological disasters and epidemics
(b) Pest attacks
(c) Cattle epidemics
(d) Food poisoning

Source: High Powered Committee Report-1999

Note: After 2004, Tsunami has also been included in the list of disasters.

Disaster Management is an applied science which seeks by the systematic observation and analysis of disasters to Improve, measures relating to prevention, mitigation, preparedness, emergency response and recovery.

Disaster Management Cycle

(1) Mitigation : Disaster scholars and emergency management professionals generally define mitigation as actions that are taken well in advance of disasters that are designed either to avoid or reduce disaster related damage. Mitigation activities can take the form of specific projects such as elevating hospitals for flood protection as well as process related activities such as hazard and vulnerability analysis that are designed to lead to future mitigative actions. However some use mitigation to refer to actions taken after an event occurs that are designed to contain impacts so that they do not become more severe.

To sum up hazard mitigation consists of practices that are implemented before impact and provide passive protection at the time disaster occurs.

Risk and Hazard assessment will be a combination of the likelihood of the event and the vulnerability of a place to that event and is called Hazard Vulnerability Analysis.

Under Hazard vulnerability analysis, community needs to identify the hazards to which they are more likely to be exposed to and then they have to rank these hazards in terms of the risks they pose. Risk of a hazard depends on two factors 1) Frequency of occurrence and 2) Magnitude of impact.

In other words

Hazard Vulnerability Analysis = Frequency of occurrence X Magnitude of Impact.

Both frequency of occurrence and magnitude of Impact are given a score as under

High Frequency or Impact = 3

Moderate Frequency or Impact = 2

Low Frequency or Impact = 1

(2) Preparedness : National Fire Protection Association (NEPA) USA defines preparedness as activities, programs and systems developed and implemented prior to a disaster /emergency that are used to support and enhance mitigation of a response to and recovery from disaster. Preparedness efforts also aim at ensuring that the resources necessary for responding effectively in the event of a disaster are in place and those faced with having to respond know how to use those resources. The activities that are commonly associated with disaster preparedness include developing planning process to ensure readiness, formulating disaster plan; stockpiling resources necessary for effective response and developing skills and competencies to ensure effective performance of disaster related tasks. The concept of disaster preparedness encompasses measures aimed at enhancing life safety when a disaster occurs. It also includes actions designed to enhance the ability to undertake emergency actions in order to protect property

and contain disaster damage and disruption, as well as the ability to engage in post- disaster restoration and early recovery activities.

The elements of disaster preparedness are

(1) Hazard Knowledge.

(2) Management, direction and coordination of emergency operations.

(3) Formal and Informal response agreements.

(4) Resource acquisition aimed at ensuring that emergency functions can be carried out smoothly.

(5) Life safety Protection.

(6) Property protection.

(7) Emergency coping and restoration of key functions.

(8) Initiation of recovery activities.

(3) Response: Response to a disaster is actually handling of situation when mass casualties actually report to hospital. When information about a disaster is received in a hospital, the disaster plan has to be activated.

CHAIN OF INCIDENT COMMAND AT EMERGENCY IN CASE OF MULTIPLE /MASS CASUALITY INCIDENT (MCI)

The information of MCI is received in control room/ medical Supdt/Directors office. After confirmation the senior most senior resident in control room attains the position of incident commander and sees to it that information starts flowing as per information flow chart.

⇩

The faculty on call from hospital administration on that day reaches emergency after getting the call and assumes the charge of incident commander taking charge from the senior resident

⇩

Medical Supdt, HOD emergency Medicine, Surgical Incharge Emergency reach emergency. Medical Supdt takes over as incident commander in coordination with faculty on call from Hospital Administration. HOD emergency medicine and surgical Incharge emergency take control of Clinical work at this time.

Information flow in mass causalities

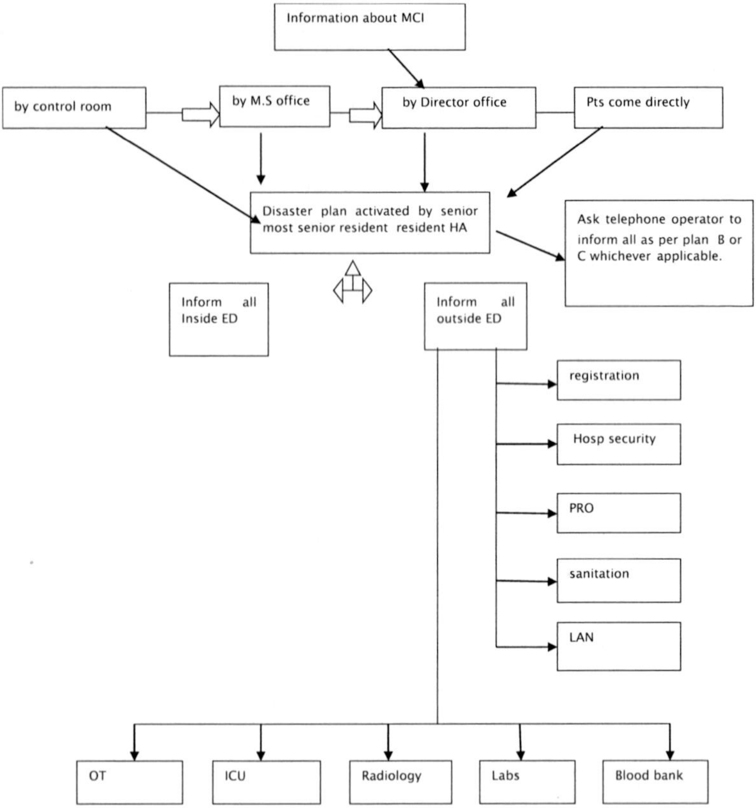

Fig. No. 25.1

Management has to clearly define in disaster manual the staff which will be responsible for handling disaster and area where patients will be kept depending upon whether patient load is moderate or heavy.

Disaster Manual is a written statement of a disaster plan which is to be activated during disasters. It should incorporate the following:

- Central Control Location (Control room).
- Disaster Alert.
- Responsibilities of individuals and departments.

- Action Card.
- Chronological action plan.
- Details of Resource mobilization for logistics and manpower.
- Triage parameter and reception centers.
- Networking including capabilities and capacities of health facilities.
- Documentation details.
- Communication.
- Quick reaction teams.
- Pre-hospital transport.
- Security arrangements.
- Evacuation details.
- Medicolegal responsibilities.
- Disposal of dead.

Disaster Management Committee consists of:

- Medical Superintendent as Chairman
- Heads of Department of following specialities
  - Emergency Medicine.
  - Orthopedics
  - Surgery
  - Medicine
  - Anaesthesiology
  - Neurosurgery
  - Cardio-Thoracic Surgery
  - Radiodiagnosis
  - Transfusion Medicine
  - Laboratory Medicine
- Nursing Superintendent
- Security Officer
- House keeping/ sanitation services
- Executive Engineers (civil, Mechanical, Electric).

TRIAGE is a dynamic process that is constantly influenced by changes in Casualty needs, Scene conditions, Resource availability and Time. Triage system should focus on Minimum morbidity and Mortality of the Critically Injured.

Two components of Triage:

1. Sorting causalities and prioritizing their care on the basis of the severity of Injuries and Illnesses.
2. Optimizing the allocation of available recourses by directing those resources to casualties who are most likely to benefit.

Triage Priorities: medical team triage patients into four priorities i.e. T1, T2, T3 and T4

Immediate Priority (T1): are the casualties who require immediate life saving procedures (airway obstruction, cardio respiratory distress, shock ….)

Urgent Priority (T2): are the casualties who require surgical or medical intervention within 1-2 hours (open chest injury without respiratory distress, abdominal injury without shock, fractures……..)

Delayed Priority (T3): are the casualties whose treatment can be safely delayed beyond 2-4 hours (walking wounded like victims suffering from sprains, strains and minor injuries)

Expectant Priorities (T4): are the casualties whose condition is so severe that they cannot survive despite the best available care and whose treatment would divert medical resources from salvageable patients (massive head injury with signs of impending death)

Responsibility of triage team will be

(1) **priority one**: Needing immediate resuscitation. (Red Category)
(2) **Priority two**: Immediate surgery. (Yellow Category)
(3) **Priority three**: Needing first aide and possibly surgery. (Green Category)
(4) **Priority four**: Needing only first aide.

Disaster Management Cycle

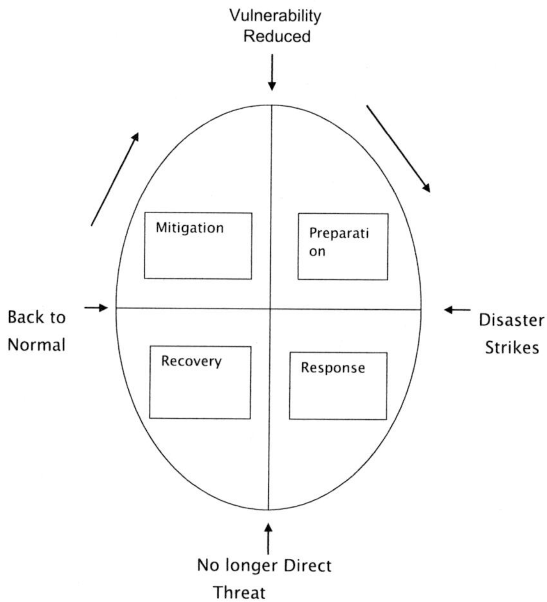

Fig : 25.2

Recovery: When initial phase of disaster is over, the work is half done. Getting a community back on its feet after a disaster is a monumental task. The goal of recovery is to ensure the economic sustainability of a community and the long term physical and mental well being of its citizens to rebuild and repair the physical infrastructure and to implement mitigation activities to reduce the impact of future disasters. The key to recovery starts during emergency preparedness planning even before an event occurs. The role of recovery planning is quite large. It is important to think how hospital and essential non – hospital services which have been overrun in an incident, can be restored. Hospital services would include in-patient, out-patient, day care services dietetics, laundry services, manifold etc while as non hospital services would include suppliers, vendors, contractors who are not in a position to maintain supply chain. So efforts are directed to restore hospital services and try to look for suppliers from outside of the affected area. Additionally with preapproved and pre-negotiated contracts vendors can begin work as soon as disaster passes. The health care system outside the hospital may be in shambles which will further complicate the picture. Therefore while a hospital is evacuating patients presenting to the emergency department need also to be provided care.

The hospital can recover only if the staff are mentally free of their family responsibilities. Therefore programs that support family and personal preparedness are very important. Staff require personal support during and after an incident.

The Medical Severity Index of Disaster

Mass casualty incident (MCI) is any incident in which emergency medical services and resources such as staff and equipment are overwhelmed by the number and severity of casualties. Due to these extensive casualties and massive disruption, there is a need for improving MCI response capacity.

Currently three evaluation methods for MCI assessment are available.

1. Medical Severity Index (MSI).
2. Potential Injury Creating Index.
3. Disaster Severity Scale.

Medical Severity Index makes it possible to immediately assess the medical size of a disaster. Here we will be more focused on this method of assessment.

Considering the definition of Medical severity Index, the parameters needed to quantify a disaster are

1. Casualty load (number of Patients).
2. Severity of Incident (severity of injuries sustained).
3. Capacity of medical services.

Casualty Load : When first notification is received about the incident, it is difficult to make anything about the number of casualties, however rough idea is got depending on the magnitude of the incident. When ambulance service reaches the site a fairly accurate estimate is made by medical personal. The original estimate by member of public tends to be overestimated, but in disasters eg earthquake the initial estimate is underestimated. Casualty load is designated as N and subsequent estimates made at intervals of 1hr, 2hr and 3hr etc are designated as N1, N2, N3 etc.

Severity of Incident: The severity of incident is represented by symbol S . Patients treated at the scene by simple triage and rapid treatment (START) program are divided into four classes.

T1 : Life Threatening cases demanding immediate attention.

T2: Non- life threatening cases requiring hospital treatment.

T3: Casualties not necessarily requiring hospitalization but rather less demanding single point care and

T4 : DOA ie Dead on arrival.

The severity of incident is expressed as

$$S = (T1 + T2)/T3$$

Since categories T1 and T2 are the casualties which need medical attention and those who have to be admitted to hospitals, they form the crucial group.

It is known that in most earthquake, railway accidents, fires, terrorist bombings and air crashes T1, T2 and DOA comprise more than 50% of total casualties. In floods many more are killed than injured. In civil disturbances on the other hand, many are slightly wounded and a few are heavily wounded.

It has been seen that if more T1 and T2 are expected S is scored as 1.5 . If only many slightly injured are expected S is scored as 0.5. Major traffic accidents usually result in figure between these two ie S=1.

Capacity of Medical Services: The capacity of medical services is divided into three phases

(a) Medical Rescue Capacity (MRC).

(b) Medical Transport Capacity (MTC).

(c) Hospital Treatment Capacity (HTC).

Medical Rescue capacity depends on the amount of professional help at the site and depends on the number of doctors, nurses, paramedics and material and equipment available at the disaster site. It is assumed that a team comprising a surgeon, anesthesiologist and two nursing staff can deal with 10 casualty categories 1 & 2 per hour.

Medical Transport Capacity depends on number of ambulances with drivers, the ease of evacuation. It is assumed that a ambulance can transport two casualties per hour if terrain and weather is okay, otherwise the capacity is going to drop.

Hospital Treatment Capacity depends on the total number of surgeons, anesthesiologists, operating rooms, intensive care beds, residents etc. HTC refers to number of casualties category 1 and 2 that can be treated during one hour. If the disaster takes place at night or weekend, the HTC will be lower . AS a rough guide HTC for general hospitals can be estimated as 3% of the total number of beds.

The capacities are expressed per unit of time, that is per hour. Under disaster conditions medical and paramedical staff can probably work efficiently for 8 hours at the most. Therefore capacities should be multiplied by 8 in order to obtain the total capacity of medical services.

Lowest capacity in any one of the above determines the capacity of the whole chain.

Once the casualty load (N), the severity of incident (S) and the total capacity (TC) of medical services are quantified

Medical Severity Index = NXS/TC.

If medical severity index is > 1, the calamity is called a disaster.

An MSI can be applied to evaluate the disaster itself and estimate the medical requirements in the disaster preparedness phase. The proposed methodology is of practical importance for handling disasters.

Fire Safety in Hospitals

Fire in hospitals can be disastrous as it can result in loss of lives due to suffocation as well as due to burns. Prevention of fires becomes even more important in hospitals as good percentage of admitted patients are non ambulatory.

National Accreditation Board for Hospitals and Health Care Providers (NABH) has provided minimum essential fire safety measures check list for hospitals. These are applicable to hospitals and health care facilities for purposes of certification and accreditation. These guidelines are meant to ensure patient safety and in no way absolves the organization of fulfilling its statutory obligation with regard to fire safety.

If organization has a valid fire safety NOC verify that minimum essential fire safety measures are in place.

If organization does not have a valid fire safety NOC

- Check for approval / registration from local health authority.
- If fire NOC is not applicable to the organization justify the same.
- If fire NOC is applicable confirm that the organization has applied for the same and that there is regular correspondence between health facility and fire department (at least once in three months) which is acknowledged. Any correspondence received from fire department has to be submitted.
- Third party inspection certificate should be available. Third party audit should provide evidence that statutory norms are adhered to. Third party inspection certificate is valid for a period of one year.
- Any observation by third party has to be addressed.
- Head of the organization has to give in writing on organizational letter head stating that fire safety norms are in place and adhered to at all times.
- During assessment verify that points in check list are in place and functioning.

Checklist

1. Firefighting equipment like wet riser, hydrants, auto sprinkler, fire alarm system, fire extinguishers of all types and sizes should be available .
2. Operational and maintenance plan for firefighting equipment including refilling of extinguishers.
3. Up to date fire drawings to be available. Where applicable, the fire drawings should also specify the location of fire dampers.

4. Fire detection and smoke detectors exist across all floors. The detectors shall be tested for functionality at regular intervals, and records maintained. 5. Central fire alarm systems installed at a location which is staffed 24/7.
6. Fire exit plan for each floor. Exit door should be openable and free from any materials which will obstruct way.
7. Fire Exit signage on all floors well illuminated/ self-glowing, as per NBC guidelines.
8. Emergency illumination system in case power goes.
9. Designated place for assembly of patients and staff in case of fire.
10. Mock fire drill records and schedule of conduct of drills.

Minimum Requirement for fire fighting installations

Type of Hospital	Wet Riser	Automatic Sprinkler	Manually operated electric fire alarm	Auto detection and fire alarm system
Hospitals less than 15 meters in height, with plot area upto 1000 square meters and upto G + 1 floor	NR	R	R	NR
Hospitals less than 15 meters in height, with plot area upto 1000 square meters and G + 2 floors	R	R	R	R
Hospitals less than 15 meters in height with plot area more 1000 square meters	R	R	R	R
Hospitals 15 meters and above but not exceeding 24 meters in height	R	R	R	R
Hospitals above 24 meters but not exceeding 45 meters in height	R	R	R	R

R stands for Required and NR for Not Required.

(Sufficient water storage (underground and/or terrace) should be provided to ensure fire-fighting).

(Adapted from *National Accreditation Board for Hospitals & Healthcare Providers(NABH)*)

Reference

1. Management of Hospitals during health crisis. Essential services package. WHO Draft (3) June 2009.
2. Ramping down and recovery from a Mass Casualty Incident. National Academy of Sciences Institute of Medicine (US) forum of Medical Health

Preparedness for catastrophic events. Medical Surge Capacity. Workshop Summary Washington (DC). National Academics Press(US); 2010. www.ncbi.nlm.gov (searched on 13/5/19).

3. Jeannette Sutton and Kathleen Tierney. Disaster Preparedness: Concepts Guidance and Research. Natural Hazards Centre. Institute of behavioral science, University of Colorado. 2006 (report prepared for Fritiz Institute Assessing Disaster Preparedness). www.colorado.edu/hazards.
4. Jan de Boer, Do Brismar, Reuben Elder, William H. Rutherford. The Medical Severity Index of Disasters. Selected Topics. Disaster Planning. The Journal of Emergency Medicine, vol 7, pp. 269-273, 1989.
5. Takahashi A, Ishii N, Kawashuma T, Nakao H. Assessment of medical response capacity in the time of disaster: the estimated formula of Hospital Treatment Capacity (HTC), the maximum receivable number of patients in hospital. Kobe J Med Sci. 2007; 53(5): 189-98.
6. Wei-feng Shen, Li-Bing Jiang, Guan-Yu –Jiang, Mao-Zhang, Yue-Feng Ma and Xiao-Jun He. Development of the Science of mass casualty incident management: reflection on the medical response to the Wenchuan earthquake and Hangzhou bus fire. J.Zhejiang Univ Sci B. 2014 Dec; 15 (12): 1072-1080.
7. Minimum Essential Fire Safety Measures Checklist. National Accreditation Board for Hospitals & Healthcare Providers(NABH). Dated 31st July 2018.

26

Disaster Evacuation Protocol

Need of evacuation of a hospital arises when the hospital itself is under threat which can be from varied reasons like earthquake, fire, bomb threat, flood etc. Deciding whether or not and when to evacuate a hospital during an emergency situation can be a daunting task. Goal of evacuation is to move patients to safety. It is important to recognize that routine care and processes will not be optimal during an evacuation scenario. Full evacuation of a hospital should generally be considered as a last resort when mitigation or other emergency response efforts are not expected to maintain a safe care environment. Evacuation plan should be simple and flexible so that it can adapt to variety of situations. The primary consideration when deciding whether to evacuate a hospital is the safety of both patients and staff. How patient and staff safety is evaluated will drastically affect whether or not a hospital evaluates. Hospital should strive to develop a clear, comprehensive and consistent decision making matrix that can be used when they are considering whether to evacuate or not. Hospital Emergency operations plans should anticipate the possibilities of catastrophic failures of their communication system and develop appropriate contingency strategies. Once the decision to evacuate has been made, then the process of evacuation is fairly linear.

Authority to Evacuate

Authority to evacuate should rest with appropriate authority may be CEO, administrator, administrator on call or Incident Commander available on site as designated in the pre-established plan. In case where an external threat to the hospital is the cause for implementing the evacuation plan, it is likely that local or state authorities will participate if not guide, the decision regarding the type or schedule of evacuation. The final decision as to the type or scale of evacuation rests with the hospital administration. All hospital evacuation plans must designate the authority to evacuate to a leader who is on–site 24hrs a day, 7 days per week so that he can immediately respond to an extraordinary situation.

The decision to evacuate is for the safety of patients and the staff, however it will not always be clear whether the decision to evacuate would be the safest course of action. Full time evacuation is not always needed and should be the last resort. Hospital authorities should carefully weigh the benefits of evacuation with the risks associated with evacuation. During the time when decision is being made hospitals should consider issuing a "Prepare only" order as long delaying the decision does not place patients and staff at risk. During "prepare only": hospital staff should prepare for evacuation ie packing patients, important records, and medication. Subsequently if evacuation is required we would be saving time and if evacuation is not required we have had a good experience. Once the decision for evacuation is made, hospital employees and state public health agencies need to be notified of the decision.

Evacuation

The person who has to take decision of evacuation and then control various activities of evacuation is called as "Incident Commander". Biggest problem which is faced is failure of communication systems during disaster and administration should anticipate this and act accordingly. Various decisions to be taken are:

- Level of Evacuation.
- Type of Evacuation.
- Evacuation time frame.
- Patient Prioritization.
- Assembly and Discharge site location.
- Labour pool activation.

- Evacuation coordinator assignment.
- Patient destination team activation.

Level of Evacuation

Evacuation can range from

Shelter in place.

Horizontal evacuation.

Vertical Evacuation.

Total or Full Evacuation.

Shelter in place : When a decision for shelter in place is taken it means the place where patients are presently situated is still safe, however have to be kept ready for evacuation along with records, medication and anytime may have to be shifted. During this stage windows, doors can be closed which will keep smoke, fire and other hazards away.

Horizontal Evacuation: The patients whom administration thinks are in danger can be moved to an area of refuge in the same floor in an adjacent smoke free zone. This is the fastest option and saves lives. This option also helps in returning back easily once the threat is over.

Vertical evacuation : This level of evacuation refers to evacuation of a specific floor of a building. This evacuation can be towards upper stories or lower stories depending upon the cause of evacuation but usually the evacuation is towards lower floors. While one floor is evacuating other floors can be used to shelter in.

Total or Full Evacuation : Total evacuation involves complete evacuation of a building or whole campus . This decision has to be taken very carefully after analyzing the situation and identifying the destination. Local State authorities also need to be taken in confidence for such a decision.

Type of Evacuation

In addition to level of evacuation, type of evacuation is also very important which means whether the evacuation has to be made on the basis of the area to be evacuated first (Geographic model), on the basis of the resources available for evacuating (Resource model) or on the basis of criticality of patient. (acuity model).

In geographic model the areas which are at greatest risk are evacuated first . Geographic model allows for partial evacuation which will not disrupt the entire hospital and does not disrupt continuity of care, however this model requires considerable time. Patient prioritization would be linked directly to resource availability, however it requires good logistical management to best allocate scarce resources at a time of crisis. In acuity model the critically sick patients are to be shifted last during evacuation, with the idea that these patients remain on ventilator and other life support equipment for maximum time as their chance of death during evacuation is maximum. However if these patients are in an area which is under maximum threat then these patients need to be moved first. Patients are evacuated in an order that ensures the greatest good for the greatest number of patients.

Evacuation Time Frames

Depending on the type of the threat administration will have to declare within how much time to evacuate;

(a) Immediate/Urgent: No time for preparation – evacuate immediately.

(b) Rapid/Urgent : Limited time for preparation (1-2 hrs) – everyone out in 4-6 hrs.

(c) Gradual/Planned : Extended time for preparation – phased evacuation to occur over many hours or even days.

Patient Prioritization

As already stated the most critical patients ie patients in ICU's should be shifted last; the idea is that most critical patients should remain most of the time with ventilator support under proper monitoring and once they are shifted to assembly area they should be the first to go to destination site. However if ICU is the area which is the most vulnerable then this area should be the first to be evacuated.

If elevators are available and can be used then patients in upper stories should be the one who are evacuated first, however if elevators are not available or cannot be used patients in lower stories should be evacuated first.

Assembly and Discharge Site location

For evacuation assembly site and discharge site locations need to be identified. Assembly site is a location where patients from patient care units are shifted before being shifted to final destination sites ie other hospitals or re-entry back into the hospital. The assembly sites are not full fledged hospitals but sites where patients receive basic care till they are shifted. It is ideal that individual patient care units remain separate at assembly sites under supervision of nurse incharge and do not mix with other units. The idea is that nurse incharges of individual patient care units know best about medical needs of patients of that unit.

Discharge sites are areas around the hospital where patients wait for being discharged home. Several locations for assembly sites and discharge sites should be located around the hospital and final decision for one taken depending upon the cause of evacuation . Assembly sites and Discharge sites should be located at distance from each other to avoid mixing.

Labour pool Activation

At each step manpower is required right from shelter in, evacuation to assembly and discharge sites, monitoring patients while shifting and at assembly sites and transportation to final destination sites.

The labour pool has to be identified in advance for different timings and may even have to be called from home. Stand by lists include both clinical and general shift.

Evacuation Coordinator Assignment

Role of evacuation coordinator is to shift patients to assembly site and discharge sites. He has to have coordination between incident commander and Unit leader. Evacuation coordinator has to clarify following : how much time is available for patients to pack, location of assembly and discharge sites, in what order evacuation of individual patient care units will take place, whether elevators would be used or not, whether fire exits are to be used, deployment of staff for evacuation. Depending upon the size of the hospital, number of evacuation coordinators could be more than one. This decision will have to be taken by Incident Commander.

Patient Destination Team activation

If the hospital authorities have decided to fully evacuate the hospital and patients are being shifted to assembly and discharge sites, patient destination team needs to be activated. Patient destination team comprises of administrators, senior nurses, officials of Medical Record Department. Role of patient destination team is to look out and shift patients on beds in other hospitals. It would be in the fitness of things if a hospital has pre-disaster agreement with destination hospitals. It is important to the success of the Patient destination Team that individual physicians do not circumvent the patient destination team and attempt to arrange beds on their own. This would unnecessarily create confusion.

Evacuation Routes

Hospitals should have pre-defined evacuation routes which should have illumination independent of regular electrification of hospital and should work even when lights have been put off. Evacuation routes should be prominently identified by signage which will illuminate even when lights are off. These routes also need to be manned by Hospital security.

Patient Tracking

While the patients are being evacuated it is important to keep their track which can be done at the time of check in and check out at various stations like patient care unit, assembly point, discharge site and at destination hospitals. This activity is important to minimize confusion and avoid panic among patient attendants and relations. Patient tracking system should tell about the location of various patients as well as their status. Patient tracking can simply be done at various points by writing on paper. Electronic tracking always has its advantages however. During evacuation or shifting patients number of hospitals loose costly and vital equipment, therefore record of equipment like transport ventilators, Spinal Boards etc which accompany patients while shifting also needs to be maintained.

Studies have shown that in a tertiary care hospital around 45-50% of patients are ambulatory, 25-28% require stretcher and wheel chairs each.

References

1. MDPH Hospital Evacuation Tool Kit: Evacuation Planning Guide. Hospital Emergency Preparedness and Response Exercise Program. HARVARD School of Public Health . 2014.
2. New AHRQ Guides offer hospitals advice on emergency evacuation, assessment and recovery. American Hospital Association. http: // www. ahrq.gov/prep/.

27

Drug Utilization

Drugs are a critical component in the modern health care system. Past two decades have witnessed introduction of myriad of new pharmaceutical products that have revolutionized medicine and this has resulted in growth of their share in overall spending in health. Are these increased health expenditures getting translated into improved health outcomes?

Some of the drug utilization indicators related to expenditure are:

- Total drug expenditure as a percentage of total health care spending
- Prescribed drug expenditure as a percentage of total drug expenditure
- Non- prescribed drug expenditure as a percentage of total drug expenditure
- Hospital drug expenditure as a percentage of total hospital expenditure
- Prescribed drug expenditure per capita
- Publicly insured drug expenditure as a percentage of prescribed drug expenditure.
- Privately insured drug expenditure (excluding out-of-pocket) as a percentage of prescribed drug expenditure nationally
- Out-of-pocket drug expenditure as a percentage of prescribed drug expenditure nationally.

Drug utilization research has been defined by WHO as "the marketing, distribution, prescription and uses of drugs in a society with special emphasis on the resulting medical, social and economic consequences."

Pharmacoepidemiology is defined as " The study of the use and effects/side effects of drugs in large numbers of people with the purpose of supporting the rational and cost-effective use of drugs in the population thereby improving health outcomes."

Pharmacosurveillance and pharmacovigilance are terms used to refer to the monitoring of drug safety such as spontaneous adverse effect reporting systems, case-control and cohort studies. Descriptive drug utilization research describes pattern of drug utilization and identifies problems deserving more detailed studies. Analytical studies try to link drug utilization data to figures on morbidity, outcome of treatment and quality of care with the ultimate goal being to assess whether drug therapy is rational or not.

Drug utilization and pharmacoepidemiology is useful for:

- Studying patterns of drug use, i.e. extent and trends in drug use and costs overtime
- Comparing actual use to prescribed guidelines, choice of drug, combinations, dosage, etc
- Studying outcomes of use.

Prescribing and dispensing data are useful for determining some of the quality indicators of drug use recommended by WHO. These include:

- Average number of drugs per prescription.
- Percentage of drugs prescribed by generic name.
- Percentage of encounters with an antibiotic prescribed.
- Percentage of encounters with an injection prescribed.
- Percentage of drugs prescribed from national list of essential drugs.
- Average drug cost per encounter.

Drug use evaluation assesses actual process of medication, i.e. indication, drug selection, dose, route of administration, duration of

Table 27.1: Causes of drug therapy problems

Drug therapy problem	Cause
Unnecessary drug therapy	– No medical indication
	– Additional/ recreational drug use
	– No drug therapy more appropriate
	– Duplicate therapy
	– Treating avoidable adverse reaction
Wrong drug	– Dosage form inappropriate
	– Contraindication present
	– More effective drug available
Dosage too low	– Wrong dosage
	– Frequency inappropriate
	– Duration inappropriate – Incorrect administration
Adverse drug reaction	– Unsafe drug for patient
	– Allergic reaction
	– Incorrect administration
	– Drug interaction
	– Dosage increased or decreased too quickly
	– Undesirable effect
Dosage too high	– Wrong dose
	– Frequency inappropriate
	– Duration inappropriate
	– Drug interaction
Inappropriate compliance	– Drug product not available
	– Cannot afford drug
	– Cannot swallow or otherwise administer drug
	– Does not understand instructions
	– Patient prefers not to take drug
Need additional drug therapy	– Untreated condition
	– Synergistic therapy
	– Prophylactic therapy

Adapted from Tomechko MA, Strand LM, Morley PC, Cipolle RJ. Q and A from Pharmaceutical Care Project in Minnesota. AM Pharm. 1995; N s 35 (4): 30-9.

PRESCRIPTION REGISTER

Number of countries keep a record of data on drug use in the form of a prescription register. Such information is useful in clinical as well as administrative discussions concerning rational use of drugs. The prescription register is based on computerized prescriptions from all the pharmacies. Main objective of a prescription register is to improve knowledge of the drug utilization in the general population after the drug has been marketed.

This can be undertaken by:

- Identifying benefits and potential problems to the public health linked to utilization of given drugs or drug groups
- Assessing the safety and effectiveness of medications
- Making drug utilization data available to the prescribing doctors as part of an audit
- Method to improve the quality of prescribing practices
- Doing health economic analysis
- Developing and validating procedures for collection, analysis and interpretation of drug utilization data
- Comparing drug utilization data across countries.

BIBLIOGRAPHY

1. Canadian Institute for Health Information. Road Map Initiative. Launching the process, 1999.
2. Developing of Drug utilization Indicators: A feasibility study using existing aggregated administrative databases. C1H1, 2002.
3. Furu K. Drug utilization is a public health perspective: Establishing a national prescription register in Norway. Norwegian Journal of Epidemiology. 2001; 11 (1): 55-60.
4. Goel V, et al. Patterns of use of specific drugs in the elderly. Patterns of Health care in Ontario. The ICES practice Atlas. 2nd edn. Canadian Medical Association, Ottawa, 1996; pp. 323-8.
5. Introduction to Drug Utilization Research. WHO publication, 2003.
6. Macleod S. The optimal drug therapy national symposium 2001: A call for action. Can J clin Pharmacol. 2001; 8 (suppl A): 2A-5A.
7. Tomechko MA, Strand LM, Morley PC, Cipolle RJ. Q and A from the pharmaceutical care project in Minnesota. Am Pharm. 1995; Ns35 (4) :3-9.
8. World Health Organisation collaborating centre for drug statistics methodology. ATC classification and DDD assignment. Oslo, Norway: World Health Organisation, 2001.

28

Energy Efficiency in Hospitals

Health care is one of the fastest growing sectors throughout the world and hospitals are an inseparable part of the health care delivery system. There is a huge requirement of energy in hospitals in the form of lighting, heating, cooling, running of machinery/Equipments and thus there is a huge energy saving potential in hospitals and health care institutions. The lighting demands of hospitals are complex due to their round the clock nature and the effects of lighting on patients and staff. A critical element for the adequate functioning of the hospital center is that of energy sources, generally electricity and fuels. In the past, the cost of these sources of energy was such that their impact on functioning costs of a center was not significant. Low prices of petroleum and petroleum products as well as subsidized electricity costs were the norm in the past century. But the situation has changed radically . The rational and efficient use of energy is ultimately aimed at reducing consumption, while maintaining the energy services of the institution. When considering energy efficiency in hospitals, it is important to keep in mind that it is not the end use of energy alone, but also the need to control the indoor climate, that is one of the principal requirements. The indoor climatic requirements are determined by the hospital activities in the buildings. Once these are established, it is necessary to provide the required climate, ideally in the most economical way. In practice energy efficiency is increasingly becoming important but medical considerations remain the top priority in the hospitals.

In hospitals, energy brought in is converted by a number of conversion systems into several internal energy streams to meet heating, cooling, and other medical equipment requirements and there are energy streams categorized as under:

Electricity: Major electricity consumers in a hospital are cooling, heating equipment, lighting, air compressors, water pumps, fans and ventilation. Other applications include laundry equipment, kitchen and canteen equipment, ovens and geysers and medical equipment including autoclaves, office facilities such as computers and photocopiers, utilities such as lifts, refrigerators, water coolers etc.

Heat Stream: is used in the form of steam and hot water. Steam is used in kitchens and for humidification in HVAC and Sterilization process. In addition steam is used to transport heat over longer distances. In many cases heat is transported from the heat generating station in the form of steam and then converted locally into central heating or hot tap water. Oil/ gas fired boilers are used to generate steam and hot water.

Compressed air: can be divided into two main categories, namely medical air and technical air. Medical compressed air refers to the direct treatment and care of patients. The technical compressed air is used for HVAC control systems, workshop applications or keeping containers under pressure.

Cold Stream: mainly takes the form of chilled water and is used for indoor climate control systems, for cooling and drying the ventilation air. In many cases cold stream is generated centrally by means of compression coolers.

Energy performance of a building can be evaluated by recording its Energy Performance Index (EPI). Energy Performance Index is defined as total energy consumption per unit of build up area of the building per year (kwh/sq mts/year). In other words it can be referred as Specific Energy Consumption of the building per annum.

EPI can be used to evaluate

- Energy efficiency of the building.
- Track improvements compared to other buildings.
- Recognize the top performers.

CII Western Region Health care Sub- committee along with SL Raheja and Schneider Electric conducted an exclusive survey on energy efficiency of hospitals. The data collected from different hospitals is analyzed primarily targeting the EPI calculation and bench mark the results with reference to ECBC standard (Energy Conservation Building Codes). The surveys conducted among the hospitals were in different climate zones as per ECBC guidelines. The minimum EPI for this zone was 200kwh/sq.mt/annum (average). More than 60% hospitals and health care facilities fail to meet the minimum EPI criteria leading to a huge potential of energy performance improvement.

The main contributors of energy consumption were found as HVAC, Medical Equipment and lighting.

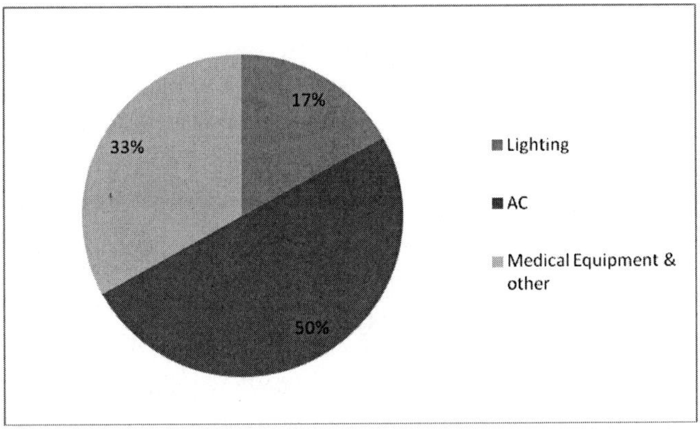

Fig. 28.1: Showing main sources of energy consumption in Hospitals

HVAC System

In many large and centrally air-conditioned hospitals, HVAC systems consume 40-50% of total electricity. Air conditioning and ventilation system in hospitals is required for

- Maintaining the requisite indoor temperature, air distribution and humidity levels for thermal comfort.
- Maintaining indoor air quality, particularly in areas requiring prevention of infection. Stringent indoor air quality levels must be maintained especially in operating rooms, emergency

rooms, intensive care units and laboratories. Certain types of rooms have special HVAC pressurization requirements. ORs, ERs, and ICUs generally run over pressure for protective isolation from airborne infection. Quarantine rooms require negative pressure. Indoor climate must be strictly regulated for temperature, humidity and quality. This increases the need for proper heating and cooling.

Lighting

Lighting is a sector with great energy saving potential. Requirement of light in a hospital varies widely depending upon the activity, time of day and the occupancy level.

Medical equipments

These include medical equipment that use energy for their normal functioning in different hospital areas. Other than medical equipment motors working in different service areas also consume lot of energy.

Steps for Saving Energy

1. The first thing that hospital manager has to do is to know how much he is spending on energy and what would be the consequences of bad and inadequate use of energy resources. This helps in identifying the critical points.
2. The hospital needs to have in place key points where energy is measured to be able to control it. It is necessary to put in place measurement equipment to monitor consumption of electricity and also identify RUE (Rational Use of Energy) opportunities. In the case of fuel consumption, the purchase data are the initial base and it is also recommendable to have places where consumption is controlled.
3. The hospital manager must be committed and involved in energy saving plans and programs. This activity will motivate others in the process and this will be the first step to start energy saving program and to generate or strengthen the RUE culture at his institution. Managers must seek the support of the employees, practical knowledge to identify and chose the most profitable energy efficiency measures to be implemented.

4. It is important to work on the evaluation method in order to determine and verify the existence and benefits of the performance improvements by monitoring and verifying. Before a project is implemented, a specification of the follow up must be developed so that it ensures the success of the project, and that the measures that are implemented are sustainable in time. Depending on the nature of the project, and the needs of the hospital, the performance follow-up on a project may be extensive or may comprise simple systems or parts of the most critical equipment.
5. Performance indicators must be identified. These may include indexes based on the measurement of a performance factor which has been agreed on, or the measurement of changes in the performance of the whole facility.
6. Carry out audits: Audits may be carried out directly by qualified personnel from the hospitals, or through a contracting firm with expertise in the field. The methodology is intended to give the hospital center personnel a guide and basic tools for its execution and for the follow-up of energetic behavior of the system or of a particular subsystem. The recommendations of an audit may be classified in two types: those which require immediate implementation, which generally comprised modifications in process and operational habits or minor maintenance of equipment and systems and those that comprise a longer execution time, which generally imply major modifications of equipment and facilities and which imply a higher investment level.

Energy Conservation Measures

Lighting: First and foremost measure to control lighting is launching an awareness campaign to train staff to turn off lights when rooms are not in use. Beyond that, high performance lighting systems significantly reduce energy usage by ensuring electric lighting is used only when needed in the amount necessary. The following options can save energy without affecting patient care or facility functionality.

- Incorporating day lighting controls in patient rooms and public spaces with large window areas.

- Integrating controls that enable continuous dimming (100to 5% lamp power).
- Installing occupancy sensors in spaces that are frequently unoccupied such as rest rooms, stairwells, service areas and mechanical plants.
- Using sensors that include dimming and stepping options for spaces that utilize day lighting.
- Incorporating exterior motion sensors which save energy and can enhance security.

Proper utilization of day lighting involving architectural designs intended to take advantage of natural light offers many benefits such as day lighting in combination with energy efficient lighting can lessen lighting power density in office areas without a reduction in measured light levels, day light produces less heat per unit of illumination thereby reducing cooling loads, a well-configured patient room can result in cost reductions. Day lighting enhances quick recovery of patients, 2.5% lower staff absenteeism, increased productivity and job satisfaction and heightened psychological well-being. Hospitals tend to have a lot of windows, particularly in wards and in consulting areas. This provides a good opportunity to maximize day light. Wire lights so that those close to the windows can be switched off, while the rest remain on with separate controls. This is called "Switching in Parallel" and enables staff and patients to make the most of natural day light which is usually preferred. As a result less lighting is used, reducing energy consumption and additional heat generated by the lights, which in turn means less cooling is required.

- Further other measures which can be made to improve energy efficiency viz-a-viz lighting are
- Specify and provide multiple levels of light; both general ambient and task lighting in patient and examination rooms. In patient rooms, bright lights can be turned on during examinations but remain off the rest of the time.
- Consolidate lamp inventories by eliminating unnecessary bulb types. LED lights need to be preferred.
- Light colored surfaces need to be encouraged.

HVAC system : The big volume of the rooms that have to be cooled and heated makes this a very high energy consuming process. High Efficiency particulate air (HEPA) filtration is required to prevent the spread of nosocomial infection in the ventilation system. HEPA filters that achieve 99.7% efficiency place greater elective demand on fans for proper air circulation.

It is possible to reduce the amount of energy that ventilation systems consume by focusing on some key energy saving opportunities . As simple as it sounds, natural ventilation and cooling relies on natural airflow between openings on opposite sides of a room or building- or rising warm air being replaced with air sucked in through windows or vents. It is also possible to use windows and doors to provide good levels of natural ventilation in some areas within a hospital, allowing mechanical ventilation to be switched off or turned down to save energy. Do not let heating and cooling operate at the same time. This can be avoided by setting a temperature "dead band" – a wide gap between the temperatures at which heating and cooling cut in. Energy consumption in HVAC system can increase substantially if regular maintenance is not undertaken. Dirty or faulty fans, air filters, air ducts and components directly affect system efficiency and increase running costs and risks of break down. Some hospitals use what is known as "Mixed Mode" system which uses a combination of both natural and mechanical systems . Fans do not need to operate at full speed all of the time and variable speed drives (VSDs) can help to reduce costs by enabling the output speed of the fans to match requirements at different times of the day. This reduction in speed saves energy. Use of Building Energy Management System (BEMS) also helps. This is based on a network of controllers and offers closer control and monitoring of building services performance including cooling, heating, ventilation and air conditioning. This is shown on a computer screen in real time and allows settings to be changed quickly and easily. BEMS can reduce total energy costs by 10% or more. Energy Management Systems have been installed in a number of hospitals in India.

Two thirds of energy from a hospital is lost through the building envelope, with the remaining third being lost through air filtration and ventilation. The rate at which the energy is lost depends on temperature difference between inside and outside, insulation properties of the building envelope and amount of fresh air entering the building either by controlled ventilation or through poorly fitting windows, doors or joins in walls.

A building envelope is the physical separator between the conditioned and unconditioned environment of a building including the resistance to air, water, heat light and noise transfer. It is comprised of all the elements of the outer shell that maintain a dry heated or cooled indoor environment and facilitate its climate control. Common measures of the effectiveness of a building envelope include physical protection from weather and climate, indoor air quality, durability and energy efficiency. In order to achieve these objectives, all building enclosure systems must include a solid structure, a drainage plane, an air barrier, a thermal barrier and may include a vapor barrier. Moisture control is important in all climates but cold climates and hot humid climates are especially demanding. The physical components of the envelope include the foundation, roof, walls, doors, windows, ceiling and their related barriers and insulation. The dimensions, performance and compatibility of materials, fabrication process and details, connections and interactions are the main factors that determine the effectiveness and durability of the building system. Building fenestration includes all envelope penetrations used for access and egress or lighting such as windows, doors, skylights. Infiltration is the unintentional or accidental introduction of outdoor air into a building typically through cracks in the envelope. Infiltration is also called air leakage.

Examples of building envelope and interior wall constructions

Windows:

Double Pane

Solar Heat Gain coeff	0.39
U fenestration	0.57

Exterior wall construction @ percast concrete panel

5 inch precast concrete panel.

2 ½ inch continuous semi-rigid mineral fiber insulation.

1 inch air space.

5/8 inch gypsum board.

3-1/8 inch metal studs.

5/8 gypsum board.

U- factor: 0.077.

Exterior wall constructions @ metal panel

Resinous coated metal panel.

1 inch air space

5/8 gypsum board.

3-1/2 mineral fiber insulation between steel studs.

5/8 gypsum board.

U-factor : 0.110 (includes air films)

Exterior wall construction – below grade

Damp soil

16 inch poured concrete foundation.

2 inch extruded polystyrene insulation.

Effective U-factor : 0.04

Slab on Grade with Terrazzo

Damp soil.

Gravel.

6 inch Concrete Slab.

Terrazzo

Effective U factor: 0.02.

Roof Construction

Gravel

4 inch Extruded polystyrene insulation.

Rutherized asphalt membrane.

4 inch concrete slab.

Steel deck.

(adapted from Energy Efficiency strategies for treatment hospitals to obtain energy savings vs The green guide for Health care Version 2.2. New York State Energy Research and Development Authority).

Energy Consuming Machines and equipment: Medical machines which are necessary for a hospital's operation also contribute to the high energy consumption of hospitals. The energy cost can be controlled during the purchase process by taking into consideration the life cycle cost analysis, the energy consumption, the energy efficiency etc. Besides measures can be taken for improving the power factor through the use of capacitors for the reduction of power loss due to harmonic currents. Some medical equipment are fixed and have regulated load while as others are portable ie plug in and process loads. While being both convenient and cost effective portable medical equipment can cost hospitals in terms of energy use. Besides awareness needs to be made regarding energy management techniques such as switching off devices when they are not in use or to make use of built-in-standby or power down modes.

Energy Management of refrigeration equipment can be reduced by regular defrosting and proper maintenance.

Provision of Hot water and Steam: Hot water use, which is very energy consuming is high in hospitals. Also because of the big size of the buildings, there is important loss of heat in the pipeline. Proper insulation must be provided in these pipelines to minimize heat loss.

Great needs of steam in laundry, sterilization process and kitchen also warrants long pipes and need to be insulated properly.

Motors and drivers : Motors are generally running out of sight sometimes for long periods. The value of the electricity consumed by an electric motor over its life is typically 100 times the purchase price of the motor itself. It is therefore important to ensure that motors are as efficient as possible.

Identifying and Repairing Problems Quickly

Two thirds of energy from a hospital is lost through the building envelope, with the remaining third being lost through air filtration and ventilation. The rate at which energy is lost depends on temperature difference between inside and outside, the insulation properties of the building envelope, and amount of fresh air entering the building either by controlled ventilation or through poorly fitting windows, doors or joins in walls. This necessitates regular maintenance of building envelope, particularly repair of gaps or holes in walls, windows, doors and skylights immediately. Compile a regular checklist to address areas where energy is lost via the building structure. Regularly check the buildings for dampness and moisture damage. Moisture can cause significant damage to the building structure and reduce its insulating properties. Make sure that insulation is in good condition and replace it if required. Water is consumed in different sections of the hospitals for various requirements. In most hospitals, water pumping systems account for 5-15% of total electricity consumption and offer scope for reducing energy consumption. This further makes prevention of leaks important.

Indian Scenario

Bureau of Energy Efficiency (BEE) has launched a program for energy conservation in the building sector. A meeting was held in the office of Indian Medical Association (IMA) under the auspices of BEE to prepare a document that can help doctors, administrators and engineering staff to

- Monitor energy usage and consumption in hospitals.
- Understand energy efficient practices and technologies in simple language.
- Launch energy efficiency and conservation awareness program.
- Implement energy conservation measures and realize the cost savings.

In majority of hospitals in India, the energy managers do not have an easy way to gauge the energy performance of their hospitals or for that matter a destination to go for. Energy benchmarking has been undertaken for comparing the energy use in commercial facilities in a few countries with a view to compare the energy performance of a building with an established norm or standard. Two indicators most commonly used internationally for benchmarking in hospitals are

(a) annual energy consumption per square meter of the hospitals building area.

(b) annual energy consumption per inpatient bed in the hospital.

Both indicators have their own particular disadvantages. When taking the built up area into consideration, the hospital management need to decide which areas of the hospital building are included in the benchmark or not eg outdoor gardening, car parts, roads, corridors and specific floors. Secondly how much of the hospitals built up or the carpet area is air conditioned or not – conditioned in real situation. When taking beds into consideration, the hospitals built up or carpet area per bed is the critical factor. This factor is determined by the type of the hospital and design criteria of its construction. One needs to take into consideration whether these are open type /rig pattern wards or individual rooms and if there is independent metering of outdoor, inpatient and diagnostic areas. Further benchmarking can be internal (comparing with previous years performance) or external. Energy performance improvement trends were seen in number of government and multi-specialty hospitals falling in various climate zones. Climate has impact on energy performance of hospitals. Energy performance in government hospitals varied from 20-269kwh/sqm/year and 321-8026 kwh/bed/year, while as in private hospitals it varied from 84 to 2610kwh/sqm/year and 5415 to 25781 kwh/bed/year.

Bibliography

1. Ravi Kapoor, Satish Kumar. Energy Efficiency in Hospitals . Best Practice Guide. USAID Eco – III Project. International Resources Group. 2011. www.eco3.org.
2. A prescriptive path to Energy Efficiency Improvements for Hospitals. Development of a prescriptive package of Energy Efficiency measures to obtain energy savings and earn points under The Green Guide for Health Care Version 2.2. Newyork State Energy Research and development authority. 2007. www.gghc.org.
3. Jim Jofferson; Energy Efficiency Opportunities in Ontario Hospitals. OHA Energy Efficiency 2006. www.oha.com.
4. Guia Para Desarrollar Proyectos de Ahorro de Energia en centros Hospitalatios. Guide for developing Energy saving Projects at Hospital Centers. Unidad de Planeacion minero. Energetic. Republica de Columbia.
5. Building technologies program. Energy efficiency and Renewable Energy. U.S Department of Energy. 2011. www.eere.energy.gov/information center.
6. Guidelines for energy efficiency in hospitals. Life- environment "EMAS, and information technology in hospitals LIFE04 ENV/GR/000114. EPTA environmental engineers. 2007. www.ec.europa.ev.
7. Eric Bonnema, Daniel Studer, Andrew Parker, Shantipless and Paul Torcelline. Large Hospital 50% Energy savings: Technical Support Document. Technical Report NREL/TP-550-47867. U.S Department of Energy. 2010. www.nrel.gov.

8. A Report on Energy Efficient Hospitals visiting the realities. www.cii.in
9. Ishburek, Joseph W, John Car Mody. Moisture control handbook: Principles and practices for residential and Small Commercial buildings. Newyork : VanNostrand Reinhold, 1993.